Contemporary Surgical Clerkships

Series Editor
Adam E. M. Eltorai, Marlborough, MA, USA

This series of specialty-specific books will serve as high-yield, quick-reference reviews specifically for the numerous third- and fourth-year medical students rotating on surgical clerkships. Edited by experts in the field, each book includes concise review content from a senior resident or fellow and an established academic physician. Students can read the text from cover to cover to gain a general foundation of knowledge that can be built upon when they begin their rotation, or they can use specific chapters to review a subspecialty before starting a new rotation or seeing a patient with a subspecialty attending.

These books will be the ideal, on-the-spot references for medical students and practitioners seeking fast facts on diagnosis and management. Their bullet-pointed format, including user-friendly figures, tables and algorithms, make them the perfect quick-reference. Their content breadth covers the most commonly encountered problems in practice, focusing on the fundamental principles of diagnosis and management. Carry them in your white coat for convenient access to the answers you need, when you need them.

Thomas Ng • Travis Geraci
Editors

Thoracic Surgery Clerkship

A Guide for Senior Medical Students

Springer

Editors
Thomas Ng
Eastridge Cole Chair of Thoracic Surgery
University of Tennessee Health Science
Center, College of Medicine
Memphis, TN, USA

Travis Geraci
Division of Thoracic Surgery, Department
of Cardiothoracic Surgery
New York University Langone Health
New York, NY, USA

ISSN 2730-941X ISSN 2730-9428 (electronic)
Contemporary Surgical Clerkships
ISBN 978-3-031-44644-3 ISBN 978-3-031-44645-0 (eBook)
https://doi.org/10.1007/978-3-031-44645-0

This Springer imprint is published by the registered company Springer Nature Switzerland AG
The registered company address is: Gewerbestrasse 11, 6330 Cham, Switzerland

Paper in this product is recyclable.

Preface: Thoracic Surgery—Welcome

General thoracic surgeons care for patients with diseases involving the lungs, esophagus, mediastinum, pleura, chest wall, trachea, and diaphragm—essentially any disease of the thorax except for the heart and great vessels. Despite this anatomic focus, however, surgeons must also be familiar with the neck and abdomen, as these areas are natural extensions of the thorax and are often involved with disease processes that originate in the chest.

The specialty of thoracic surgery is constantly evolving. New advances in the field continue to develop and improve outcomes for patients. From a surgical perspective, the evolution of minimally invasive surgery has resulted in shorter hospitalization, decreased morbidity, and faster recovery after surgery. Surgery that once required an open thoracotomy are now amenable to robotic and/or single-port approaches. From an oncologic perspective, new therapies for lung cancer, including immunotherapy, drugs targeted at specific molecular targets, and novel ablative technology have all improved overall survival for patients. In the modern era, successful patient care is truly a multidisciplinary effort, involving pulmonologists, radiologists, oncologists, and surgeons.

In the United States, training in thoracic surgery is combined with cardiac surgery; however in practice, the specialties are substantially different and often practiced independently. Both cardiac and thoracic surgery have become increasingly complex and highly specialized. In Canada, where the specialty first emerged, training in thoracic surgery continues to be distinct from cardiac surgery. Dr. Griffith Pearson, affectionately known as the "Father of Thoracic Surgery," started a training program at the University of Toronto in the late 1960s. His students, now giants in thoracic surgery, have continued to pass on his teachings. Dr. Pearson's legacy will live on, as the training of many thoracic surgeons can always be traced back to him.

In honor of our teachers, and their teachers before, we have written a book intended for medical students and trainees on their thoracic surgery rotations. This book is designed to be concise, straightforward, and to the point; but at the same time, it covers the majority of thoracic surgery, both medical and surgical. In addition, we also aim to provide important insights, tips, and pitfalls, gained through our years of practice, information which may not be found in standard texts. Although targeted for senior medical students, this book is also appropriate for general surgery residents and advanced practitioners, and detailed enough for thoracic fellows/residents to utilize as a reference when reviewing for a specific topic.

We would like to express our gratitude to all the authors who contributed to this project, devoting much time and effort in providing us with high-quality chapters. Finally, our careers, including this book, is only possible through the extraordinary support of our families. Much love and thanks go to our children, Jax, Caroline, and Elizabeth, and to our loving wives, Katie and Amy, for their unwavering support.

Memphis, TN, USA Thomas Ng, MD, FRCSC, FACS
New York, NY, USA Travis Geraci, MD

Contents

1 **Imaging in Thoracic Surgery** 1
John Scaringi and Michael S. Furman

2 **Chest Tubes** 15
Lindsey Moran and Thomas Ng

3 **Thoracic Anesthesiology** 27
Jenny Han, Joshua Potvin, Andrew Winegarner, and Andrew Maslow

4 **Lung Cancer Screening** 47
Kena Vyas and Terrance Healey

5 **Lung Cancer Diagnosis and Staging** 57
Hannah L. McMullen and Natalie S. Lui

6 **Early-Stage Non-small Cell Lung Cancer (Stages I and II)** 73
Les James and Amie Kent

7 **Surgery for Advanced-Stage Non-small Cell Lung Cancer (Stages III and IV)** 85
Nikia T. Toomey and Thomas Ng

8 **Superior Sulcus (Pancoast) Tumors** 91
Brenden P. Sheridan and Thomas Ng

9 **Neuroendocrine Tumors of the Lung** 101
Nidhi Desai and Thomas Ng

10 **Pulmonary Function Testing and Preoperative Assessment** 111
Angel G. Doño, Travis Geraci, and Thomas Ng

11 **Pulmonary Resection, Approaches and Techniques** 121
Benjamin R. Zambetti and Thomas Ng

12 **Pulmonary Metastasis and Metastasectomy** 133
Tanvi Subramanian and Jessica Donington

13 Mesothelioma and Solitary Fibrous Tumor of the Pleura 141
David Chen and Harvey Pass

14 Thoracic Oncology 153
Christopher G. Azzoli

15 Radiotherapy for Primary and Metastatic Lung Cancer 167
David L. Schwartz and Stephen G. Chun

16 Massive Hemoptysis 175
Joseph R. Slaughter and Thomas Ng

17 Infections of the Lung 187
Les James and Travis Geraci

18 Congenital Malformations of the Lung 199
Travis Geraci and T. K. Susheel Kumar

19 Chronic Obstructive Pulmonary Disease 217
Travis Geraci and Andrew J. DeMaio

20 Spontaneous Pneumothorax 229
Darren S. Bryan and John S. Young

21 Pleural Empyema and Effusions 237
Michael A. Wright and Thomas Ng

22 Chylothorax 249
Haley Leesley and Steven Milman

23 Thoracic Trauma 255
Aaron Zuckerman and Leslie S. Tyrie

24 Thoracic Outlet Syndrome 269
Jason C. Zhang and Michael E. Barfield

25 Hyperhidrosis 281
Melanie P. Subramanian and Stephanie H. Chang

26 Lung Transplantation 287
Shair Ahmed and Lara Schaheen

27 Esophageal Reflux and Barrett's Esophagus 297
Andrew Hawkins and Philip Carrott

28 Hiatal Hernias 311
Ashley J. McCormack, Costas Bizekis, and Travis Geraci

29 Esophageal Motility Disorders 323
Travis Geraci and Thomas Ng

30 Benign Esophageal Tumors 337
Mohammad Abdallat and John S. Young

31 **Esophageal Perforation and Caustic Injury** 345
Dana Ferrari-Light and Oliver S. Chow

32 **Esophageal Cancer** 357
Jacques P. Fontaine and Jose M. Pimiento

33 **Esophagectomy: Approaches and Surgical Techniques** 373
Mohamed El Zaeedi and Travis Geraci

34 **Tracheal Stenosis** 397
Marcus Alvarez and Thomas Ng

35 **Tracheal Malignancies** 407
Natalie Ostro, Travis Geraci, and Michael Zervos

36 **Tracheostomy and Tracheoinnominate Fistula** 415
Jennifer Nishimura

37 **Chest Wall Tumors** 431
Hamza Durrani and Adam Bograd

38 **Chest Wall Deformities** 447
Christina Bi and Travis Geraci

39 **Thymic Disorders and Malignancies** 461
Camille C. Yongue, Travis Geraci, and Robert Cerfolio

40 **Mediastinal Tumors** 477
Ashley N. Miller and Thomas Ng

Index 493

Chapter 1
Imaging in Thoracic Surgery

John Scaringi and Michael S. Furman

Introduction to Imaging Modalities

- Medical imaging occupies a vital role in the diagnosis and management of thoracic diseases.
- Chest radiography is often the initial study of choice given its practicality and broad, macro view of the chest.
- Computed tomography (CT) scan offers advanced diagnostic information and imaging detail.
  - A low-dose CT scan of the chest is the preferred study for lung cancer screening.
  - CT scanning may be augmented with intravenous or oral contrast to highlight vascular or gastrointestinal structures.
- Fluoroscopy provides real-time evaluation of the aerodigestive tract, often in the perioperative period or in patients with chest trauma.
- Positron emission tomography (PET) is used for assessment of pulmonary nodules and to assess regions of locoregional or distant metastasis for lung cancer staging.
  - PET scans provide information regarding the cellular activity of a lesion by its avidity for fluorodeoxyglucose (FDG).

J. Scaringi · M. S. Furman (✉)
Department of Diagnostic Imaging, Warren Alpert Medical School of Brown University, Providence, RI, USA
e-mail: jscaringi@lifespan.org; mfurman@lifespan.org

T. Ng, T. Geraci (eds.), *Thoracic Surgery Clerkship*, Contemporary Surgical Clerkships, https://doi.org/10.1007/978-3-031-44645-0_1

Radiography

- Electromagnetic radiation in the form of x-rays are passed through a patient, some of which are attenuated based on tissue density (tissues appear white), and then collected on a detector, resulting in a two-dimensional projection of a three-dimensional object.
- Standard views include posteroanterior (PA), anteroposterior (AP), and lateral projections.
- Limited sensitivity and specificity when compared to CT given suboptimal soft tissue resolution.
- Most useful as the initial study of the chest (in most cases), postoperative assessment, pneumothorax, and pleural effusion.

Computed Tomography (CT) Scan

- Utilizes x-rays similar to radiography; however, the x-ray source and detector spin around the patient generating cross-sectional data.
- CT scans may be obtained at different slice thickness, commonly 1–2 mm.
  - High-resolution scans, producing 0.5 mm thickness images, require more radiation, but provide greater anatomic detail.
  - Low-dose CT scans in the chest are recommended for select patients for lung cancer screening (Chap. 5).
- Hounsfield units (HU) are an arbitrary assignment of value to assess tissue attenuation from air (−1000) to water (0) to bone (1000). This information is useful in delineating structures in the chest such as fluid, fat, and soft tissue.
- CT images may be augmented with intravenous iodinated contrast (CT-Angiogram, CTA), which increases the density of blood vessels and hypervascular structures.
  - Useful for patients with suspected pulmonary embolism (CT-PE protocol), with suspected pulmonary arteriovenous malformation, or when pathology involves or abuts critical vascular structures.
  - Contrast agents may cause renal impairment, so should be used with caution in patients with renal insufficiency or injury.

Fluoroscopy

- Real-time imaging using low-dose x-rays.
- A contrast material is usually required; in the chest, barium and water-soluble contrast are typical contrast media.
  - Water-soluble contrast, while less opaque than barium, may be preferred if there is suspected extraluminal contrast accumulation, as it is more easily

reabsorbed. However, water-soluble contrast must be avoided if there is a risk for aspiration as the resultant pneumonitis can be morbid.
  - Barium provides superior images over water-soluble contrast, is inert if extravasated, but will be difficult to entirely remove if it does.
- Limitations include patient ability to participate in the examination.

Ultrasound (US)

- Real-time multiplanar imaging utilizing high-frequency sound waves without ionizing radiation.
- Typically used to assess the volume and complexity of pleural effusion (fluid will appear dark, whereas the lung tissue will appear white). Although technically challenging, evaluation of mediastinal vascular and soft tissue anatomy can be performed.
- Air significantly attenuates sound-wave quality. Therefore, ultrasound cannot be relied upon for evaluation of intrapulmonary pathology.

Magnetic Resonance Imaging (MRI)

- Multiplanar imaging without ionizing radiation that can identify unique characteristics of soft tissues and fluids that are not delineated by CT.
- While not a prerequisite, the use of intravenous gadolinium contrast is highly beneficial in demarcating tissue planes, tissue enhancement, and angiography (MRA).
- Typically used for assessment of vascular anatomy, neuroanatomy, and pathology in the mediastinum and chest wall. Can serve as an alternate modality to assess pleural pathology.
  - MRI is an important imaging modality for thoracic outlet syndrome, pleural mesothelioma, and Pancoast tumors.
- Quality is significantly compromised by respiratory motion, which can limit the study or necessitate sedation for adequate imaging.
- Air causes artifact; as a result, more subtle intrapulmonary pathology is not well evaluated with this modality, and CT is generally preferred.

Nuclear Medicine

- Positron emission tomography (PET) is used for assessment of growing pulmonary nodules, chest wall lesions, pleural abnormalities, and for lung cancer staging.

- A PET scanner measures the emission of positrons from a radiopharmaceutical glucose mimicker, fluorodeoxyglucose (FDG), which is taken up by metabolically active tissue (most commonly, neoplastic tissue, infection, or inflammation).
- A PET scan can help characterize the physiologic behavior of a nodule, which may inform further workup and/or management decisions.
- Typically, pulmonary nodules greater than 8 mm can be reliably evaluated. Smaller nodules are often not detected accurately.
- The standard uptake value (SUV) relates to the concentration of activity of a given tissue and correlates to the biologic nature of the process; often a higher SUV reflects a more aggressive neoplastic process.

  In general, inflammatory and infectious processes typically have a low-to-moderate SUV (1–3), and neoplastic processes have a higher SUV (3–15). Notable expectations include tuberculoma (SUV 20s) and adenocarcinoma in situ (no/minimal SUV) and carcinoid tumor (no/minimal SUV).

- Practically requires relatively long preparation. With rare exceptions (vasculitis, fever of unknown origin), can be considered reserved for oncologic imaging.

• Split ventilation-perfusion imaging (V/Q scan) uses radiopharmaceutical agents to assess matching or mismatching of ventilation and perfusion of the lung (essentially, to assess for pathology involving gas exchange of oxygenation supply and carbon dioxide release).

  - Historically, this was used to assess pulmonary embolism as it was a noninvasive alternative to catheter angiography. It has fallen into disuse, however, with the advent of CTA, which is faster, is more accurate, and provides additional diagnostic information outside of the pulmonary arterial system.
  - There remains some diagnostic usefulness for chronic illnesses with impaired gas exchange, most notably chronic thromboembolic pulmonary hypertension (CTEPH).
  - Split lung function can be used to objectively quantify the function of specific lung regions by measuring ventilation or perfusion activity of that region and expressing this as a percentage of total lung activity.

Findings and Diagnoses: Lungs

Pulmonary Nodules and Masses

• An opacity within the lung that is less than 3 cm is defined as a pulmonary nodule, while an opacity greater than 3 cm is referred to as a pulmonary mass (Fig. 1.1).

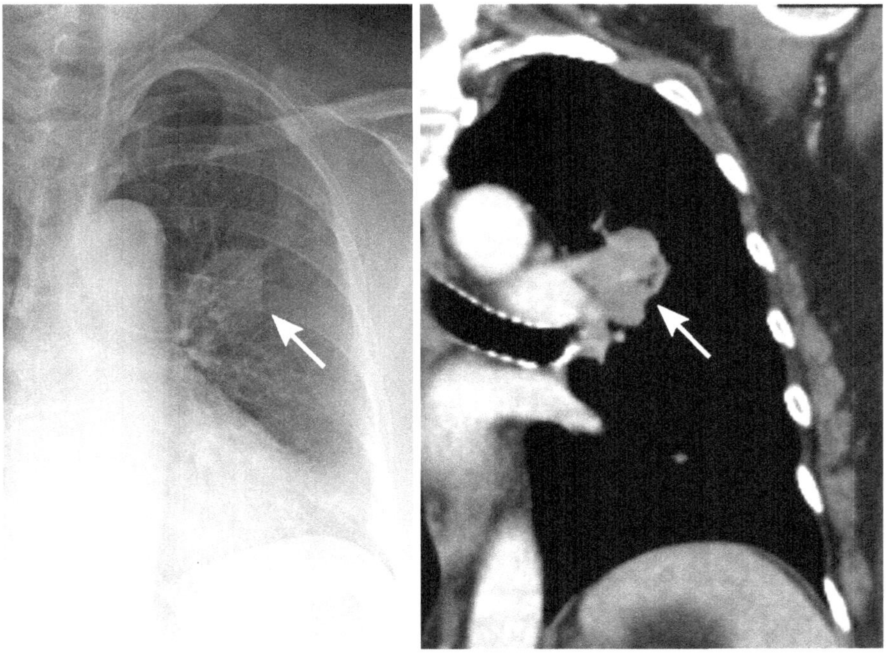

Fig. 1.1 Lung mass. (Left) Chest radiograph demonstrating a perihilar mass (arrow). (Right) Coronal CT demonstrating same perihilar mass (arrow)

- Both nodules and masses can represent benign or malignant etiologies. Characteristics are variable, but often have discernible patterns:
  - Granuloma: smooth margins, often with calcifications
  - Hamartoma: lobulated margins, ringed or arced calcifications
  - Arteriovenous malformation: lobulated margins, feeding vessels
  - Carcinoid tumor: rounded, lobulated margins, with eccentric calcifications, may have an endobronchial component
  - Lung cancer: spiculations, heterogeneous, may have areas of cavitation
  - In situ lung cancer: ground-glass appearance, part-solid, cystic areas
  - Pulmonary metastasis: round, smooth margins
- Large nodules and masses may be identified on radiograph; small nodules can be occult on radiograph. In both cases, CT is often needed for further characterization.
- Three-dimensional reconstructions may be obtained for further visual understanding of pulmonary anatomy and/or the relationship of target nodules/masses to the surrounding anatomy (Fig. 1.2).

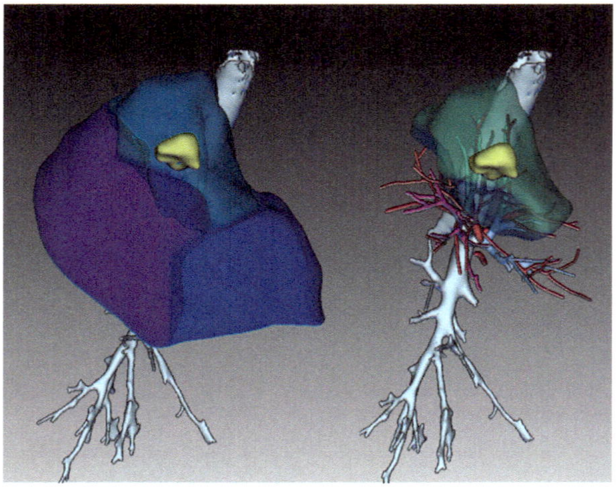

Fig. 1.2 Lung mass. CT scan 3D reconstruction delineating the segmental anatomy. Note the yellow mass in the apical (S1) segment of the right upper lobe

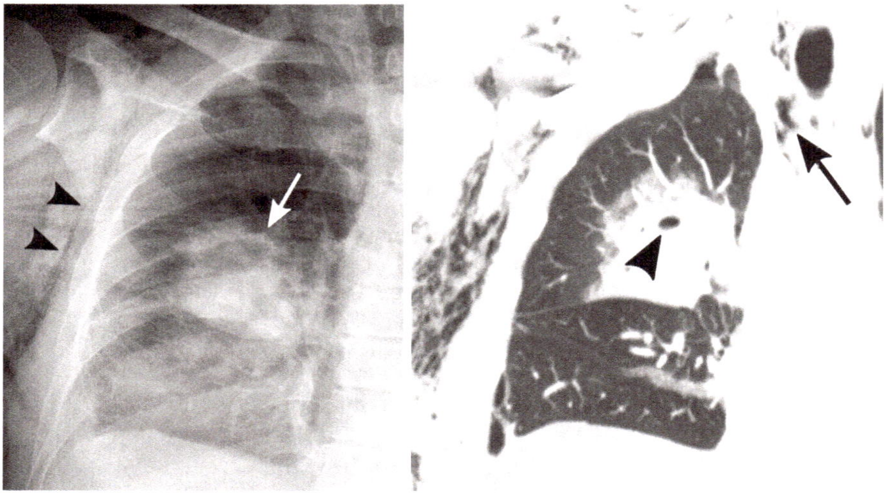

Fig. 1.3 Pulmonary laceration and contusion. (Left) Chest radiograph demonstrating a right mid-lung opacity with an area of central lucency consistent with laceration and contusion (white arrow). Soft tissue gas within subcutaneous tissues and outlining the pectoralis major muscle (black arrowheads). (Right) Coronal CT demonstrating soft tissue emphysema as well as pulmonary contusion and laceration (arrowhead). Pneumomediastinum is better appreciated on CT (long arrow)

Trauma

- Traumatic injuries in the chest include pulmonary contusion or laceration and pulmonary vascular injury.
- Pulmonary contusion results from hemorrhage of the alveolar capillary network with blood filling the alveoli and interstitium (Fig. 1.3).

- A laceration is a tear of the pulmonary interstitium.
- A pulmonary hematoma is a focal collection of blood within the lung parenchyma.
- Pulmonary vascular injury ranges from disruption of an intrapulmonary vessel to transection of the pulmonary hilum.
- The American Association for the Surgery of Trauma grades injuries from I to VI, with higher grades often requiring surgical management.

Diffuse Lung Disease

- A spectrum of predominantly chronic diseases, affecting the entire pulmonary interstitium. These include the idiopathic interstitial pneumonias, connective tissue disorders, cystic lung diseases, and drug-induced lung disease (Fig. 1.4).
- There is considerable overlap of the radiologic features of these disorders.
- Accurate diagnosis typically requires evaluation with high-resolution CT and pulmonology workup.

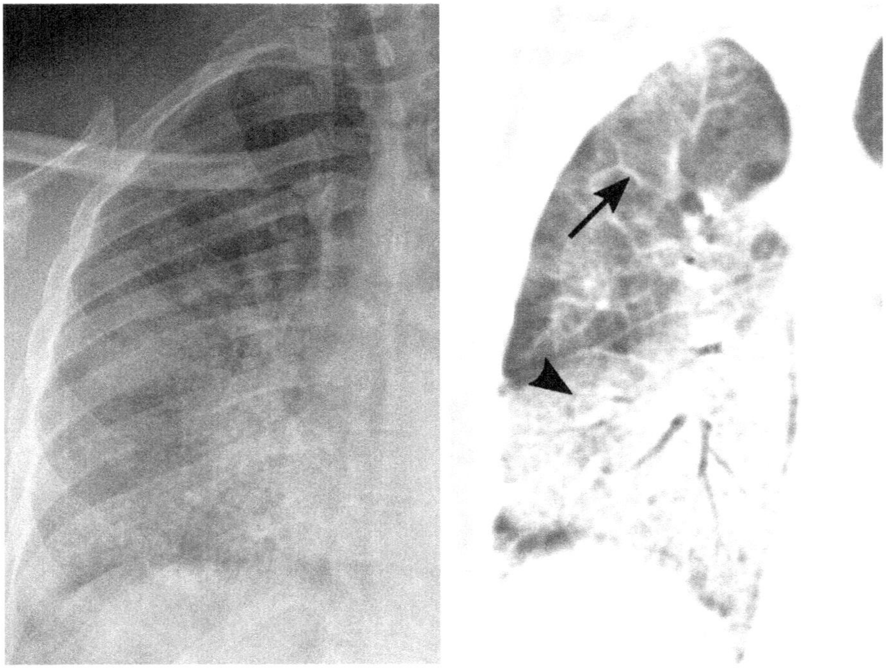

Fig. 1.4 Pulmonary alveolar proteinosis. (Left) Chest radiograph demonstrating right greater than left basilar predominant ground-glass opacities. (Right) Coronal CT demonstrating basilar predominant ground-glass opacities with interlobular (black arrow) and intralobular (black arrowhead) septal thickening consistent with a "crazy paving" pattern

Findings and Diagnoses: Pleura

The pleura includes both the visceral and parietal pleura as well as the potential pleural space between them.

Effusion

- Pleural effusions may be transudative or exudative (see Chap. 22). An exudative effusion may be suggested on imaging by regions of fluid heterogeneity or thickened pleura (inflammation).
- Transudative effusions are unassociated with pleural disease and are often seen in conditions such as congestive heart failure or cirrhosis (Fig. 1.5).
- Exudative effusions result from an underlying condition which causes increased pulmonary capillary permeability, with common causes including pleural infection or neoplasm.

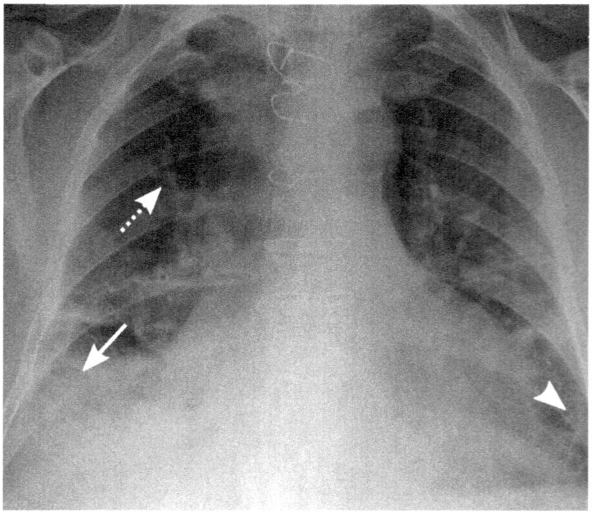

Fig. 1.5 Alveolar pulmonary edema. Findings of pulmonary edema with an enlarged cardiomediastinal silhouette, Kerley B lines (arrowhead), right pleural effusion (arrow), vascular redistribution (dotted arrow), and scattered perihilar opacities

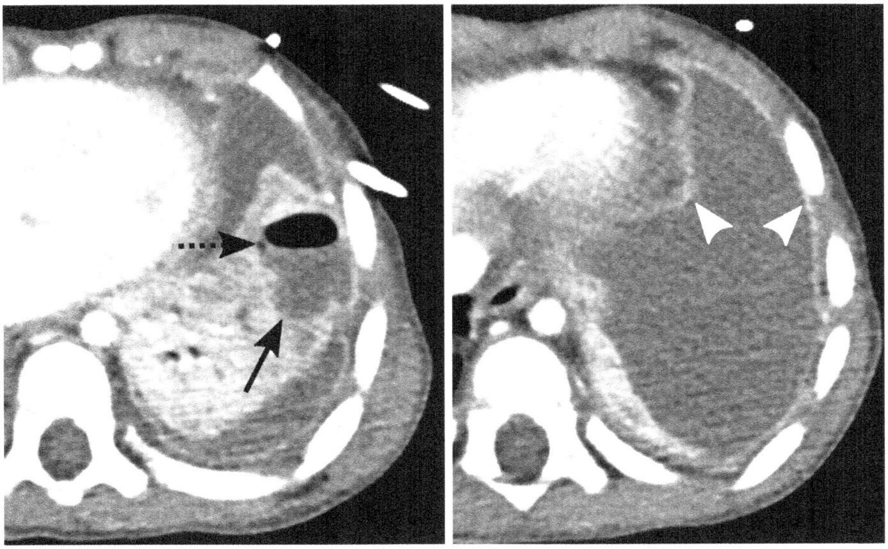

Fig. 1.6 Empyema and pulmonary abscess. (Right) Intrapulmonary abscess (solid arrow) with an air-fluid level (dotted arrow). (Left) Empyema with enhancing pleura (split pleura sign, arrowhead)

Infection

- An infected pleural effusion is referred to as an empyema. The most common cause of empyema is infection of an exudative parapneumonic effusion caused by an adjacent pneumonia (Fig. 1.6).
- On CT scan, an empyema appears as a fluid collection with thickened and enhancing surrounding pleura. If directly involving the chest wall, this collection is termed an empyema necessitans.
- Treatment of empyema involves a combination of antibiotics with catheter drainage, the installation of pleural lytic agents, and/or surgical decortication (see Chap. 22).

Trauma

- Traumatic injury may

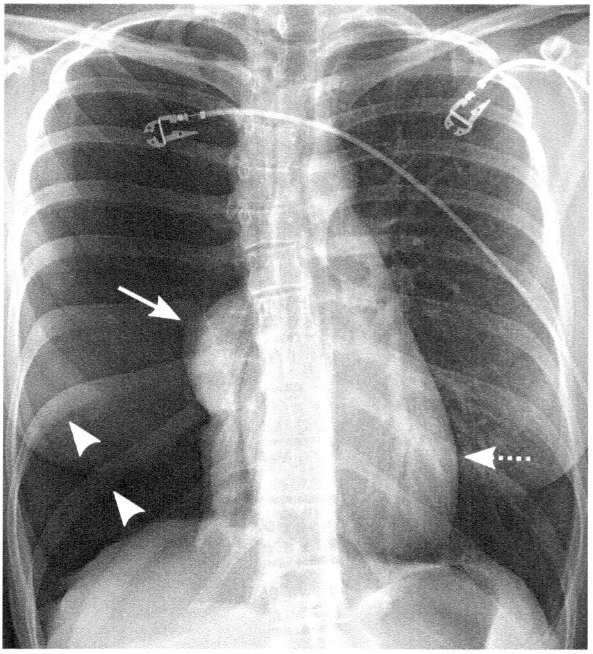

Fig. 1.7 Pneumothorax. Large right-sided pneumothorax with radiographic findings suggestive of tension physiology (although tension pneumothorax should be diagnosed clinically in a patient with hypotension and pneumothorax, not radiographic). The right lung is collapsed (solid arrow) with right to left shift of the mediastinum (dotted arrow). There is asymmetric widening of the right ribs (arrowhead)

- result in filling of the pleural space with air, fluid, or blood.
- Pneumothorax is air within the pleural space and can be seen on imaging as a lucent region within the thorax with adjacent compressed lung (Fig. 1.7).
  - In a tension pneumothorax, the intrapleural pressure exceeds atmospheric pressure; this along with mediastinal shift compromises cardiopulmonary function. The diagnosis is made clinically with the additional finding of hypotension and may be suggested radiographically by contralateral shift of mediastinal structures and flattening of the ipsilateral hemidiaphragm (Fig. 1.7).
- Fluid within the pleural space is termed a hydrothorax; blood product within the pleural space is a hemothorax.
  - These entities look similar on radiography.
  - On CT, these conditions may be differentiated by their density, with hydrothorax having a density similar to water (0 Hounsfield units) and hemothorax having a density similar to blood and soft tissue (40 Hounsfield units).
- A combination of air and either fluid or blood within the pleural space is referred to as a hydropneumothorax or a hemopneumothorax, respectively.

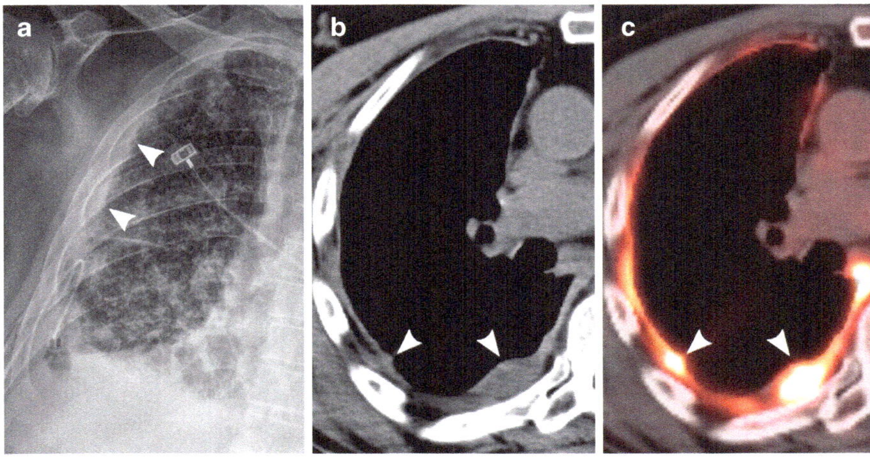

Fig. 1.8 Mesothelioma. (**a**) Radiograph demonstrating thickened pleura (arrowheads) and scattered opacities; (**b**) CT demonstrates circumferentially thickened pleura; (**c**) on PET/CT the thickened pleura is metabolically active with areas of more focal nodular thickening in keeping with mesothelioma

Masses

- Common benign pleural masses include solitary fibrous tumors of the pleura and lipoma.
- Malignant pleural masses are most likely pleural metastases. Other more common lesions include malignant mesothelioma and lymphoma (Fig. 1.8).

Findings and Diagnoses: Mediastinum

The mediastinum is composed of the structures between the lungs, demarcated superiorly by the thoracic inlet and inferiorly by the diaphragm. This compartment includes the anterior or prevascular compartment, the middle or visceral compartment, and the posterior or paravertebral compartment. The anterior and middle mediastinum are divided by the anterior aspect of the pericardium. The posterior mediastinum begins at the anterior margin of the vertebral body.

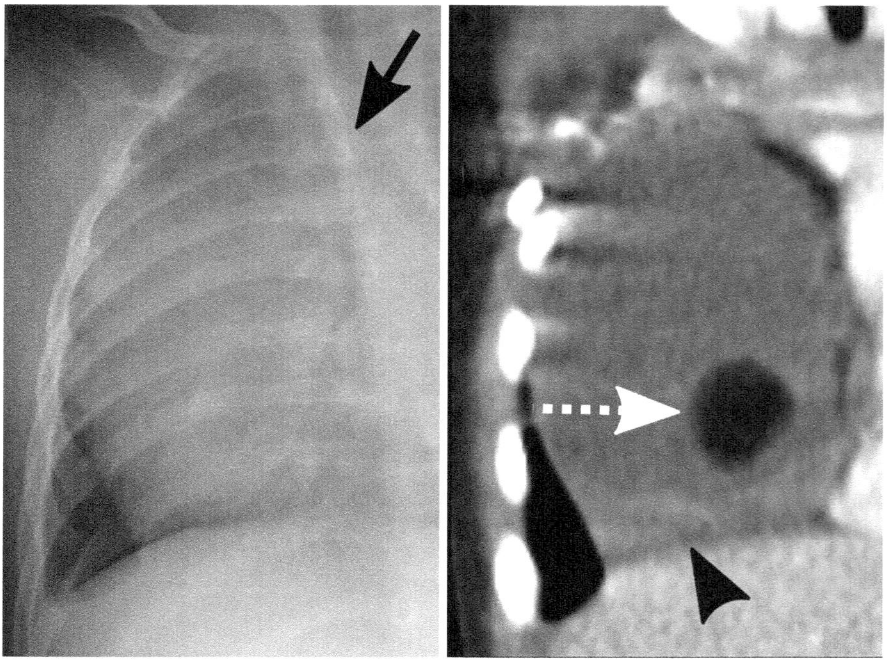

Fig. 1.9 Mediastinal teratoma. (Right) Pediatric radiograph with a large anterior mediastinal mass that exerts mass effect on the distal trachea and mainstem bronchi (arrows). Coronal CT demonstrating the mass which contains fat (dotted arrow), fluid, and soft tissue density (arrowhead) in keeping with a teratoma

Masses

- Each area within the mediastinum is composed of different structures, with different corresponding masses found within each compartment (see Chap. 4).
- The classic differential diagnosis for anterior mediastinal masses includes the four "Terrible T's" (Fig. 1.9):
  - Thymoma (thymic malignancies)
  - Thyroid malignancies, thyroid goiter, parathyroid
  - Teratoma, seminoma, and non-seminomatous germ cell tumors
  - "Terrible" lymphoma
- The most common middle mediastinal mass-like lesion is lymphadenopathy. This finding may be secondary to infection, inflammation including granulomatous inflation, or malignancy.
- Posterior mediastinal masses may also represent lymphadenopathy. Additional more common masses include neurogenic tumors such as neurofibroma and schwannoma.

Trauma

- Trauma to the mediastinum may result in blood or air within the mediastinal space, known as a mediastinal hematoma or pneumomediastinum, respectively.
- Presence of mediastinal hematoma (widened mediastinum, apical cap, depressed left main bronchus, deviated esophagus or trachea, and blunted aortopulmonary window seen on chest radiograph) mandates workup to rule out aortic injury.
- On radiograph pneumomediastinum appears as linear lucencies projecting over the mediastinum and often the lower neck. Pneumomediastinum is most often from lung rupture or an esophageal injury. When the etiology of pneumomediastinum is unknown (no recent surgery or instrumentation, major trauma), further evaluation for occult esophageal rupture with either a CT chest with oral contrast or an esophagram should be considered. Spontaneous pneumomediastinum (air originating from bronchopulmonary source) is a diagnosis of exclusion, made only when esophageal perforation has been ruled out.

Findings and Diagnoses: Chest Wall

The chest wall is composed of cutaneous and subcutaneous soft tissues, the thoracic cage, muscles, and neurovascular structures.

Masses

- Chest wall masses include benign and malignant neoplasms which either arise from the thoracic cage or soft tissue (see Chap. 38).
- Common benign osseous lesions include fibrous dysplasia and bone cysts.
- Benign soft tissue masses include tumors of fat (lipoma) and vascular (hemangioma) origin. Elastofibroma dorsi is an additional common soft tissue tumor. This tumor has a characteristic location between the inferior scapula and chest wall and appears as a soft tissue mass on CT.
- Malignant masses include chondrosarcoma, osteosarcoma, rhabdomyosarcoma, and osseous metastasis.

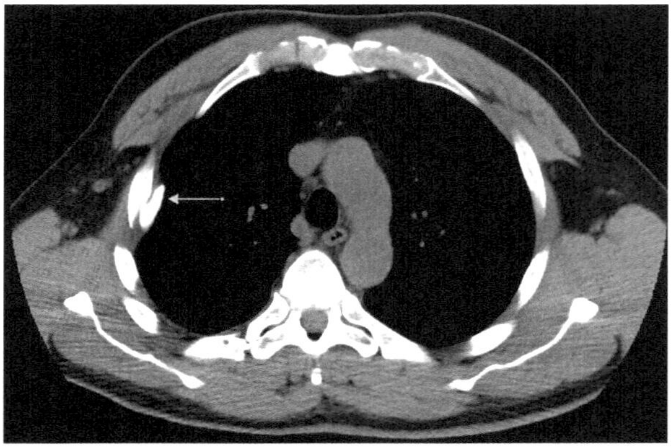

Fig. 1.10 Rib fracture. Axial CT scan of the chest demonstrating a displaced right third rib fracture (arrow)

Trauma

- Rib fractures are common in the setting of chest trauma (Fig. 1.10), and the location of the patient's pain can guide the search for fractures. A chest radiograph is the best first test; however, if there is a strong clinical suspicion for rib fractures, a negative chest x-ray does not exclude fracture, and CT is more sensitive.
- Flail chest is fracture of at least three contiguous ribs in two or more places and results in paradoxical movement of the affected chest wall segment with respiration. Flail chest may lead to ventilation difficulties and often elevates the patient's level of care.
- High-energy trauma may result in sternal fracture, which is best evaluated on CT. In the setting of sternal fracture, it is important to evaluate for associated injuries such as mediastinal hematoma, cardiac and pericardial injuries, and injuries to the great vessels.

Key Reference

- Webb WR, Higgins CB. Thoracic imaging: pulmonary and cardiovascular radiology. Philadelphia: Wolters Kluwer; 2017.

Further Reading

Golding RP. Fundamentals of body CT, 4th edition. Radiology. 2014;181(1):224.

Hansell DM, Bankier AA, MacMahon H, McLoud TC, Müller NL, Remy J. Fleischner society: glossary of terms for thoracic imaging. Radiology. 2008;246(3):697–722. https://doi.org/10.1148/radiol.2462070712.

Moore EE, Malangoni MA, Cogbill TH, et al. Organ injury scaling. IV: thoracic vascular, lung, cardiac, and diaphragm. J Trauma. 1994;36(3):299–300.

Rosado-de-Christenson M, Martinez-Jimenez S. Diagnostic imaging: chest. 3rd ed. Amsterdam: Elsevier; 2021.

Chapter 2
Chest Tubes

Lindsey Moran and Thomas Ng

Introduction

Chest tubes (also referred to as thoracostomy tube, chest drain, or intercostal drain) are routinely used to remove air or fluid from the pleural space, in order to promote expansion of the lung. There are a variety of indications for chest tubes which must be considered prior to tube placement. The type of tube, insertion technique, location of tube, and duration of treatment all depend on a multitude of factors that will be discussed in more detail here.

Indications

- Pneumothorax
- Hemothorax
- Pleural effusion (symptomatic and/or recurrent)
  - Symptomatic/recurrent transudative/exudative effusion
  - Empyema/parapneumonic effusion
  - Chylothorax
  - Malignant effusion
- Traumatic injuries involving the chest

L. Moran
Department of Surgery, Warren Alpert Medical School of Brown University, Providence, RI, USA

T. Ng (✉)
Division of Thoracic Surgery, University of Tennessee Health Science Center, College of Medicine, Memphis, TN, USA
e-mail: tng4@uthsc.edu

T. Ng, T. Geraci (eds.), *Thoracic Surgery Clerkship*, Contemporary Surgical Clerkships, https://doi.org/10.1007/978-3-031-44645-0_2

- Postoperative (cardiac and thoracic surgery)
- Rewarming a hypothermic patient

Contraindications

There are no absolute contraindications to chest tube insertion. Several factors should be considered along with a thoughtful risk versus benefit analysis. Special consideration should be given to the following:

- Patients at risk for excessive bleeding (coagulopathies, bleeding disorders, medications)
- Previous thoracic surgery, especially pneumonectomy and pleurodesis
- Diaphragm hernia (risk of abdominal viscera injury)
- Skin or soft tissue malignancies in the area of tube insertion

Chest Tube Selection

- Three types of tubes: large bore (Fig. 2.1), pigtail catheter (Fig. 2.2), and tunneled catheter (Fig. 2.3).
- Large-bore tubes are often used in emergent/traumatic situations and after thoracic and cardiac surgery, for drainage of air and blood. They can also be used for any other indication listed above; however, since it may be difficult to place these tubes in a precise location, large-bore tubes may be less effective for located effusion such as parapneumonic effusion/empyema.
- Pigtail catheters are often used in the management of pneumothorax and pleural effusions, with less traumatic insertion and less discomfort (due to smaller caliber) compared to large-bore chest tubes. They are not optimal for hemothorax as the small caliber of these tubes will not successfully evacuate clotted blood. However, although counterintuitive due to the thick loculated nature, pigtail

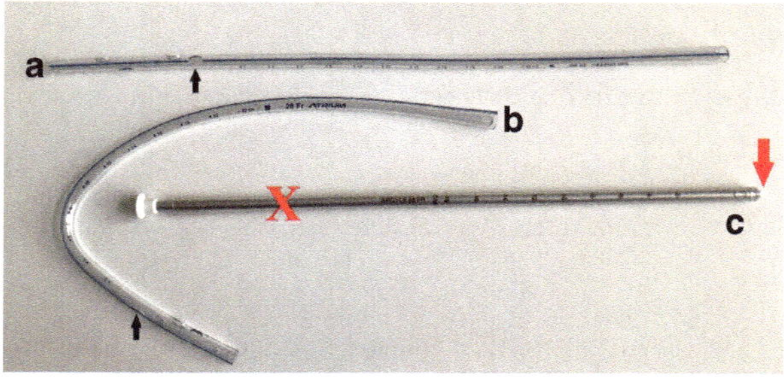

Fig. 2.1 Large-bore chest tubes. Notice the last hole is always in line with the radiopaque stripe (black arrow) so that the position of this hole can be identified on X-ray (see Fig. 2.4b). A is straight, B is curved, C is straight with trocar for insertion, and this type is not recommended for use (red x) as the sharp tip (red arrow) can cause extensive damage to internal structures

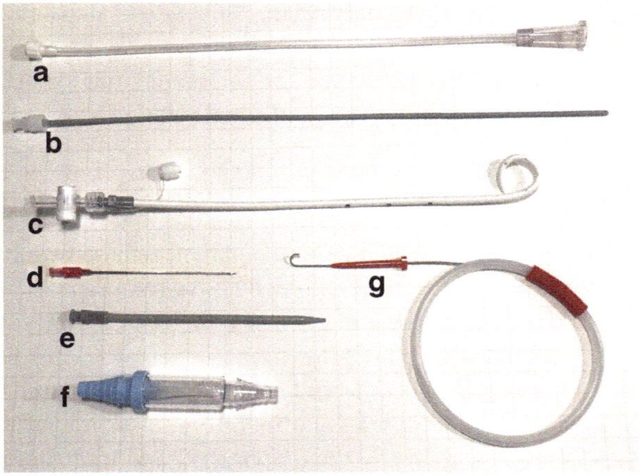

Fig. 2.2 Pigtail chest catheter insertion. A is Luer lock connector from catheter to drainage system, B is pigtail catheter trocar, C is pigtail catheter with Luer lock, D is large-bore needle through which guidewire is advanced, E is tract dilator, F is Heimlich valve, and G is guidewire

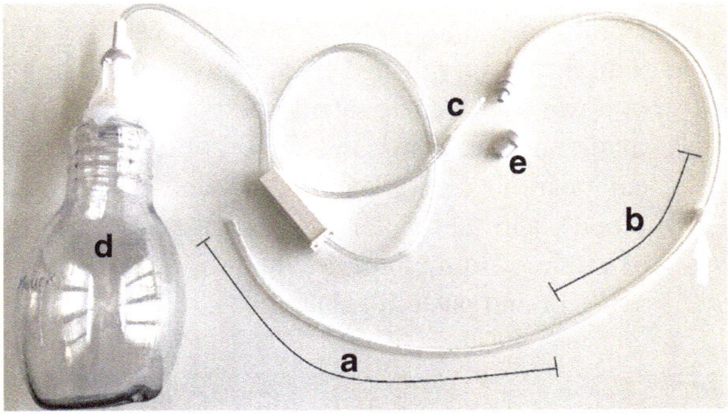

Fig. 2.3 Tunneled chest tube for long-term placement. **A** is portion in pleural space; **B** is subcutaneous portion, with cuff (arrow) that holds this in place; **C** is connector from vacuum bottle to tunneled catheter; **D** is vacuum bottle; **E** is catheter cap when tube not in use

catheters are ideal for parapneumonic effusion/empyema as they can be placed the precise location of the loculated effusion using image guidance (ultrasound or computed tomography scan, CT), allowing for the delivery of lytic therapy into the middle of the effusion for effective lyses and drainage (see Chap. 22).
- Indwelling tunneled catheters are used in the long-term management of chronic pleural effusions, most commonly malignant effusions (see Chap. 22).

Insertion Technique

- Overview (common to all insertion techniques)
  - All insertion techniques require consent, patient identification, surgeon/proceduralist identification, procedure identification, and site identification.
  - Pre-procedure antibiotics and full skin preparation.
  - Full patient draping.
  - Full mask, gown, and gloves for the surgeon/proceduralist.
  - Time-out.

  - Adequate local anesthesia, at the site of incision, intercostal blocks at, above, and below the intercostal entry.
  - Only in life-threatening or emergent situations can the above be omitted.
  - Placement should be confirmed with a chest X-ray following insertion.

- Large-bore chest tube (Fig. 2.1)
  - Lateral decubitus position is ideal, but may not be feasible if the patient is unstable, in which case, the patient will be in supine position. Commonly, the ipsilateral arm is positioned above the head.
  - Site of incision is in the mid to anterior axillary line at the level of the nipple, as this is the area of the thinnest chest wall muscle, the serratus anterior; other sites on the chest would encounter the much thicker pectoralis major or latissimus dorsi muscles. Furthermore, insertion site below the level of the nipple may risk injury to the diaphragm, and insertion site much above the level of the nipple may risk injury to axillary structures. Make a skin incision that is large enough for the provider to insert a finger.
  - Gently spread the subcutaneous tissues using a blunt clamp down to the chest wall; however, during this maneuver it is important to tunnel in the direction you want your chest tube to be positioned (Fig. 2.4a, b). In the case of traumatic pneumothorax and hemothorax, tunnel superiorly and posteriorly (apical position for pneumothorax and posterior position to drain dependent blood), and then enter the pleural space with the clamp and spread (in this example of tunneling, the intercostal entry into pleural space is much more superior and posterior than the skin incision).

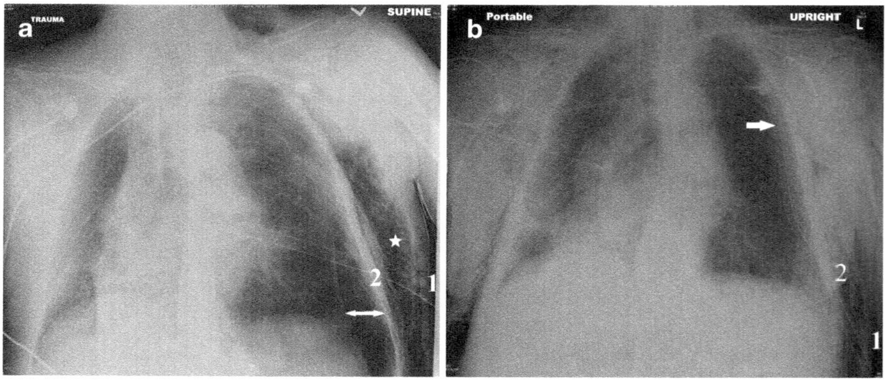

Fig. 2.4 Effect of proper tunneling in the placement of large-bore chest tubes. (**a**) Minimal tunneling, as indicated by the similar level of the skin incision site (1) and the intercostal entry site (2), resulting in a chest tube directed straight toward the mediastinum and likely buried in the fissure, with subcutaneous air (star) and failure to expand the lung (double arrow) due to poor positioning; (**b**) the same patient now with full lung expansion after revision of chest tube placement, effective tunneling toward the apex as indicated by the distance between the skin incision (1) and the intercostal entry site (2), results in a trajectory that facilitates positioning of the tube into the apex. Note the last hole is always in line with the radiopaque stripe so that the position of this hole can be identified on X-ray (arrow)

– Always enter the pleural space with a blunt clamp directly above the rib to avoid the intercostal neurovascular bundle.
– Perform a finger sweep by inserting a finger through the wound and into the pleural space, to confirm that you are in the correct space and that there are not excessive adhesions preventing tube insertion. You may gently separate adhesions with your finger if they break down easily although there is a risk of bleeding with this maneuver.
– Chest tube insertion into pleural space may be by partial guidance with the blunt clamp or by simply advancing the tube through the incision (with a properly tunneled path, the chest tube should end up in the desired position). The distance that a chest tube is to be advanced can be estimated, but never advance if there is resistance.
– Connect chest tube to chest drainage system (described below).
– Secure the drain using heavy nonabsorbable stitch.
– Cover the chest tube with dressing.

• Pigtail chest catheter (Fig. 2.2)

– Patient position depends on the location of the target as pigtail catheters can be placed almost anywhere in the chest:

  Supine for anterior chest access
  Lateral decubitus or supine with the arm above the head for lateral chest access
  Lateral decubitus, prone, or sitting up while leaning forward with support for posterior chest access

– A small skin incision of 5 mm or less is made over or close to the site of pathology. Staying above the rib, advance the large-bore needle into the pathology while drawing back on the connected syringe to aspirate fluid/ air, often under image guidance (ultrasound or CT).
– Hold the needle in place while removing the syringe and insert guidewire through the needle. As long as there is no resistance, advance until approximately 20 cm of wire is remaining; this allows for enough external length to keep constant control of, minimizing the risk of accidental loss of the entire wire into the chest.
– Increase the skin incision with the knife, large enough for the dilator to pass (5 mm or so), but make sure this incision is contiguous with the skin incision of the guidewire (no skin bridge).
– Dilate the tract with the dilator over the guidewire; do not insert the full length of the dilator, as its rigidity can injure internal structures. The distance the dilator is advanced should only be the thickness of the patient's chest wall. Always have one hand on the guidewire during dilation to prevent accidental loss of the entire wire into the chest.
– Remove the dilator, assemble the internal trocar with the pigtail catheter (this straightens out the curl of the catheter and makes it more rigid), and over the guidewire, insert this assembly into the chest. Unless there is CT guidance, do

not insert the full length of the pigtail catheter/trocar assembly as the trocar is rigid and can injure internal structures. Advance this assembly slightly more than the thickness of the chest wall, followed by only advancing the pigtail catheter, while keeping a hold of the internal trocar and guidewire to prevent these from advancing. Once the pigtail catheter is advanced, remove trocar and guidewire. Again, always have one hand on the guidewire during catheter advancement to prevent accidental loss of the entire wire into the chest.

- Connect the pigtail catheter to the drainage system connector and then to the drainage system (see below).
- Secure the pigtail catheter with a heavy nonabsorbable suture.
- Cover with dressing.

Drainage Systems

- Three-chamber drainage systems: two types, wet suction (Fig. 2.5a) or dry suction (Fig. 2.5b)
  - First chamber: collection chamber

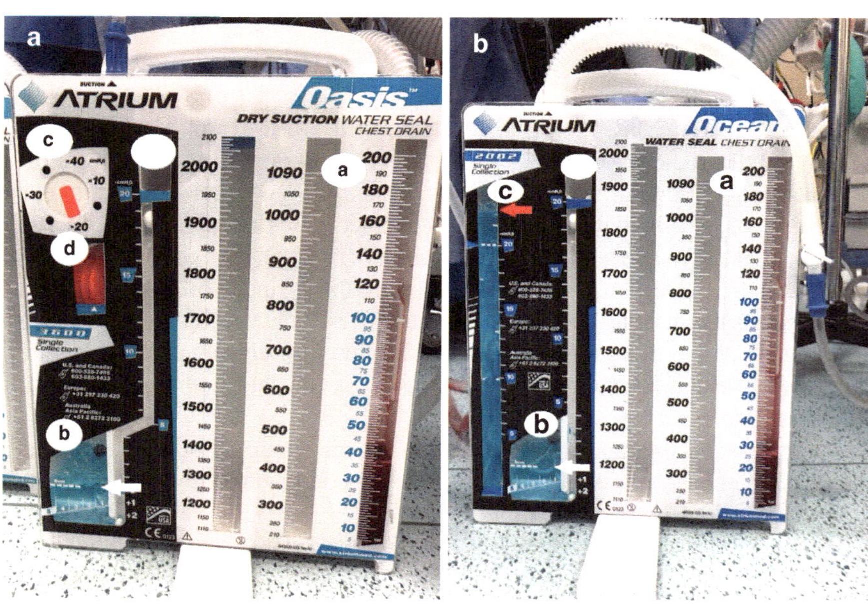

Fig. 2.5 Three-chamber drainage system. (**a**) Wet suction: A is collection chamber, B is waterseal chamber with air leak noted (white arrow), and C is wet suction chamber regulated by the height of the water with "bubbling" in this chamber indicating adequate suction applied (red arrow). (**b**) Dry suction: A is collection chamber, B is waterseal chamber with air leak noted (arrow), C is dry suction chamber regulated by dial, and D is red corrugated balloon that indicates adequate suction applied

Directly connected to patient's chest tube.
Volume and quality of draining fluid can be assessed.

- Second chamber: waterseal chamber

  The small amount of water added to this chamber acts as a one-way valve.
  Look for air leak here by asking patient to cough: if present then determine if this is a system leak or patient leak by clamping the tube at the skin level; if leak ceases, then this is a patient leak; if leak persists, then this is a system leak (last hole of chest tube outside of patient, loose connection, hole in tubing, crack in the drainage system), in which case you can determine the site by marching the clamp distally until leak ceases or just replace with entire new tubing and drainage system.
  Look for tidaling; this reflects changes in intrapleural pressure: large amounts of tidaling may reflect large residual space (post-resection or non-expanded trapped lung) or respiratory distress; no tidaling may represent clogged/kinked tube or tube not located in the pleural space.
  If this chamber is overfilled, use a needle and syringe to pull out water from the access port, which may be located in front or behind.

- Third chamber: suction chamber

  Wet suction (Fig. 2.5a): The amount of suction is regulated by the height of the column of water you fill in this chamber. Wall suction is applied to this chamber; once wall suction exceeds the height of the column of water, then there is "bubbling," which represents equilibration of the excess suction from the wall so that the patient only sees the pressure you set by the height of the water you fill. The maximum water height filled is usually −20 cm H_2O; to decrease the suction/level of fluid, remove water out of this third chamber with a needle and syringe via the access port located behind.
  Dry suction (Fig. 2.5b): The amount of suction is regulated with a simple dial, without the need to fill (increase suction) or remove water (decrease suction). A higher amount of suction (up to −40 cm of H_2O) can be applied compared to wet suction. Also unlike the noise of the wet suction, the third chamber of the dry suction emits no noise.
  There is controversy after lung resection regarding the routine use of suction versus waterseal, with some studies showing waterseal to result in quicker resolution of air leak while others did not. However, since there seems to be no disadvantage and that a patient is more likely to get out of bed and ambulate, early waterseal seems appropriate.

• Heimlich valve (Fig. 2.6)

  - Usually utilized for outpatient chest tube management.
  - Heimlich valve is a one-way valve, acting much like to waterseal chamber, to prevent fluid or air returning into the patient.

  - The Heimlich valve is connected to the chest tube, which is then connected to a drainage bag to collect fluid, with a hole punched on the superior aspect of the bag to allow egress of air (Fig. 2.6).
  - Fluttering of the valve suggests air leak, but precise determination of leak requires disconnection of the drainage bag from the valve and submerging the valve under water to look for air bubbles on cough.
- Digital drainage system (Fig. 2.7)
  - Digital drainage systems report numeric values of air leak rate and fluid loss volume.
  - Digital systems have a number of advantages over traditional analogue chest drains, such as reporting objective and continuous data, portability, precision adjustments, and overall ease of operation.

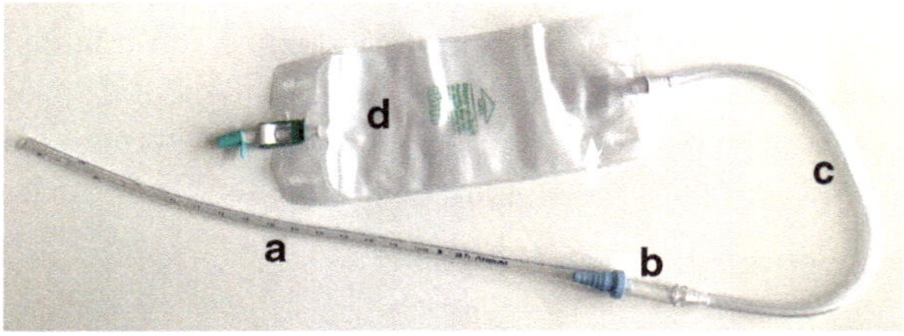

Fig. 2.6 Outpatient chest tube management with Heimlich valve. A is chest tube, B is Heimlich valve, C is tubing connecting valve to drainage bag, and D is drainage bag with a hole punched in its superior aspect to allow egress of air (arrow)

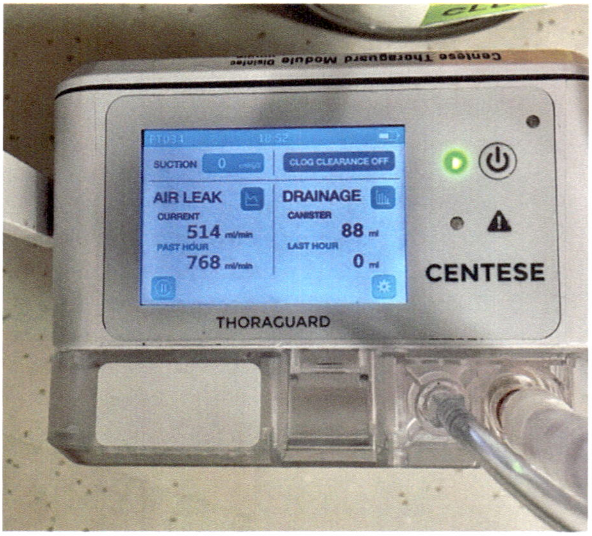

Fig. 2.7 Digital interface of digital drainage system on a waterseal setting (0 suction) reporting an air leak of 514 mL/min and total fluid output of 88 mL

Chest Tube Removal

- Timing of removal: There are several factors that must be considered, and be aware that each care provider may have different criteria for tube removal. Note that X-ray appearance plays a less central role in this decision, so long as the below criteria are met (i.e., if there is a persistent pneumothorax on X-ray and the chest tube has no leak and with the appropriate drainage, then chest tube may still be removed).
  - Presence of an air leak

    Regardless of the indication, presence of an air leak is a contraindication to chest tube removal. There must be no air leak to be considered for removal, or the patient will develop pneumothorax, possibly tension. After major pulmonary resection, it may be difficult to differentiate true parenchymal leak vs air from residual/post-resection space (the former you would leave tube in while the latter you would remove tube); here experience of the provider will be important; alternatively the use of a digital drainage system may help (air leak rate of <15–20 mL/min during normal respiration would suggest that tube is ready for removal).
  - Quantity of drainage

    For empyema, drainage should be minimal, "single digits" in 24 h, prior to removal. One may consider managing "empyema tubes" by serially "inching the tube out" to allow for the distal tract to collapse.
    After lung resection and most other indications, 24 h output of 400 mL or less is acceptable for removal, provided the drainage is not purulent, chyle, or pure blood.
  - Quality of drainage

    Chest tubes with chylous or purulent output should not be removed until further workup is completed.
    Chest tubes with bloody output should not be removed if there is any concern for ongoing bleeding.
- Technique for removal
  - The most effective removal technique has been long debated, without clear superiority of one technique over another.
  - Theoretically, as pleural pressure is positive, removal of tube during Valsalva maneuver, regardless of the phase of respiration, should minimize the risk of the patient drawing in air to result in pneumothorax post removal.
  - Steps for removal

    Remove occlusive dressing.

Free the tube by cutting any sutures securing it in place.
Some pigtail catheters have a string that keeps the catheter curled; it is important to open the lock mechanism to release tension on that string so that the tube can be removed smoothly without force and that the string does not snap and risk retaining a piece in the patient.
Remove the tube as described above, but remove and cover as quickly as possible to minimize the risk of patient drawing in air. Some may have pre-placed suture to close the chest tube site, in which case remove the tube and tie the stitch as quickly as possible; this may require two persons to achieve.
Apply clean occlusive dressing.
Obtain follow-up chest X-ray 4–6 h later.

Complications

- Injury to organs/structures
  - Lung (Fig. 2.8)
  - Intercostal artery (Fig. 2.9)
  - Cardiac
  - Esophageal
  - Great vessels
  - Diaphragm
  - Abdominal viscera: stomach, liver, bowel, spleen
- Re-expansion pulmonary edema

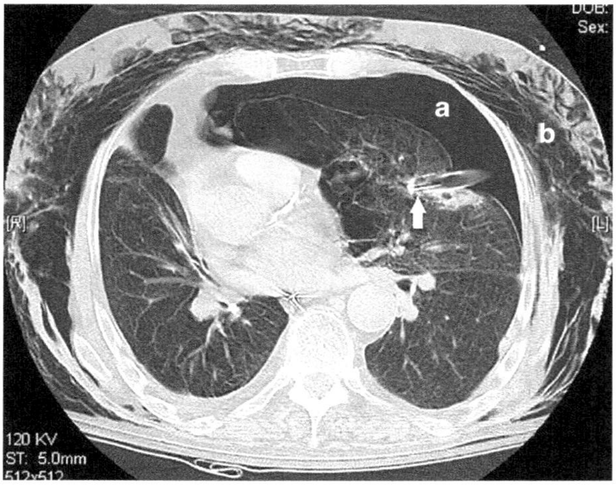

Fig. 2.8 Chest tube placed into the lung parenchyma (arrow), with persistent pneumothorax (A) and subcutaneous air (B)

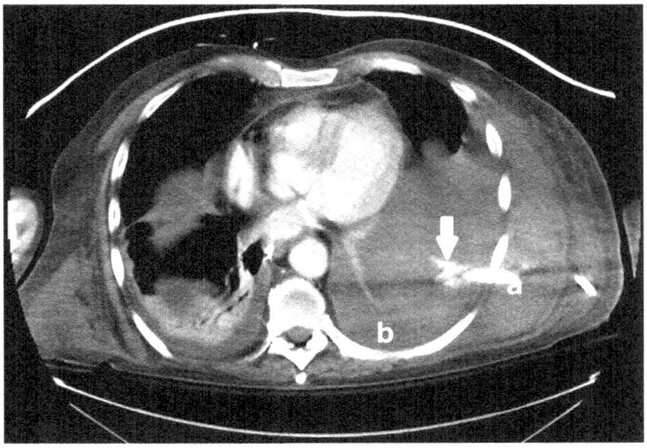

Fig. 2.9 Intercostal artery injury from chest tube (A), with arterial blush (arrow) on contrast CT and hemothorax (B)

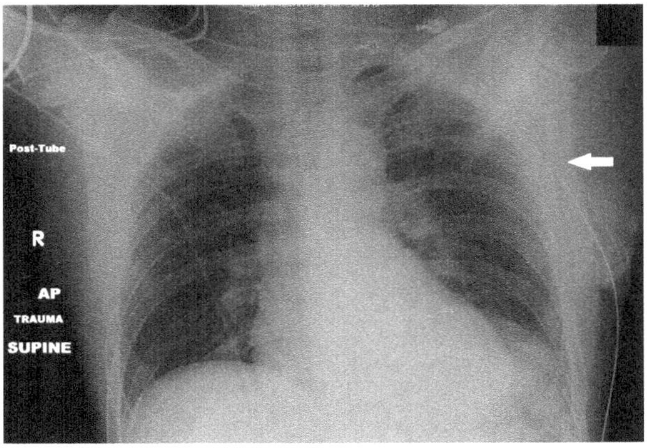

Fig. 2.10 Chest tube incorrectly placed, subcutaneous position (arrow)

  - Occurs when chronic large effusions are drained too rapidly, especially if active suction is applied.
  - If chronic large effusion is encountered, clamp chest tube immediately after insertion, release 1 L at a time (i.e., every 6 h) and re-clamp, and never place tube on suction.
  - Similar can occur with chronic large pneumothoraces.

- Empyema
  - Break in sterile technique.
  - Leaving chest tube in place too long.

- Malposition
  - Intraparenchymal (Fig. 2.8)
  - Subcutaneous (Fig. 2.10)
  - Intra-abdominal (Fig. 2.11)
  - Accidental dislodgement

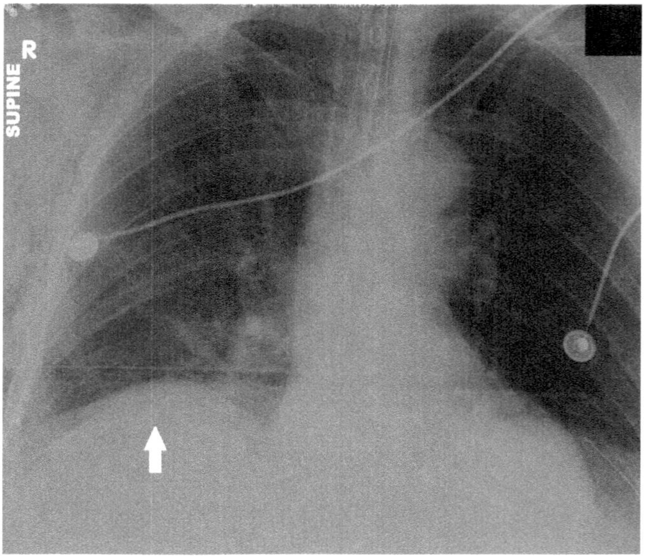

Fig. 2.11 Chest tube incorrectly placed, intra-abdominal position (arrow), likely through the diaphragm

- Retained chest tube from fracture

Key Reference
- Thoracic surgery clinics: clinical management of chest tubes. 2017;27(1):1–72.

Further Reading

Cerfolio RJ, Bryant AS, Skylizard L, Minnich DJ. Optimal technique for the removal of chest tubes after pulmonary resection. J Thorac Cardiovasc Surg. 2013;145(6):1535–9.

French DG, Dilena M, LaPlante S, Shamji F, Sundaresan S, Villeneuve J, Seely A, Maziak D, Gilbert S. Optimizing postoperative care protocols in thoracic surgery: best evidence and new technology. J Thorac Dis. 2016;8(Suppl 1):S3–S11.

McElnay PJ, Lim E. Modern techniques to insert chest drains. Thorac Surg Clin. 2017;27(1):29–34.

Novoa NM, Jiménez MF, Varela G. When to remove a chest tube. Thorac Surg Clin. 2017;27(1):41–6.

Venuta F, Diso D, Anile M, Rendina EA, Onorati I. Chest Tubes: Generalities. Thorac Surg Clin. 2017;27(1):1–5.

Chapter 3
Thoracic Anesthesiology

Jenny Han, Joshua Potvin, Andrew Winegarner, and Andrew Maslow

Introduction

The following chapter introduces concepts that the modern-day anesthesiologist faces when caring for a thoracic surgical patient. Care begins with the preoperative evaluation of lung function and comorbidities to predict the patient's ability to tolerate the impact of anesthesia and surgery. Based on this, perioperative decisions regarding the surgical procedure and conduct of anesthesia are made. Care extends into the postoperative period with emphasis on analgesia through several numbers of techniques available. At all points of care, clear communication between the anesthesiologist and the thoracic surgeon is necessary to develop an individualized plan for each patient and during the case to address nuances as they present. The coordinated care extends into the postoperative period to assure maintenance of analgesia and major organ function. This chapter also describes the anesthesia care of the patient with a mediastinal mass as these patients require very specific considerations and preparation for scheduled procedures.

Preoperative Evaluation of the Thoracic Patient

- General preoperative principles apply to the thoracic surgical patient; however, there are unique principles requiring close attention.

J. Han · J. Potvin · A. Winegarner · A. Maslow (✉)
Department of Anesthesiology, Warren Alpert Medical School of Brown University, Providence, RI, USA
e-mail: JHan3@Lifespan.org; jpotvin1@lifespan.org

T. Ng, T. Geraci (eds.), *Thoracic Surgery Clerkship*, Contemporary Surgical Clerkships, https://doi.org/10.1007/978-3-031-44645-0_3

- It is essential to obtain a focused history and physical examination prior to undergoing surgery, specifically including allergies, anesthesia history, comorbidities, and an airway exam.
- Assessment of functional capacity (physical tolerance) is paramount prior to initiating any type of anesthetic. Ideally, patients should be able to climb two flights of stairs without developing symptoms such as chest pain or shortness of breath.
- Standard laboratory data.
- Pulmonary function tests should also be obtained to define baseline lung function and responsiveness to bronchodilator therapy (delineate reversal vs nonreversible causes of obstructive lung disease).
- The decision to proceed with surgery is based on a variety of factors including patient functional capacity, type of pulmonary pathology, extent of disease, the possibility of cure, and feasibility of surgical correction/management of pathology.

Age

- There is no maximum age cutoff prior to thoracic surgery or pulmonary resection.
- Respiratory complications following surgery increase with advanced age (>80 years).
- Pneumonectomy carries a higher risk of mortality when compared to lobectomy in patients of advanced age (>70 years).

Common Comorbid Conditions

- Pulmonary
  - Chronic obstructive pulmonary disease (COPD) is the most common comorbid condition among patients undergoing noncardiac thoracic surgery.

    Severity of lung dysfunction secondary to COPD is a predictor of perioperative outcome. Severity of disease can be best defined by the FEV1 (see Chap. 11).

    Of note, when high FiO_2 is given to patients with severe COPD, it may cause a decrease in alveolar ventilation and an increase in alveolar dead space by redistributing perfusion away from lung areas with "normal" V/Q matching to areas of very low V/Q matching. This could ultimately result in severe hypercarbia. Oxygen should be titrated carefully to prevent hypoxemia without causing hypercapnia.

    COPD can commonly result in pulmonary hypertension and right ventricular (RV) dysfunction in up to 50% of patients.

All COPD patients should receive maximal bronchodilator therapy prior to their procedure.
Smoking cessation should be encouraged both preoperatively for at least 4 weeks prior to the procedure and indefinitely postoperatively.

- Cardiac
  - Cardiac complications are the second most common cause of perioperative morbidity and mortality in the thoracic surgical patient.
  - Baseline cardiac function is an important contributor of perioperative morbidity and mortality.
  - Thoracic surgery is considered an intermediate risk procedure in terms of cardiac ischemia.
- Renal
- Preoperative renal dysfunction (serum creatinine >2 mg/dL) may lead to perioperative morbidity and mortality.

Airway Anatomy (Fig. 3.1)

Knowledge of the thoracic and airway anatomy is essential for a variety of reasons:

- Necessary for flexible fiberoptic bronchoscopy to diagnose/manage pathology
- Successful placement of double-lumen tubes and bronchial blockers
- Manage intraoperative pulmonary dysfunctions/problems

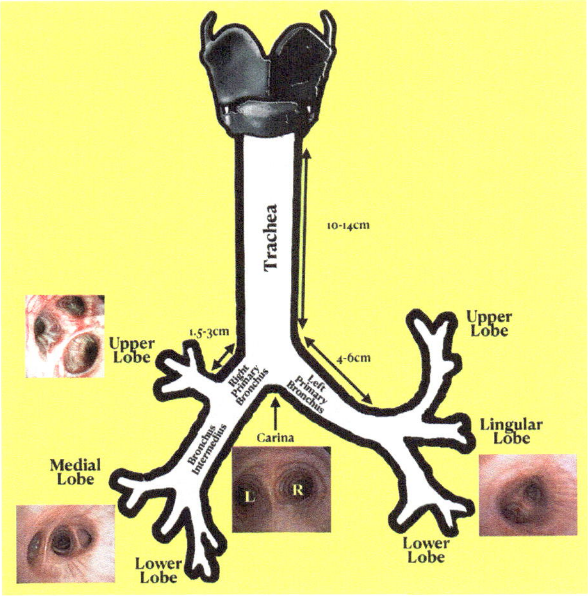

Fig. 3.1 Airway anatomy with bronchoscopic images. (Reprinted with permission from Neustein SM: The use of bronchial blockers for providing one-lung ventilation. J CardioThorac Vasc Anesth 2009;23:860–868. Falzon D, Alston P, Coley E, Montgomery K: Lung isolation for thoracic surgery: From inception to evidence-based. J CardioThorac Vasc Anesth 2017;31:678–693)

Trachea

- Approximately 11–15 cm in length (depending on sex/height) and extends from the lower end of the cricoid cartilage (C6) and divides at the carina (T5).
- Surrounded by 16–20 C-shaped tracheal cartilaginous rings which occupy the anterior two-thirds of its aspect. The C-shaped rings are joined posteriorly by the fibroelastic tissue and trachealis muscle. Identification of the rings allows for anteroposterior orientation allowing for correct delineation of the left and right mainstem bronchi during bronchoscopy.
- Diameter is about the size of an individual's index finger.

Mainstem Bronchi

- The carina is the transition point from the trachea and gives rise to the left and the right mainstem bronchi.
- The right mainstem bronchus is wider and shorter than the left mainstem bronchus. The right also comes off at a 25–30° angle as compared to the 45° angle on the left. The large opening along with the less acute angle makes pulmonary aspiration as well as endotracheal tube mainstems more likely on the right.

Lobes/Bronchopulmonary Segments

- The right lung comprises three lobes with a total of ten bronchopulmonary segments. The left lung comprises two lobes with a total of eight bronchopulmonary segments.
- The orifice of the right upper lobe lies in the lateral wall of the right main bronchus only about 2 cm from the carina. This can be identified by a trifurcation of three segmental bronchi known as the apical, anterior, and posterior divisions (as shown in Fig. 3.1). The right main bronchus continues as the bronchus intermedius for another 2.5 cm terminating in bronchi that lead to the middle and lower lobes. Less than 10% of the time, the right upper lobe bronchus may originate above the carina.

- The left main bronchus bifurcates into the bronchi of the left upper and lower lobes at its distal end. This occurs approximately 5 cm from its takeoff at the carina. The left upper bronchus consists of an upper and lingula division.
- Given the greater distance to the distal branches as compared to the right bronchus, it is easier to place a left-sided double-lumen tube or bronchial blocker as there is less risk of obstructing segmental bronchi.

Hemodynamic Monitoring

All patients undergoing thoracic surgery will have standard American Society of Anesthesiologists (ASA) monitors including electrocardiogram (ECG), pulse oximetry, noninvasive blood pressure (NIBP) cuff measurements, end-tidal capnography, and temperature.

- Monitoring oxygenation by pulse oximetry may be adequate during single-lung ventilation (SLV).
- Consider placing an arterial line in complex and/or prolonged cases, or in patients with cardiac comorbidities.

Fluid Management

Intraoperative Fluid Administration (Crystalloid)

- Restrictive administration (< 2 mL/kg/h or <1 L/case) is associated with optimal outcomes (Fig. 3.2).
- In thoracic pulmonary cases, liberal fluid administration is associated with worse outcomes (acute lung injury, cardiovascular).
- Restrictive fluid administration is not associated with renal dysfunction.

Transfusion of blood products should be preserved for patients whose hemoglobin levels (Hgb) are less than 8.0 g/dL in concern of precipitation of respiratory complications and transfusion-related acute lung injury (TRALI).

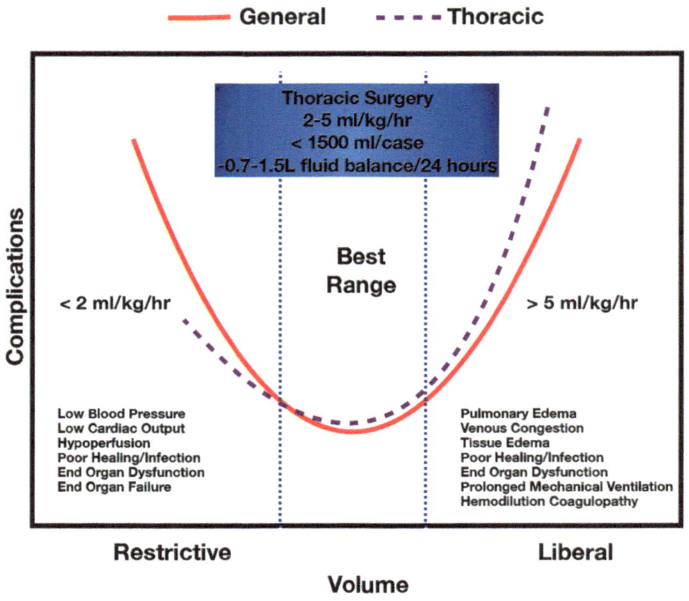

Fig. 3.2 Association of fluid administration with outcomes

Analgesia

Adequate pain management is essential in thoracic surgery to support pulmonary function and reduce postoperative complications by allowing deep breathing, effective coughing, early mobilization, and prevention of atelectasis, pneumonia, and acute lung injury.

- Multimodal analgesic approach is promoted for the enhanced recovery pathway.
- Analgesia regimen/plan depends on the extent of incision, open vs minimally invasive, and the existence of contraindications to specific regimens (regional blocks).
- Multimodal approach including opioids, acetaminophen, nonsteroidal anti-inflammatory drugs (NSAIDs), N-methyl-D-aspartate (NDMA) receptor antagonists, gabapentin, and lidocaine.

Anatomy of Pain

- Intercostal nerves: Skin and intercostal muscles and parietal pleura (all phrenic nerve)
- Vagus nerve: Lung and mediastinum

- Thoracodorsal and long thoracic (arise from C5–C7): Latissimus dorsi and serratus muscles/region
- Thoracotomy incision: Between T4 and T6
- Esophageal incision: From T3 to T7

Opioids

- Used to be the main component of postoperative analgesic regimens in thoracic surgery.
- But due to its side effects, particularly sedation, respiratory depression, and inhibition of cough, the newer approach for pain management targets minimization or sparing of opioids.

Acetaminophen

- Has been shown to decrease overall opioid consumption and has been incorporated into various enhanced recovery after surgery (ERAS) protocols.
- Oral doses are as effective as intravenous dosing.

NSAIDs

- Have been shown to reduce opioid consumption; the combination of NSAIDs and acetaminophen is effective in pain management after thoracic surgery.
- Intravenous or oral routes are employed.
- Caution is applied in elderly patients who may have occult preexisting renal or cardiovascular diseases.
- Caution is applied for patients with preexisting renal disease.
- Caution is applied for patients with increased bleeding risk.

Ketamine

- NMDA receptor antagonist, can provide potent analgesic effects and reduce inflammatory cytokine release.
- Intravenous routes are limited to the immediate perioperative use as injections.
- Has been used for PCA regimens but only under closely monitored settings.

Regional Analgesia Techniques (Fig. 3.3)

- Applied as single injection and/or continuous infusions.
- Medications include local anesthetics, opioids, steroids, and/or α-2 agonists alone or in combination.
- Techniques can be grossly divided into neuraxial (epidural and spinal), paraspinal (paravertebral and erector spinae blocks), and chest wall blocks (serratus anterior, transversus thoracic muscle plane, and pectoralis blocks).

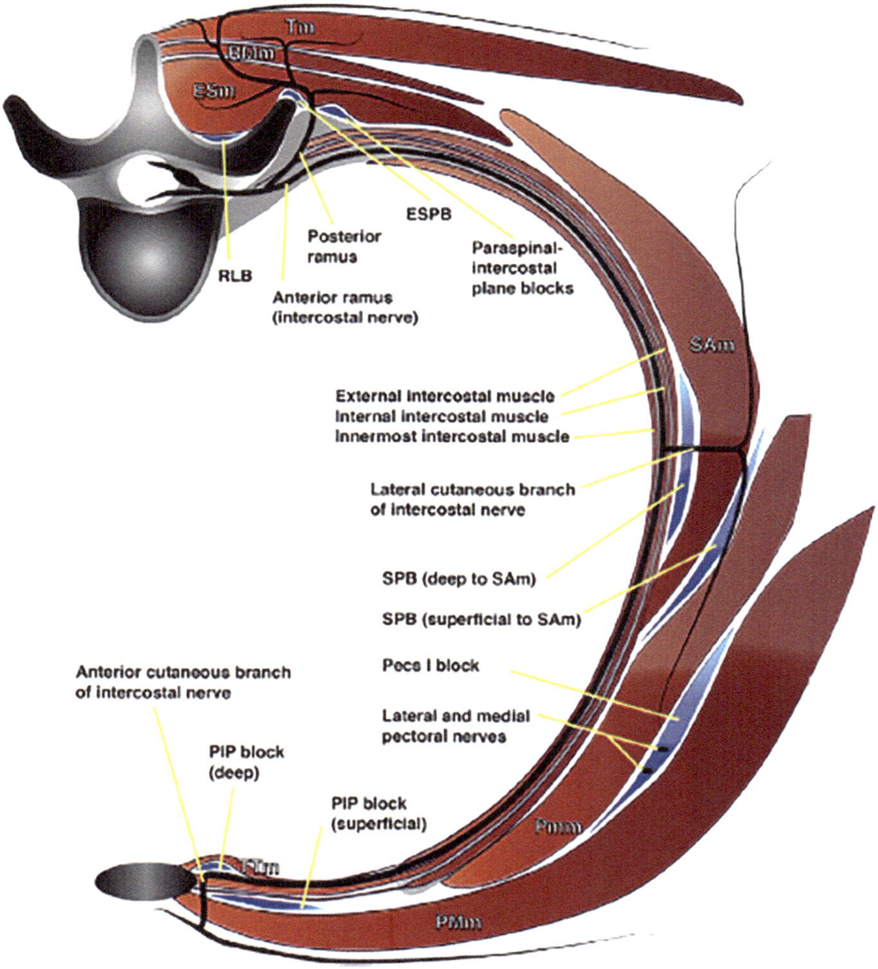

Fig. 3.3 Thoracic blocks. (Chin KJ: Thoracic wall blocks: From paravertebral to retrolaminar to serratus to erector spinae and back again—A review of evidence. Best Practice & Research Clinical Anesthesiology 2019;33:67–77). *ESm* erector spinae muscle, *RMm* rhomboid major muscle, *Tm* trapezius muscle, *SAm* serratus anterior muscle, *PMm* pectoralis major muscle, *Pmm* pectoralis minor muscle, *TTm* transversus thoracis muscle, *RLB* retrolaminar block, *ESPB* rector spinae plane block, *SPB* serratus plane block, *PIP* parasternal intercostal plane

- Chest wall blocks have an advantage in that they may be safer to perform in patients with coagulation abnormalities; however, their duration and coverage are limited.

Continuous Thoracic Epidural Analgesia (TEA)

- Typically reserved for an open thoracotomy incision.
- The insertion site is one to two spinal segments above the middle of the proposed incision.
- A large range of pharmacologic regimens can be employed.
- Advantages: good analgesic effect, minimal respiratory depression, long duration, earlier return of gastrointestinal function (compared to other medications).
- Disadvantages: bilateral effect increases hemodynamic changes; risks urinary retention, hypotension, and epidural hematoma; failure rate up to 15%.

Single-Injection Intrathecal (Spinal) Injections

- Typically opioids are injected, although clonidine has been employed in the past. Immediate preoperative injection. Lipophobic opioids like morphine (5–20 μg/kg) or dilaudid (0.5–2 μg/kg) are injected as they spread to the substantia gelatinosa of the dorsal horn prior to penetrating the spinal cord making them a better choice for thoracotomy incisions as they spread cephalad.
- Advantages: provides 12–24 h of analgesia.
- Disadvantages: slow onset, 1–2 h, variable analgesia, requires close monitoring of respiratory function for 24 h, postspinal headache.

Paravertebral Nerve Block

- Technique that injects medication (local anesthetic) at the ventral ramus of the spinal ganglion in the paravertebral space, to block ipsilateral sympathetic and somatic nerves that come off the intercostal nerve.
- Ideally performed using ultrasound; however landmark techniques are described.
- Typically plain local anesthetic solutions are employed (bupivacaine (or equivalent) 0.25–0.5% 20–30 mL injection and/or 10–15 mL/h infusion).
- Advantages: unilateral block, minimal or no sedation, avoid complications associated with epidural catheters and spinal injections.
- Disadvantages: minimal spread, requires multiple injections to block multiple levels, limited duration of effect.

Intercostal Nerve Block

- Technique that injects local anesthetic along the inferior portion of the rib where the neurovascular bundle passes.
- Advantages: can be performed intraoperatively by the surgeon under direct visualization or postoperatively using a percutaneous approach.
- Disadvantages: requires multiple single injections, possible vascular injury.

Erector Spinae Plane Block

- Technique that injects medications deep to the erector spinae muscle and superficial to transverse process.
- Medications more likely to block dorsal ramus off the spinal ganglion; however, spread to the ventral ramus also occurs.
- Ideally performed using ultrasound; however landmark techniques are described.
- Advantages: unilateral block, effective analgesia with minimal or no sedation, effective at reducing respiratory complications, does not require multiple injections, can be employed with borderline coagulation function.
- Disadvantages: $\leq$1% epidural/spinal spread, less effective block than paravertebral block, limited duration of effect.

Other analgesic approaches such as cryoanalgesia of intercostal nerves or transcutaneous electric nerve stimulation (TENS) may be considered although studies show no evidence of reduction in opioid consumption or improved pain management; further studies are needed to evaluate its role in thoracic anesthesia.

Airway Management

Specific airway and ventilator management are different for thoracic surgery patients compared to non-thoracic surgery patients. For procedures involving one side of the thorax, single-lung ventilation (SLV; only ventilating one lung) is employed to facilitate surgical exposure and the surgical procedure. While the surgeon operates on one side, the opposite lung is ventilated.

Indications for Single-Lung Ventilation

- Thoracic surgery
- Infection (avoid spilling into good lung)
- Pulmonary hemorrhage (avoid blood clot/asphyxiation of the good lung)

- Bronchopleural fistula
- Tracheobronchial disruption
- Life-threatening hypoxemia (shunting) due to unilateral lung disease

Double-Lumen Bronchial Tube

- Two lumens: the longer one ideally extends into either the left or right bronchus, and the shorter lumen terminating in the trachea like a normal endotracheal tube.
- A cuff for each lumen (tracheal cuff and bronchial cuff) which can facilitate isolated ventilatory systems of either right or left regardless if a right or left double-lumen tube is used.
- Closing off either lumen will selectively deflate the lung on the closed offside, while the other side is able to continue ventilating.
- Double-lumen endotracheal tube (DLETT) is much larger than a single-lumen endotracheal tube (ETT) so as to accommodate two lumens.
- Although examination using a stethoscope can help position and confirm proper positioning of airway devices, a fiberoptic bronchoscope is extremely useful (Fig. 3.4).

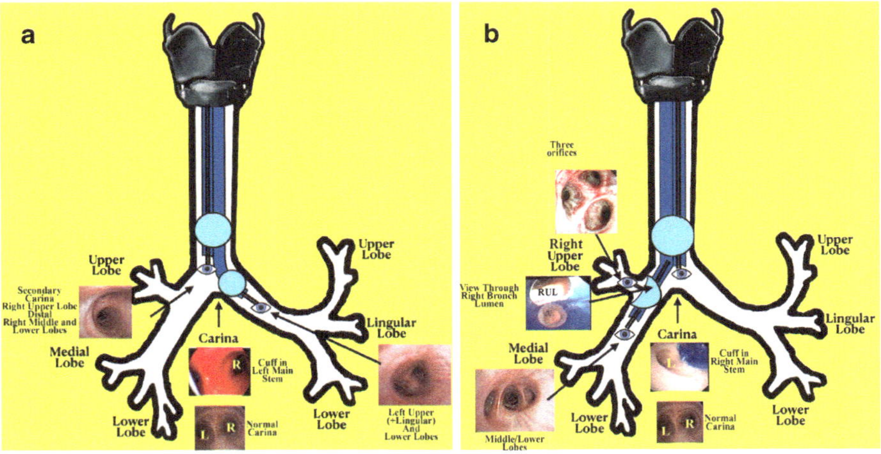

Fig. 3.4 Bronchoscopic view of an appropriately double-lumen tube. (**a**) Left-sided double-lumen endotracheal tube; (**b**) right-sided double-lumen tube. (Bronchoscopic images reprinted with permission from: Falzon D, Alston P, Coley E, Montgomery K. Lung isolation for thoracic surgery: From inception to evidence-based. J CardioThorac Vasc Anesth 2017;31:678–693. Neustein SM. The use of bronchial blockers for providing one-lung ventilation. J CardioThorac Vasc Anesth 2009;23:860–868. Bustamante S, Shravan Cheruku MD. 3D Printing for Simulation in Thoracic Anesthesia. J Cardiothorac Vasc Anesth. 2016 Dec;30(6):e61–e63. Failor E, Bowdle A, Jelacic S, Togashi K: High-Fidelity Simulation of Lung Isolation With Double-Lumen Endotracheal Tubes and Bronchial Blockers in Anesthesiology Resident Training. J CardioThorac Vasc Anesth.2014;28;865–869)

- While both left and right DLETT can be used to isolate either lung, left-sided DLETT is preferred over right, due to the longer length of the left main bronchus which allows for easier positioning. For right-sided DLETT, the short right main bronchus requires more precise positioning, specifically of the bronchial lumen, such that the bronchial lumen distal orifice is toward the bronchus intermedius and the side orifice of the bronchial lumen is toward the right upper lobe bronchus (note that bronchial lumen of left DLETT does not have a side orifice).
- Right-side DLETT is utilized during surgical procedures involving the left main bronchus, such as left main sleeve resection, left upper or lower sleeve lobectomy, or left pneumonectomy.

Placement

- With the tip of the bronchial lumen facing up, the bronchial portion of the DLETT is passed through the vocal cords. The entire tube then needs to be rotated 90° toward bronchus the tube is designed for (for a left-sided DLETT, rotate 90° to the left after passing the bronchial lumen through the cords), whereafter continue advancing the tube as you would a normal ETT.
- After passage of the DLETT, either by examination and selective closure of a lumen or by using a fiberoptic bronchoscope, the position of the DLETT is facilitated. Initially, placement via the larger tracheal lumen and identification of the carina determines the position of the bronchial lumen. If not clear, the placement of the FOB via the bronchial lumen and withdrawing the DLETT to view the carina will help facilitate passage into the desired bronchus.
- Regardless of how the operator places the DLETT, use of a FOB will confirm placement and repositioning of the DLETT as needed. Under this visualization, the bronchial cuff can then be inflated and confirmed to be seated correctly without herniating back into the trachea.

Bronchial Blockers

- A variety of bronchial blockers exist, but their fundamental design remains the same (Fig. 3.5).
- There are adult and pediatric bronchial blockers (4–5 mm and 2–3 mm).
- Placement through a single-lumen ETT (although can be placed via DLETT if needed for special circumstances).
- The small lumen within the bronchial blocker allows for air to escape the operative lung to facilitate deflation/collapse, allows suction, or administration of continuous positive airway pressure, the latter described below in management of hypoxemia.
- Lung deflation occurs during apnea.

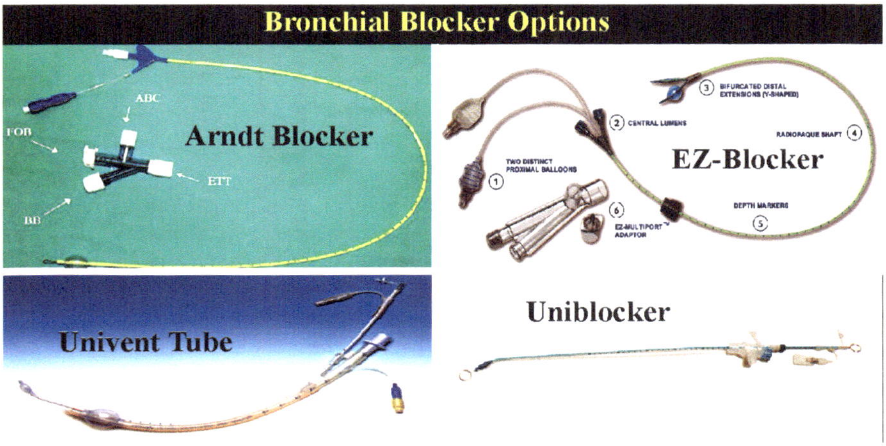

Fig. 3.5 Bronchial blockers. (Reprinted with permission from: Iyer MH, Kumar N, Hussain N et al.: Airway management during anesthesia for lung transplantation: Double-lumen tube or endobronchial blocker? J CardioThorac Vasc Anesth. 2021;35:1286–1291. Heir JS, Sekhon AK, Thakar DR, Jackson TA, Lasala JD, Purugganan RV: External tracheal manipulation maneuver (ETMM) to facilitate endobronchial blocker placement. J CardioThorac Vasc Anesth. 2016;30:1061–1063). *FOB* fiberoptic bronchoscopy, *BB* bronchial blocker, *ABS* airway breathing circuit, *ETT* endotracheal tube

- When finished, the blocker is removed, while the single-lumen ETT is left in place.
- Drawbacks of bronchial blockers are they do not stay in place as readily as a double-lumen tube, more easily herniate back from the bronchus into the trachea especially with repositioning, and no access to the blocked lung.
- Placement depends on the type of bronchial blocker being used, but general principles remain the same:
  - Intubate the patient a single-lumen endotracheal tube (preferably 8.0 for adult).
  - Place/advance the bronchial blocker through the endotracheal tube under direct visualization with a fiberoptic bronchoscope (Fig. 3.6).
  - Guide the bronchial blocker into the bronchus of the operative lung.
  - Lock the bronchial blocker into place once it is confirmed in the correct bronchus; then position the patient for the surgery (place in lateral decubitus position as if often needed for thoracic cases).
  - For single-lung ventilation:

    Open the lumen to room air and deflate the operative lung during apnea; suction can be applied to the lumen to hasten the process.
    Inflate the bronchial blocker cuff under direct visualization with the fiberoptic bronchoscope.
    Expect cuff to herniate proximally during inflation.
    Position bronchial blocker just below the carina.

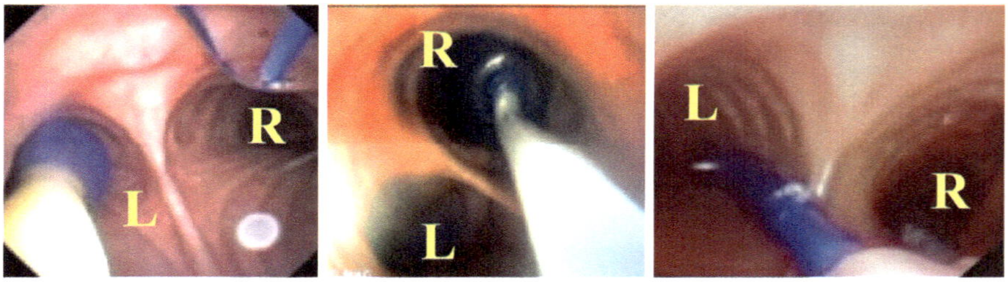

Fig. 3.6 Bronchoscopic view of the placement of bronchial blockers. (Reprinted with permission from: Iyer MH, Kumar N, Hussain N et al.: Airway management during anesthesia for lung transplantation: Double-lumen tube or endobronchial blocker? J CardioThorac Vasc Anesth. 2021;35:1286–1291. Heir JS, Sekhon AK, Thakar DR, Jackson TA, Lasala JD, Purugganan RV: External tracheal manipulation maneuver (ETMM) to facilitate endobronchial blocker placement. J CardioThorac Vasc Anesth. 2016;30:1061–1063)

Normal Endotracheal Tube

1. Used for smaller pediatric patients who need single-lung ventilation, wherein double-lumen tubes bronchial blockers are too large.
2. Intentionally mainstem intubate the nonoperative lung.
3. Use a fiberoptic bronchoscope to place (Seldinger technique) and confirm a mainstem intubation.

Single-Lung Ventilation

- Tidal volume; 5–8 mL/kg (ideal body weight).
- PEEP 5–10 cm H_2O to reduce atelectasis.
- Desired airway pressures: peak <35 cm H_2O; plateau <25 cm H_2O.
- Intermittent recruitment maneuvers to reduce atelectasis.
- Adjust FiO_2% (typically >50%) to increase blood oxygen levels.

Physiologic Changes During Single-Lung Ventilation: Shunts and Hypercarbia

Shunt

- Upon initiation of single-lung ventilation, a large shunt is created as blood continues to flow to the deflated lung, where it is not being oxygenated at all.
- Hypoxic pulmonary vasoconstriction (HPV) attenuates shunt as the pulmonary vessels constrict in response to regional hypoxemia.

- Small amount of shunt (10–15%) persists due to bronchial arterial flow.
- Many anesthetic drugs (inhalation anesthesia; propofol) and nonspecific pulmonary vasodilators cause pulmonary vasodilation and reduce HPV and increase shunt and hypoxemia.
- High airway pressures and high pulmonary artery pressures to the nonsurgical lung may redirect blood to the surgical non-ventilated and non-oxygenated lung and increase shunt.

Hypercarbia (>50 mmHg)

- Need to maintain minute ventilation to prevent hypercarbia.
- Hypercarbia increases pulmonary vascular resistance and pulmonary artery pressure.
- Mild hypercarbia (<50–55 mmHg) may have benefits:
  - Accentuate HPV.
  - Increase oxygen delivery.
  - For patients with baseline pulmonary hypertension, mild hypercarbia may reduce pulmonary artery resistance.
- Replaces oxygen from Hgb.

Troubleshooting Desaturation Events While on Single-Lung Ventilation

- DLETT or bronchial blocker malpositioned
- Low FiO_2 (relative issue)
- Hypoventilation (displace oxygen from hemoglobin: Bohr effect)
- Ventilation/perfusion mismatching (loss of lung units)
- Shunt (above)
- Diffusion across capillary issues (less common as an acute problem)
- Low mixed venous oxygen saturation

Enhanced Recovery After Surgery (ERAS) or Enhanced Recovery After Thoracic Surgery (ERATS)

Preoperative Phase

- Preoperative visit and assessment
- Patient education and explanation of ERAS
- Smoking cessation

- Preoperative rehabilitation or prehabilitation
  - Exercise
  - Incentive spirometry
  - Pulmonary toilet medications
  - Anemia evaluation
- Preoperative carbohydrate drink (up to 2 h before surgery)
- Avoidance of preoperative sedating medications
- Preoperative analgesics
  - Tylenol
  - NSAIDs/Cox-2 inhibitors
  - Gabapentin

Perioperative Phase

- Prophylactic antibiotics
- Regional anesthesia
  - Intercostal blocks
  - Erector spinae plane block
  - Paravertebral block
- Minimal use of narcotics/opioid sparing techniques
  - Ketamine
  - Steroids
  - Tylenol
  - NSAIDs
  - Gabapentin
  - Magnesium
  - Dexmedetomidine
- Protective lung ventilation
- Fluid control (avoid fluid overload)
- Intraoperative warming
- Venous thromboembolism prophylaxis
- Postoperative nausea and vomiting (PONV) prophylaxis
- Atrial fibrillation prophylaxis
- Avoid urinary catheters
- Avoid arterial lines
- Minimally invasive surgery
- Single chest drain with early removal

Postoperative Phase

- Avoidance of postoperative fluids
- Multimodal analgesia/minimize opiates
  - Tylenol
  - Cox-2 inhibitor
  - Gabapentin
  - Oral narcotics
- Early feeding/drinking
- Early mobilization
- Early removal of chest drains and catheters
- Early discharge

Mediastinal Masses

- Surgeries and procedures for mediastinal masses are unique due to risk of cardiovascular and pulmonary collapse from compression by the mass.
- Life-threatening airway obstruction and/or cardiovascular collapse in patients with mediastinal masses are known to occur with induction of anesthesia, during the procedure, and in the post-procedure period.
- Mediastinal mass syndrome (MMS) is due to compression or infiltration of otherwise normal mediastinal structures by the mass. Patients complain of dyspnea, cough, and/or syncope with position changes. Presentation with swelling/edema of the head and neck with or without swelling of upper body vasculature hints toward superior vena syndrome.
- Aside from general cardiopulmonary history and exam, imaging is the cornerstone of the preoperative evaluation to guide subsequent care. Computed tomography (CT) is the standard imaging technique to define disease, mass size/position, anatomy, and relationship to surrounding cardiopulmonary structures and its extent of compression.
- For the patient considered at risk for airway compression, flow volume loops, sitting and supine, can be obtained; extrathoracic mass causes inspiratory compression, while intrathoracic mass causes expiratory compression.
- For the patient considered at risk for cardiac involvement, echocardiography at baseline and with position change may be useful to predict risk and plan care.
- Proper care requires a coordinated multidisciplinary effort. Given how quickly complications can happen, the pre-procedure communication between the anesthesiologist and the surgeon regarding the procedure and formation of a plan to address complications are crucial to the care of these patients.

- Anesthetic strategies for patients with large compressive mediastinal mass include upright positioning, spontaneous ventilation, rigid bronchoscopy available, minimize sedation (utilize local or regional techniques), use short-acting agents, avoid paralytics, lower extremity IV access for superior vena cava (SVC) syndrome, and have available vasoactive drugs, helium-oxygen, and extracorporeal membrane oxygenation/cardiopulmonary bypass.

Key Reference

- Foley KA, Slinger P. Fiberoptic bronchoscopic positioning of double-lumen tubes. Anaesth Intensive Care Med. 2017;18:602–5.

Further Reading

Batchelor TJP, Rasburn NJ, Abdelnour-Berchtold E, Brunelli A, Cerfolio RJ, Gonzalez M, Ljungqvist O, Petersen RH, Popescu WM, Slinger PD, Naidu B. Guidelines for enhanced recovery after lung surgery: recommendations of the enhanced recovery after surgery (ERAS®) society and the European Society of Thoracic Surgeons (ESTS). Eur J Cardiothorac Surg. 2019;55(1):91–115. PMID: 30304509. https://doi.org/10.1093/ejcts/ezy301.

Campos JH. Update on tracheobronchial anatomy and flexible fiberoptic bronchoscopy in thoracic anesthesia. Curr Opin Anaesthesiol. 2009;22(1):4–10. Epub 2009/03/20. PubMed PMID: 19295287. https://doi.org/10.1097/ACO.0b013e32831a43ab.

Campos J. Fiberoptic bronchoscopy for positioning double-lumen tubes and bronchial blockers. In: Slinger P, editor. Principles and practice of anesthesia for thoracic surgery. Cham: Springer; 2019. https://doi.org/10.1007/978-3-030-00859-8_17.

Chin KJ. Thoracic wall blocks: from paravertebral to retrolaminar to serratus to erector spinae and back again—a review of evidence. Best Pract Res Clin Anaesthesiol. 2019;33:67–77.

De Decker K, Jorens PG, Van Schil P. Cardiac complications after noncardiac thoracic surgery: an evidence-based current review. Ann Thorac Surg. 2003;75(4):1340–8. https://doi.org/10.1016/s0003-4975(02)04824-5.

Dulu A, Pastores SM, Park B, Riedel E, Rusch V, Halpern NA. Prevalence and mortality of acute lung injury and ARDS after lung resection. Chest. 2006;130(1):73–8. https://doi.org/10.1378/chest.130.1.73.

Edrich T. Bronchoscopic anatomy. In: Hartigan PM, editor. Practical handbook of thoracic anesthesia. Boston, MA: Springer US; 2012. p. 127–39.

Erdos G, Tzanova I. Perioperative anaesthetic management of mediastinal mass in adults. Eur J Anaesthesiol. 2009;26:627–32.

Falzon D, Alston RP, Coley E, Montgomery K. Lung isolation for thoracic surgery: from inception to evidence-based. J Cardiothorac Vasc Anesth. 2017;31(2):678–93. Epub 2016/09/07. PubMed PMID: 27595530. https://doi.org/10.1053/j.jvca.2016.05.032.

Fernández-Pérez ER, Keegan MT, Brown DR, Hubmayr RD, Gajic O. Intraoperative tidal volume as a risk factor for respiratory failure after pneumonectomy. Anesthesiology. 2006;105(1):14–8. PMID: 16809989. https://doi.org/10.1097/00000542-200607000-00007.

Forrest P. Thoracic anaesthesia. 2018. http://www.anaesthesia.med.usyd.edu.au/resources/lectures/pforrest/thoracic%20anaesthesia.htm.

Frendl G, Sodickson AC, Chung MK, et al. 2014 AATS guidelines for the prevention and management of perioperative atrial fibrillation and flutter for thoracic surgical procedures. J Thorac Cardiovasc Surg. 2014;148(3):e153–93. https://doi.org/10.1016/j.jtcvs.2014.06.036.

Golledge J, Goldstraw P. Renal impairment after thoracotomy: incidence, risk factors, and significance. Ann Thorac Surg. 1994;58:524.
Gothard J. Lung injury after thoracic surgery and one-lung ventilation. Curr Opin Anaesthesiol. 2008;19:5–10.
Grichnik KP, D'Amico TA. Acute lung injury and acute respiratory distress syndrome after pulmonary resection. Semin Cardiothorac Vasc Anesth. 2004;8(4):317–34. https://doi.org/10.1177/108925320400800405.
Hughes R, Gao F. Pain control for thoracotomy. Contin Educ Anaesth Crit Care Pain. 2005;5(2):56–60. https://doi.org/10.1093/bjaceaccp/mki014.
Iyer A, Yadav S. Postoperative care and complications after thoracic surgery. In: Firstenberg MS, editor. Principles and practice of cardiothoracic surgery. London: IntechOpen; 2013. https://doi.org/10.5772/55351.
Keshava HB, Boffa DJ. Cardiovascular complications following thoracic surgery. Thorac Surg Clin. 2015;25(4):371–92. Epub 2015/10/31. PubMed PMID: 26515939. https://doi.org/10.1016/j.thorsurg.2015.07.001.
Kim JA, Ahn HJ, Oh AR, Choi J. Restrictive intraoperative fluid management was associated with higher incidence of composite complications compared to less restrictive strategies in open thoracotomy: a retrospective cohort study. Sci Rep. 2020;10(1):8449. PMID: 32439944; PMCID: PMC7242459. https://doi.org/10.1038/s41598-020-65532-w.
Lee E-H. Optimal fluid therapy for thoracic surgery. J Thorac Dis. 2019;11:1753–5. https://doi.org/10.21037/jtd.2019.05.15.
Licker M, de Perrot M, Spiliopoulos A, Robert J, Diaper J, Chevalley C, Tschopp JM. Risk factors for acute lung injury after thoracic surgery for lung cancer. Anesth Analg. 2003;97(6):1558–65. PMID: 14633519. https://doi.org/10.1213/01.ANE.0000087799.85495.8A.
Licker M, Hagerman A, Bedat B, Ellenberger C, Triponez F, Schorer R, Karenovics W. Restricted, optimized or liberal fluid strategy in thoracic surgery: a narrative review. Saudi J Anesth. 2021;15(3):324–34.
Lin J, Gong C, Yu L, Gao F, Yu J, Chen J, Chen X, Zheng T, Zheng X. Regional analgesia in video-assisted thoracic surgery: a Bayesian network meta-analysis. Front Med. 9:842332. https://doi.org/10.3389/fmed.2022.842332.
Martin LW, Sarosiek BM, Harrison MA, Hedrick T, Isbell JM, Krupnick AS, Lau CL, Mehaffey JH, Thiele RH, Walters DM, Blank RS. Implementing a thoracic enhanced recovery program: lessons learned in the first year. Ann Thorac Surg. 2018;105(6):1597–604.
OpenAnesthesia. Risk stratification (thoracic anesthesia). 2022. https://www.openanesthesia.org/risk_stratification_thoracic_anesthesia/.
Rogers LJ, Bleetman D, Messenger DE, Joshi N, Wood L, Rasburn NJ, Batchelor TJP. The impact of enhanced recovery after surgery (ERAS) protocol compliance on morbidity from resection for primary lung cancer. J Thorac Cardiovasc Surg. 2018;155:1843–52.
Slinger PD, Johnston MR. Preoperative evaluation of the thoracic surgery patient. Semin Anesth Perioper Med Pain. 2002;21(3):168–81. https://doi.org/10.1053/sane.2002.34192.
Turnage WS, Lunn JJ. Postpneumonectomy pulmonary edema. A retrospective analysis of associated variables. Chest. 1993;103(6):1646–50. PMID: 8404079. https://doi.org/10.1378/chest.103.6.1646.
Wilkinson J, Pennefather SH, McCahon RA. Thoracic anaesthesia. Oxford: Oxford University Press; 2011.
Wu Y, Yang R, Xu J, Rusidanmu A, Zhang X, Hu J. Effects of intraoperative fluid management on postoperative outcomes after lobectomy. Ann Thorac Surg. 2019;107:1663–9.

Chapter 4
Lung Cancer Screening

Kena Vyas and Terrance Healey

Introduction

- Lung cancer is the number one cause of cancer mortality worldwide with the leading risk factor related to tobacco use. Studies have shown that screening with low-dose CT has resulted in earlier detection of lung cancer leading to a decrease in lung cancer mortality.
- Lung cancer mortality has been shown to be reduced by at least 20% in patients who undergo lung cancer screening with low-dose CT scan.
- Screening guidelines implemented by multiple professional organizations such as the United States Preventive Services Task Force (USPSTF), American Thoracic Society, American College of Radiology, and National Comprehensive Cancer Network have suggested using low-dose thoracic CT to screen for lung cancer.

K. Vyas (✉) · T. Healey
Department of Diagnostic Imaging, Warren Alpert Medical School of Brown University, Providence, RI, USA

T. Ng, T. Geraci (eds.), *Thoracic Surgery Clerkship*, Contemporary Surgical Clerkships, https://doi.org/10.1007/978-3-031-44645-0_4

Epidemiology

- Lung cancer is the leading cause of cancer-related mortality among men and women.
- Overall lung cancer is the second most common cancer in the United States.
- The incidence of lung cancer rises with age, with the average age being 70 years at time of diagnosis.

Risk Factors

- Smoking (accounts for 90% of all lung cancers), including secondhand smoke
- Age
  - Incidence increases with age.
- Emphysema and chronic obstructive pulmonary disease
- Interstitial lung disease
- Prior history of cancer (lung cancer, head and neck cancer, smoking-related cancers)
- Environmental exposures
  - Radon, asbestos, polycyclic aromatic hydrocarbons (tar, soot), arsenic, metals (beryllium, cadmium, chromium, nickel)
- History of radiation (e.g., breast cancer, lymphoma)
- Family history of lung cancer
- Race/ethnicity

Screening Guidelines

- The USPSTF recommends screening for lung cancer in adults 50–80 years old with a 20 pack-year smoking history, current smokers, or those who have quit within the last 15 years with low-dose computed tomography annually.
  - A pack-year is defined as smoking an average of one pack of cigarettes per day for 1 year. For example, a person could have a 20 pack-year history by smoking 1 pack a day for 20 years or 2 packs a day for 10 years.

  - Low-dose CT scanning has shown to be superior to a chest radiograph for lung cancer screening.

- Screening does not need to be performed if life expectancy is limited and the patient has turned 81 years old, has health problems that preclude lung cancer treatment and/or is unwilling to have curative surgical treatment, or has abstained from smoking for 15 years.
- Most insurance programs and Medicare pay for lung cancer screening tests.
- Guidelines currently recommend annual screening; however, reported data suggest that intervals of 2–2.5 years may be safe and effective.

Screening

- Lung cancer has better survival rates when diagnosed earlier.
- Screening goal is to detect asymptomatic disease, when treatment will be most successful.
- Screening should increase quality of life and life expectancy.
- Screening with low-dose CT scan can diagnose lung cancer earlier leading to a decrease in lung cancer-related deaths with the initiation of early treatment.
- Only test that has shown a reduction in lung cancer-related mortality in smokers.
- There are no absolute contraindications to low-dose CT screening.
- Low-dose CT scan is as accurate as standard-dose CT scan for pulmonary nodule detection.
- Low-dose CT scan is able to detect very small lung nodules (benign and malignant) by using thinner slices.
- CT findings can include a variety of findings that are classified according to the Lung-RADS classification system per the American College of Radiology.
- Lung-RADS provides a systematic approach and management guidelines for lesions suspicious for cancer (Fig. 4.1):
  - Lung-RADS 1–2: benign
  - Lung-RADS 3 (probably benign): require surveillance
  - Lung-RADS 4 (suspicious): require further evaluation

American College of Radiology™

Lung-RADS® v2022

Release Date: November 2022

Lung-RADS	Category Descriptor	Findings	Management
0	**Incomplete** Estimated Population Prevalence: ~ 1%	Prior chest CT examination being located for comparison (see note 9)	Comparison to prior chest CT;
		Part or all oflungs cannot be evaluated	Additional lung cancer screening CT imaging needed;
		Findings suggestive of an inflammatory or infectious process (see note 10)	1-3 month LDCT
1	**Negative** Estimated Population Prevalence: 39%	**No lung nodules OR**	12-month screening LDCT
		Nodule with benign features: • Complete, central, popcorn, or concentric ring calcifications **OR** • Fat-containing	
2	**Benign** - Based on imaging features or indolent behavior Estimated Population Prevalence: 45%	**Juxtapleural nodule:** • < 10 mm (524 mm³) mean diameter at baseline or new **AND** • Solid; smooth margins; and oval, lentiform, or triangular shape	
		Solid nodule: • < 6 mm (< 113 mm³) at baseline **OR** • New < 4 mm (< 34 mm³)	
		Part solid nodule: • < 6 mm total mean diameter (< 113 mm³) at baseline	
		Non solid nodule (GGN): • < 30 mm (< 14,137 mm³) at baseline, new, or growing **OR** • ≥ 30 mm (≥ 14,137 mm³) stable or slowly growing (see note 7)	
		Airway nodule, subsegmental - at baseline, new, or stable (see note 11)	
		Category 3 lesion that is stable or decreased in size at 6-month follow-up CT **OR** Category 4B lesion proven to be benign in etiology following appropriate diagnostic workup	
3	**Probably Benign** - Based on imaging features or behavior Estimated Population Prevalence: 9%	**Solid nodule:** • ≥ 6 to < 8 mm (≥ 113 to < 268 mm³) at baseline **OR** • New 4 mm to < 6 mm (34 to < 113 mm³)	6-month LDCT
		Part solid nodule: • ≥ 6 mm total mean diameter (≥ 113 mm³) with solid component < 6 mm (< 113 mm³) at baseline **OR** • New < 6 mm total mean diameter (< 113 mm³)	
		Non solid nodule (GGN): • ≥ 30 mm (≥ 14,137 mm³) at baseline or new	
		Atypical pulmonary cyst: (see note 12) • Growing cystic component (mean diameter) of a thick-walled cyst	
		Category 4A lesion that is stable or decreased in size at 3-month follow-up CT (excluding airway nodules)	
4A	**Suspicious** Estimated Population Prevalence: 4%	**Solid nodule:** • ≥ 8 to < 15 mm (≥ 268 to < 1,767 mm³) at baseline **OR** • Growing < 8 mm (< 268 mm³) **OR** • New 6 to < 8 mm (113 to < 268 mm³)	3-month LDCT; PET/CT may be considered if there is a ≥ 8 mm (≥ 268 mm³) solid nodule or solid component
		Part solid nodule: • ≥ 6 mm total mean diameter (≥ 113 mm³) with solid component ≥ 6 mm to < 8 mm (≥ 113 to < 268 mm³) at baseline **OR** • New or growing < 4 mm (< 34 mm³) solid component	
		Airway nodule, segmental or more proximal - at baseline (see note 11)	
		Atypical pulmonary cyst: (see note 12) • Thick-walled cyst **OR** • Multilocular cyst at baseline **OR** • Thin- or thick-walled cyst that becomes multilocular	
4B	**Very Suspicious** Estimated Population Prevalence: 2%	**Airway nodule,** segmental or more proximal - stable or growing (see note 11)	Referral for further clinical evaluation
		Solid nodule: • ≥ 15 mm (≥ 1767 mm³) at baseline **OR** • New or growing ≥ 8 mm (≥ 268 mm³)	Diagnostic chest CT with or without contrast; PET/CT may be considered if there is a ≥ 8 mm (≥ 268 mm³) solid nodule or solid component; tissue sampling; and/or referral for further clinical evaluation Management depends on clinical evaluation, patient preference, and the probability of malignancy (see note 13)
		Part solid nodule: • Solid component ≥ 8 mm (≥ 268 mm³) at baseline **OR** • New or growing ≥ 4 mm (≥ 34 mm³) solid component	
		Atypical pulmonary cyst: (see note 12) • Thick-walled cyst with growing wall thickness/nodularity **OR** • Growing multilocular cyst (mean diameter) **OR** • Multilocular cyst with increased loculation or new/increased opacity (nodular, ground glass, or consolidation)	
		Slow growing solid or part solid nodule that demonstrates growth over multiple screening exams (see note 8)	
4X	Estimated Population Prevalence: < 1%	Category 3 or 4 nodules with additional features or imaging findings that increase suspicion for lung cancer (see note 14)	
S	**Significant or Potentially Significant** Estimated Population Prevalence: 10%	**Modifier:** May add to category 0-4 for clinically significant or potentially clinically significant findings unrelated to lung cancer (see note 15)	As appropriate to the specific finding

Fig. 4.1 Lung-RADS scoring system for detected pulmonary nodules on low-dose CT scan for lung cancer screening

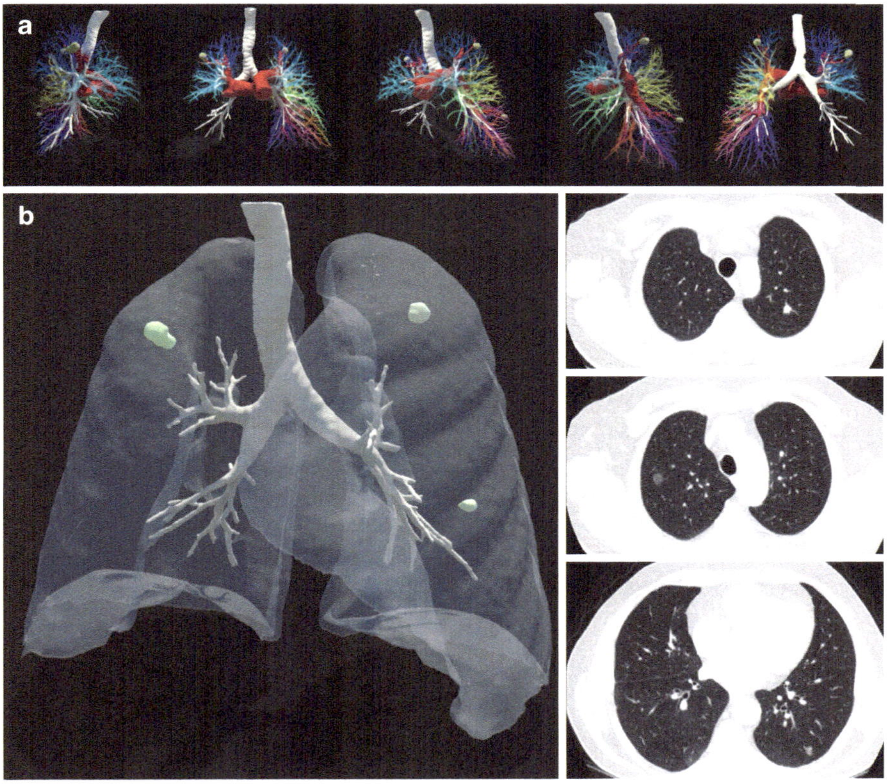

Fig. 4.2 CT scan imaging of lung nodules. (**a**) 3D reconstruction formats that demonstrate pulmonary nodules in the right upper, left upper, and left lower lobes. (**b**) These 3D reconstructions correspond to the findings in the axial reformats of the CT scan

Descriptors

- Nodules and focal lung lesions are reported according to:
  - Anatomic location such as segment or lung lobe (Fig. 4.2a, b)
  - Series/image numbers
  - Nodule size
  - Attenuation: fat, calcification, soft tissue
  - Opacity: solid, ground glass, etc.

    Solid and part solid nodules are more likely to be faster growing and invasive.
  - Margins: smooth, lobulated, spiculated
- Comparisons with prior imaging is a part of nodule evaluation.

Major Clinical Trials in Lung Cancer Screening

National Lung Screening Trial, 2011

- Randomized trial comparing low-dose CT scanning with chest radiography for lung cancer screening in 53,454 high-risk patients, over 3 years, in the United States.
  - Patients age 55–74, history of 30 pack-years of smoking, and current smokers or those who quit within 15 years.
- Data at a median follow-up of 6.5 years:
  - Positive findings were defined as a noncalcified nodule ≥4 mm. Overall, 24% of CT scans were reported as abnormal and 7% of chest radiographs were abnormal.
  - High false-positive rate of abnormal findings (a detected nodule was not lung cancer): 96% for CT and 95% for chest radiograph.
  - CT scanning detected 645 cases of lung cancer in 100,000 person-years versus 572 by chest radiograph.
- Results
  - Low-dose CT scanning reduced lung cancer mortality by 20%.
  - Reduction of all-cause mortality of 6.7% in the CT screening group.
  - Number needed to treat: for those undergoing at least 1 screening test, 320 patients required screening to prevent 1 lung cancer.

NELSON Trial, 2020

- Randomized trial of 15,789 patients of low-dose CT scanning at increasing intervals versus no screening, in Europe:
  - Patients aged 50–74 who were current or former smokers.
  - Screening intervals were performed at 1 year, 2 years, and 2.5 years.
- Results after 10-year follow-up:
  - Lung cancer mortality was reduced by 24% in men and 33% in women (results limited by smaller sample size).
  - A volume-based nodule measurement was used to define a positive finding, resulting in a detection rate of 2.1%.

Meta-Analysis, 2020

- Composite group analysis of seven randomized lung cancer screening trials with low-dose CT.
- Evaluated over 84,000 patients, who all had a greater than 15 pack-year smoking history.
- Results
  - Statistically significant 17% relative reduction in lung cancer mortality (risk ratio 0.83)
  - Nonsignificant relative reduction in overall mortality by 4%

Benefits Related to Screening

- Improved oncologic outcome due to earlier detection and therefore treatment. Lung cancer survival is directly related to the stage at time of diagnosis.
  - National Lung Screening Trial, 2011: 20% reduction in lung cancer mortality
  - NELSON European randomized trial, 2020: reduction in lung cancer mortality in men by 24% and women by 33%
- Earlier detection of lung cancer may undergo a complete surgical resection and have increased survival in comparison to patients who are treated for advanced disease with chemotherapy.
- Improved quality of life.
- Cost-effectiveness.
- Improved rate of smoking cessation.

Potential Harm to Screening

- Radiation exposure
  - Low-dose CT scanning has a lower exposure in comparison to other imaging modalities like PET or routine CT scanning.
  - A low-dose CT scan is approximately 10–30% of the dose of routine CT scan.
  - It is estimated that after 10 years of screening, for every 100 lung cancers detected, 1 major cancer would be induced by radiation.
- Physiological distress and anxiety
  - Distress from false-positive results or false-negative results
  - Distress from years-long follow-up of indeterminate nodules

- Overdiagnosis of abnormal findings
  - Detecting malignancy that would not have otherwise become significant
  - Detection of incidental findings or indeterminate nodules
- Procedure-associated complications
  - Patients who undergo further testing, including biopsy or surgery, have a low, but nonzero, rate of procedure-related complications.
  - Procedures performed for non-cancerous findings are often unnecessary and potentially harmful.
- Financial cost
  - There is a significant financial burden to the health system associated with screening, particularly follow-up over time of identified nodules, the majority of which do not represent lung cancer.

Conclusion

- Lung cancer is the leading cause of cancer-related mortality.
- USPSTF recommends screening for lung cancer in adults 55–80 years old with a 20 pack-year smoking history, current smokers, or those who have quit within the last 15 years with low-dose computed tomography annually.
- Screening with low-dose CT results in earlier detection of lung cancer leading to a decrease in lung cancer mortality.

Key Reference

- National Lung Screening Trial Research Team; Aberle DR, Adams AM, Berg CD, Black WC, Clapp JD, Fagerstrom RM, Gareen IF, Gatsonis C, Marcus PM, Sicks JD. Reduced lung-cancer mortality with low-dose computed tomographic screening. N Engl J Med. 2011;365(5):395–409.

Further Reading

American College of Radiology. Lung cancer screening resources. https://www.acr.org/Clinical-Resources/Lung-Cancer-Screening-Resources. Accessed 1 Jul 2022.

Committee on Thoracic Radiology of the ACR Commissions on Body Imaging and the Committee on Practice Parameters. ACR–STR practice parameter for the performance and reporting of lung ... In: ACR–STR practice parameter for the performance and reporting of lung cancer screening thoracic computed tomography (CT). 2019. https://www.acr.org/-/media/ACR/Files/Practice-Parameters/CT-LungCaScr.pdf. Accessed 1 Jul 2022.

de Koning HJ, van der Aalst CM, de Jong PA, Scholten ET, Nackaerts K, Heuvelmans MA, Lammers JJ, Weenink C, Yousaf-Khan U, Horeweg N, van't Westeinde S, Prokop M, Mali WP, Mohamed Hoesein FAA, van Ooijen PMA, Aerts JGJV, den Bakker MA, Thunnissen E, Verschakelen J,

Vliegenthart R, Walter JE, Ten Haaf K, Groen HJM, Oudkerk M. Reduced lung-cancer mortality with volume CT screening in a randomized trial. N Engl J Med 2020;382(6):503–13.
Jonas DE, Reuland DS, Reddy SM. Screening for lung cancer with low-dose computed tomography: an evidence review for the U.S. preventive services task force. 2021. https://www.ncbi.nlm.nih.gov/books/NBK568576/. Accessed 1 Jul 2022.
Kazerooni E, Lung CT. Screening reporting & data system (Lung-RADS). In: Lung RADS. American College of Radiology. https://www.acr.org/Clinical-Resources/Reporting-and-Data-Systems/Lung-Rads. Accessed 1 Jul 2023.
Mazzone PJ, Silvestri GA, Souter LH, Caverly TJ, Kanne JP, Katki HA, Wiener RS, Detterbeck FC. Screening for lung cancer: CHEST guideline and expert panel report. Chest. 2021;S0012-3692(21)01307–6.
Sadate A, Occean BV, Beregi JP, Hamard A, Addala T, de Forges H, Fabbro-Peray P, Frandon J. Systematic review and meta-analysis on the impact of lung cancer screening by low-dose computed tomography. Eur J Cancer. 2020;134:107–14.
Tanoue LT, Tanner NT, Gould MK, Silvestri GA. Lung cancer screening. https://www.atsjournals.org/doi/full/10.1164/rccm.201410-1777CI. Accessed 1 Jul 2022.
United States Preventive Services Taskforce. Lung cancer: screening. In: Recommendation: lung cancer: screening. 2021. https://www.uspreventiveservicestaskforce.org/uspstf/recommendation/lung-cancer-screening. Accessed 1 Jul 2022.
Wood DE, Eapen GA, Ettinger DS, et al. Lung cancer screening. JNCCN. 2012. https://jnccn.org/view/journals/jnccn/10/2/article-p240.xml. Accessed 1 Jul 2022.

Chapter 5
Lung Cancer Diagnosis and Staging

Hannah L. McMullen and Natalie S. Lui

Introduction

- Lung cancer diagnosis and staging is a multidisciplinary process often involving pulmonologists, radiologists, oncologists, and thoracic surgeons.
- Individuals may undergo diagnosis and staging of lung cancer after presenting with symptoms, incidental findings on imaging, or abnormal findings on chest CT for lung cancer screening.
- The process of diagnosis and staging is dynamic and incorporates the elements of clinical information; radiographic imaging, including chest radiograph (CXR), CT, and positron emission tomography (PET); magnetic resonance imaging (MRI); and histopathology derived by techniques of bronchoscopy, percutaneous needle biopsy/aspiration, or surgery.
- Identifying the specific cell type with its molecular and genetic profile of lung cancer helps inform treatment, especially for select patients with specific lung cancer mutations.
- For complex and/or unique clinical scenarios, multidisciplinary lung cancer tumor boards are established to help determine the relevant studies, interpretation of data, and optimal management.
- It is important to note that in clinical practice, the diagnosis, staging, and treatment are often performed together, instead of in stepwise sequence.

H. L. McMullen · N. S. Lui (✉)
Division of Thoracic Surgery, Department of Cardiothoracic Surgery, Stanford Health Care, Stanford, CA, USA
e-mail: hanmcm@stanford.edu; natalielui@stanford.edu

T. Ng, T. Geraci (eds.), *Thoracic Surgery Clerkship*, Contemporary Surgical Clerkships, https://doi.org/10.1007/978-3-031-44645-0_5

Lung Cancer Statistics, American Cancer Society 2022

- Approximately 15% of all malignancies, behind the prostate in men and breast in women.
- Accounts for 20% of all cancer deaths, more than the breast, prostate, and colon combined.
- Over 230,000 diagnosed and 130,000 deaths in the USA yearly.
- Only 25% present early stage to be considered for surgery.

Clinical Evaluation

- Presentation
  - Asymptomatic

    Found incidentally on imaging for other reasons
    Found on screening CT scan

  - Symptomatic

    Pulmonary—cough, hemoptysis, dyspnea, wheeze, pneumonia.
    Extrapulmonary intrathoracic—chest pain, hoarse voice, dysphagia, superior vena cava (SVC) syndrome, dyspnea (effusion, phrenic nerve paralysis), Pancoast's syndrome.
    Metastatic—common sites are the brain, bone, liver, and adrenal.
    Paraneoplastic:

      Metabolic: hypercalcemia, Cushing's syndrome, syndrome of inappropriate antidiuretic hormone (SIADH)
      Neurological: Lambert-Eaton syndrome, encephalopathy, subacute cerebellar degeneration
      Skeletal: clubbing, pulmonary hypertrophic osteoarthropathy
      Other: hematologic, cutaneous/muscular

- Risk Factors
  - Smoking (duration, amount)
  - Age
  - Previous history of cancer
  - Family history of cancer
  - Radon exposure (mining)
  - Asbestos exposure
  - Pulmonary fibrosis
  - Human immunodeficiency virus (HIV)

Initial Radiographic Evaluation

- Pain radiograph (Fig. 5.1a–e): nodule (defined as ≤3 cm), mass (>3 cm), infiltrate, atelectasis, effusion, elevated diaphragm (phrenic nerve invasion)

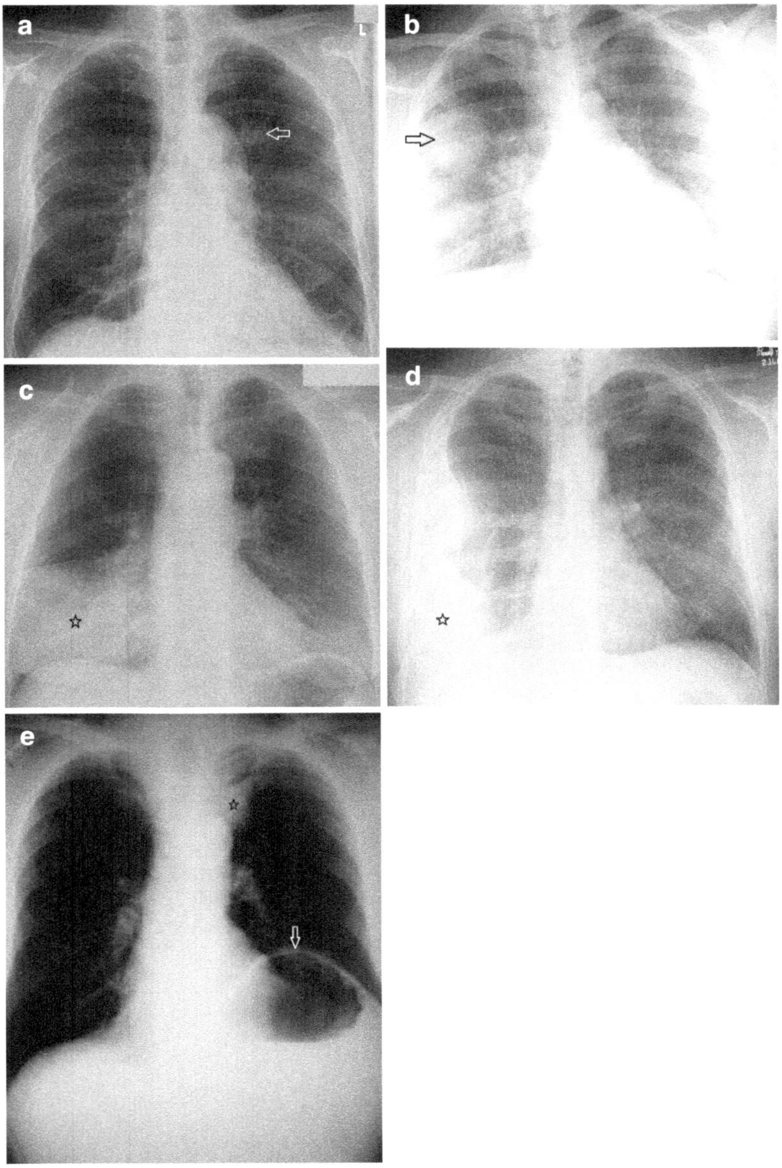

Fig. 5.1 Chest radiograph of lung cancer. (**a**) Spiculated nodule in the left upper lobe (arrow); (**b**) mass in the right upper lobe as defined by size >3 cm (arrow); (**c**) right middle lobe atelectasis/consolidation (star) due to endobronchial obstruction; (**d**) malignant pleural effusion (star); (**e**) left upper lobe mass abutting the mediastinum (star) and invading the phrenic nerve to cause hemidiaphragm paralysis/elevation (arrow)

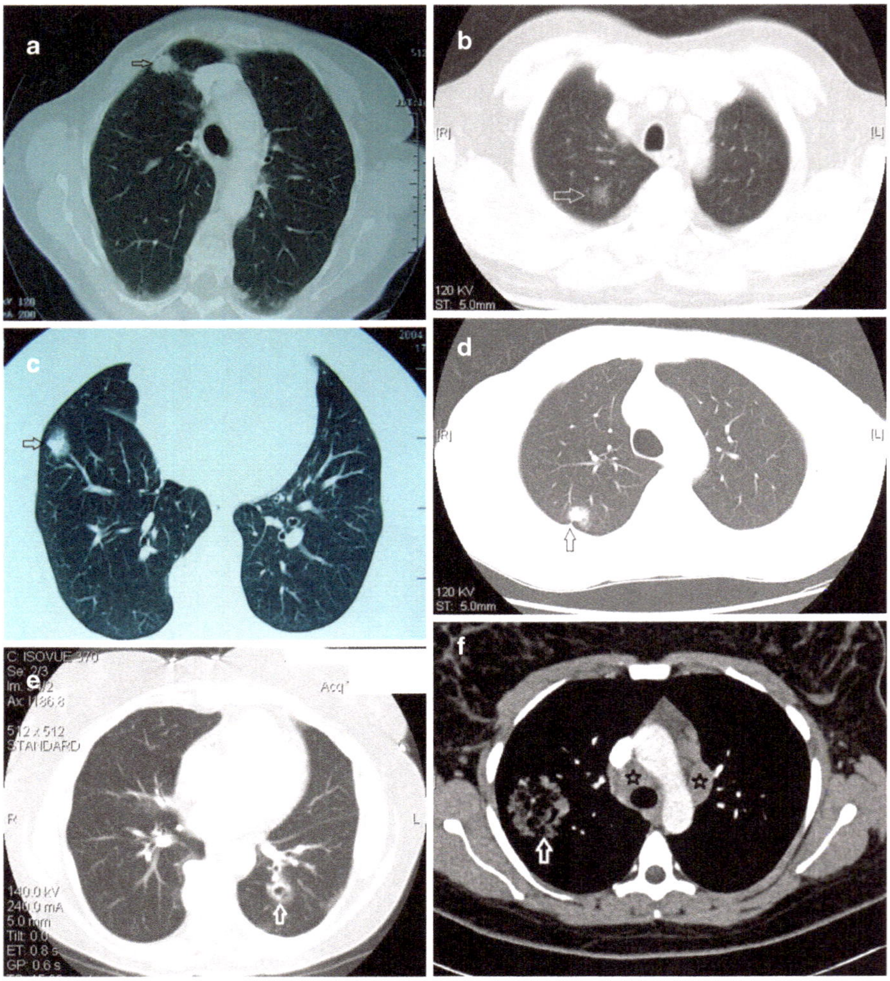

Fig. 5.2 CT scan of lung cancer. (**a**) Spiculated right upper lobe lung nodule; (**b**) right upper lobe ground-glass nodule; (**c**) right lower lobe mixed-solid and ground-glass nodule; (**d**) right upper lobe nodule with pleural tag; (**e**) cavitary left lower lobe squamous cell carcinoma; (**f**) right upper lobe mass as defined by size >3 cm (arrow) with mediastinal adenopathy as defined by nodal size >1 cm in short axis (star)

- CT scan (Fig. 5.2a–f)
  - Nodule/mass characteristics

    Size

    Growth versus stability (compare to prior imaging studies)

    Border: spiculated or lobulated versus smooth
    Internal composition: solid, ground glass, mixed solid/ground glass, cavitary (note wall thickness), calcification
    Pleural tag
    Pleura deformity and puckering/retraction
    Invasion into adjacent structures

- Lymphadenopathy
    Defined as a lymph node greater than 1 cm in the shortest dimension
    Regions: hilar (N1), mediastinal (N2), contralateral or supraclavicular (N3)
- Effusion(s)
    Pleural or pericardial
- Sites of potential metastasis
    Most common: liver, adrenal, and skeletal lesions

Diagnosis: Techniques for Lung Biopsy

- Sputum cytology
  - Limited by low sensitivity for lung cancer
  - Not valid for lung cancer screening
  - May yield diagnosis in patients with central lesions or with endobronchial tumor
- Percutaneous needle biopsy, often by CT guidance (Fig. 5.3a), but can also be performed with fluoroscopy or ultrasound (if lesion abuts the chest wall)
  - Ideal for peripherally located lesions
  - Performed using local anesthetic and conscious sedation
  - Risk of pneumothorax
- Bronchoscopic biopsy
  - Ideal for centrally located lesions, lesions that narrow/obstruct an airway seen on CT (bronchus sign, Fig. 5.3b).
  - With a navigational or robotic bronchoscopic system, peripheral lesions can also be biopsied (Fig. 5.3c).
  - Often requires general anesthesia.
  - Can be combined with endobronchial ultrasound (EBUS)-guided mediastinal lymph node for staging.
- Surgical biopsy (Fig. 5.3d)
  - Often performed by wedge resection, and is the most definitive method for diagnosis, but is also the most invasive biopsy technique.

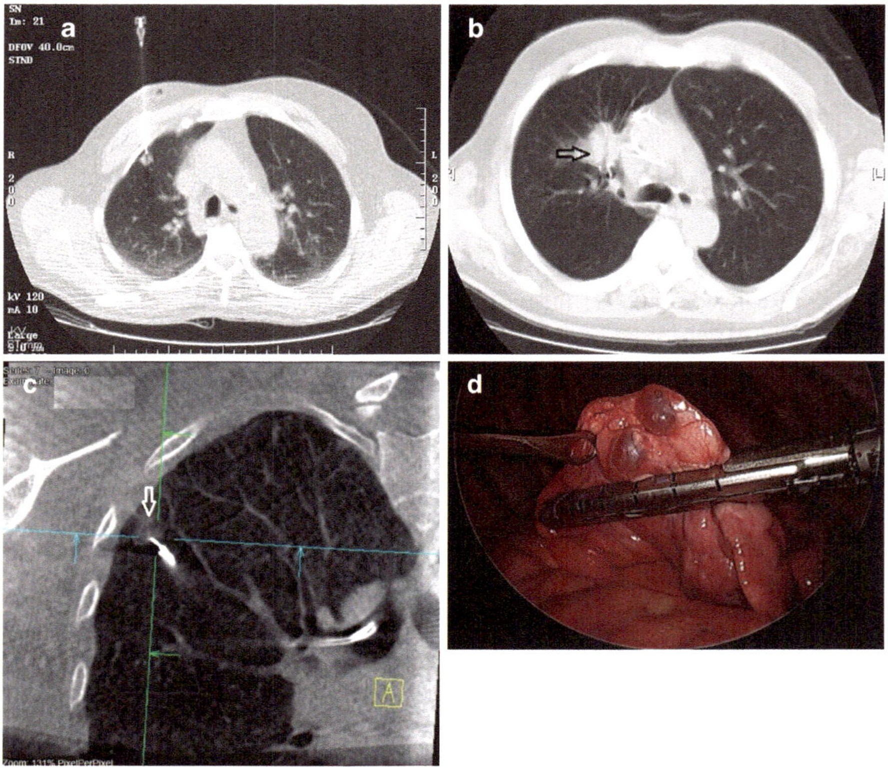

Fig. 5.3 Lung biopsy techniques for suspected lung cancer. (**a**) CT-guided needle biopsy of a peripheral right upper lobe nodule; (**b**) central right upper lobe mass with a bronchus sign thus ideal for bronchoscopic biopsy; (**c**) peripheral right upper lobe nodule successfully biopsied by navigation bronchoscopy; (**d**) video-assisted thoracoscopic surgery (VATS) wedge resection of peripheral right lung lesion

- Considered if a suspicious lesion undergoes percutaneous or bronchoscopic biopsy with nondiagnostic result.
- Considered if lesion is peripheral, but is less optimal for central lesions as such lesions may not be amenable to wedge (usually best to avoid performing diagnostic anatomic lung resection).
- If surgical biopsy is considered for a highly suspicious lesion, complete staging workup and preoperative pulmonary functional evaluation should be performed prior.
- Usually performed using minimally invasive surgical approaches: video-assisted thoracoscopic surgery (VATS) or robotic platform for excisional biopsy by wedge resection, followed by frozen section pathologic analysis, and then potential anatomic lung resection.

- For lesions that are not easily identified intraoperatively by visualization or palpation, preoperative localization techniques may be required, such as with hookwire, coil, Lipiodol, methylene blue, barium, radiotracer, or indocyanine green (ICG).
- Can be combined with definitive/curative resection during the same operation (completion lobectomy or segmentectomy) if lung cancer is confirmed by frozen section.

Diagnosis: Pathologic Cell Types

- Classifying lung cancer as non-small cell or small cell alone is no longer sufficient as specific cell types (and its subtypes) have significant implications with regard to prognosis and treatment.
- Adenocarcinoma:
  - Approximately 40% of all lung cancers, common cell type in nonsmokers.
  - Most commonly peripheral, but may also be central.
  - Cuboidal to columnar epithelial cells arranged in acinar or glandular pattern, supported by fibrous stroma; but these features may not be present when poorly differentiated.
  - Stain positive for TTF-1, Napsin A, CK7.
  - Subtypes, listed from best to worse prognosis; a given tumor may have one or more subtypes:

    Lepidic
    Papillary
    Acinar
    Micropapillary
    Solid

  - Other variants: invasive mucinous, colloid, fetal, enteric.
- Squamous cell carcinoma:
  - Approximately 30% of all lung cancers
  - May be central, cavitary
  - Polygonal cells, with stratification, intercellular bridge formation, keratinizing, formation of epithelial pearls; but these features may not be present when poorly differentiated
  - Stain positive for p63, p40, CK 5/6
- Adenosquamous:
  - Combined cell type with at least 10% of each type

- Large cell undifferentiated:
  - Diagnosis made only after extensive workup on resected specimens (should not be made on needle biopsy)
  - Finding a tumor that lacks features of small cell, adenocarcinoma, or squamous cell carcinoma
- Sarcomatoid carcinoma:
  - Pleomorphic carcinoma: at least 10% spindle and/or giant cells
  - Carcinosarcoma: mixture of carcinoma and sarcoma (rhabdomyosarcoma, chondrosarcoma, osteosarcoma) elements
  - Pulmonary blastoma: biphasic tumor of fetal adenocarcinoma and primitive mesenchymal stroma
- Neuroendocrine (see Chap. 10):
  - Small cell carcinoma: 15% of all lung cancers
  - Large cell neuroendocrine
  - Atypical carcinoid
  - Typical carcinoid

Lung Cancer TNM Staging

- The American Joint Commission on Cancer lung cancer staging system (8th Edition) was implemented in January 2018 (Tables 5.1 and 5.2).

Table 5.1 TNM definitions in the American Joint Commission on Cancer staging system (8th edition)

T_x	In sputum/bronchial washings (not on imaging/bronchoscopy)
T_0	No evidence of tumor
T_{is}	Carcinoma in situ
T_1	≤ 3 cm, surrounded by lung/visceral pleura, not involving the main bronchus
$T_{1a(mi)}$	Minimally invasive carcinoma, invasive component ≤5 mm
T_{1a}	≤1 cm
T_{1b}	>1 to ≤2 cm
T_{1c}	>2 to ≤3 cm
T_2	>3 to ≤5 cm, involvement of a main bronchus without the carina, invasion of visceral pleura, presence of partial/complete lung atelectasis or pneumonitis

Table 6.1 (continued)

T_{2a}	> 3 to ≤4 cm
T_{2b}	>4 to ≤5 cm
T_3	>5 to ≤7 cm, involvement of the chest wall/pericardium/phrenic nerve, satellite nodules in the same lung
T_4	>7 cm, invasion of the mediastinum/diaphragm/heart/great vessels/recurrent laryngeal nerve/carina/trachea/esophagus/spine, tumors in different lobe of ipsilateral lung
N_1	Ipsilateral peribronchial/hilar nodes and intrapulmonary nodes
N_2	Ipsilateral mediastinal/subcarinal nodes
N_3	Contralateral mediastinal/hilar nodes, ipsilateral or contralateral scalene/supraclavicular nodes
M_1	Distant metastasis
M_{1a}	Tumor in contralateral lung or pleural/pericardial nodule or malignant effusion
M_{1b}	Single extrathoracic metastasis, including single non-regional node
M_{1c}	Multiple extrathoracic metastases in one or more organs

Table 5.2 TNM groupings in the American Joint Commission on Cancer staging system (8th edition)

		N0	N1	N2	N3
T1	T1a	IA1	IIB	IIIA	IIIB
	T1b	IA2			
	T1c	IA3			
T2	T2a	IB	IIB	IIIA	IIIB
	T2b	IIA			
T3	T3	IIB	IIIA	IIIB	IIIC
T4	T4	IIIA	IIIA	IIIB	IIIC
M1	M1a	IVA	IVA	IVA	IVA
	M1b	IVA	IVA	IVA	IVA
	M1c	IVB	IVB	IVB	IVB

- For adenocarcinoma, it is important to note that the pathologic T size is based on the invasive component; the noninvasive component (lepidic) should not be included in the measurement.
- Location of lymph node stations is designated numerically (Fig. 5.4, Table 5.3) with single-digit nodes being mediastinal (N2 ipsilateral, N3 contralateral) and double-digit nodes being intrathoracic (N1).

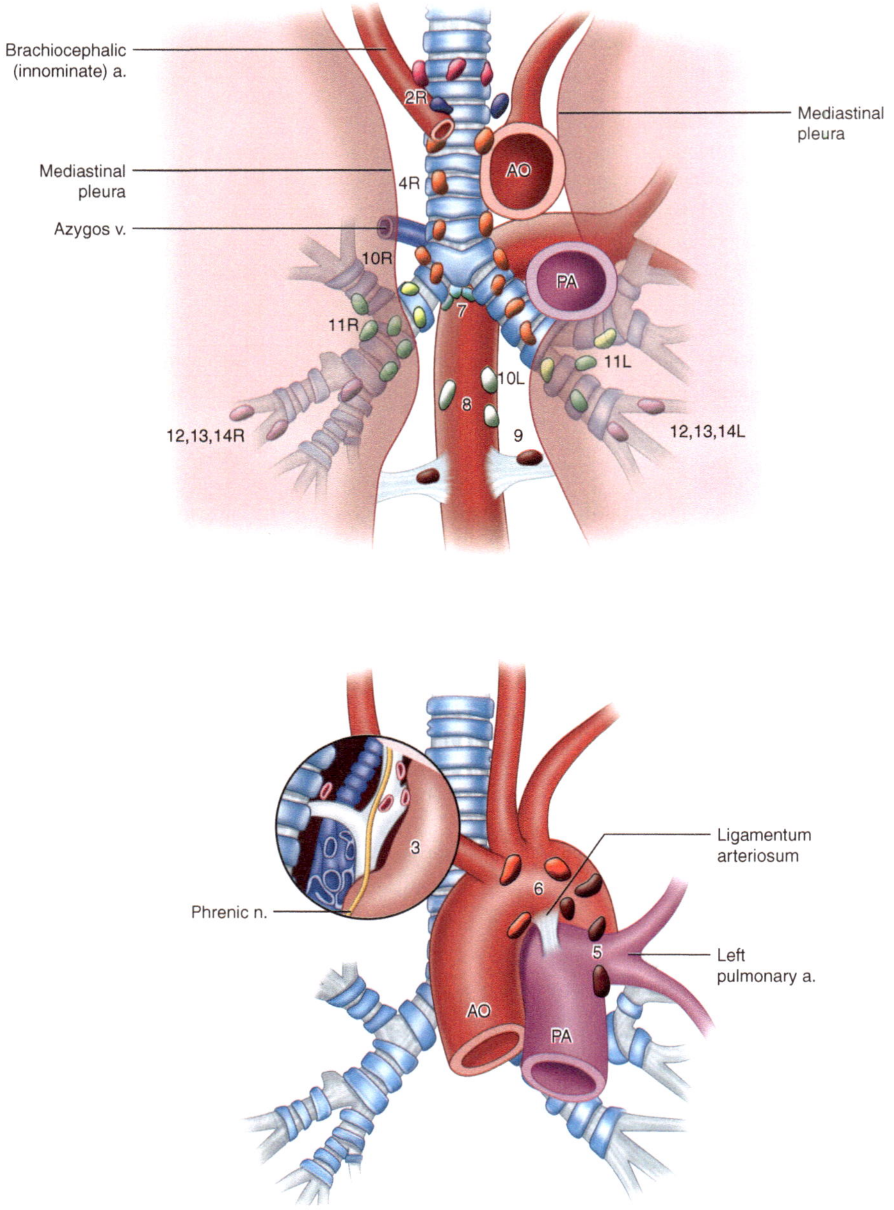

Fig. 5.4 Numeric designation of lymph node stations, anatomic map to illustrate location

Table 5.3 Description of lymph node station location; see Fig. 5.4 for anatomic map

Mediastinal nodes N2 ipsilateral, N3 contralateral	Superior mediastinal nodes 1. Highest mediastinal 2. Upper paratracheal 3. Pre-vascular and retrotracheal (also azygous nodes)
	Aortic nodes 5. Subaortic (aortopulmonary window) 6. Para-aortic (ascending aorta or phrenic nerve)
	Inferior mediastinal nodes 7. Subcarinal 8. Paraesophageal (below the carina) 9. Pulmonary ligament
Hilar/intrathoracic nodes N1	N1 Nodes 10. Hilar 11. Interlobar 12. Lobar 13. Segmental 14. Subsegmental

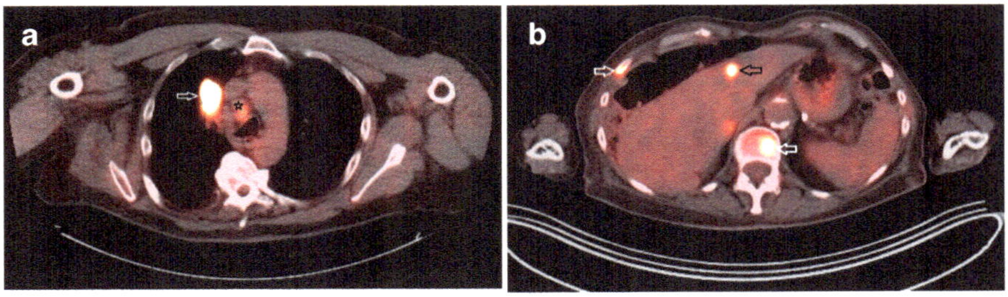

Fig. 5.5 Staging of lung cancer with PET scan. (**a**) Avid right upper lobe lung cancer (arrow) with avid right paratracheal (4R, N2) lymph node (start) therefore stage IIIA; (**b**) avid liver (black arrow) and bone (white arrow) lesions therefore stage IVB

Noninvasive Staging Tests

- CT scan (Fig. 5.2a–f)
  - Recommended for all patients with a diagnosis or high suspicion of lung cancer.
  - Scans through the chest and upper abdomen to specifically evaluate:

    Primary lesion (size, location, presence of invasion).
    Lymph nodes (hilum, mediastinum, supraclavicular) with lymphadenopathy defined as size >1 cm in the shorted axis. Of note, this criterion has low sensitivity/specificity (approximately 70%) for malignant involvement.
    Presence of effusion: pleural or pericardial.
    Distal metastasis: liver, adrenal, bone.

  - A CT completed with intravenous (IV) contrast, although not mandatory, allows for evaluation of the hilum, mediastinum, and liver:

Most commonly indicated for tumors that abut or invade the pulmonary artery, pulmonary vein, SVC, or pericardium/heart.

- FDG PET-CT (Fig. 5.5a, b)
  - Recommended for all patients with a diagnosis or high suspicion of lung cancer
  - Whole-body nuclear imaging with 18F-labeled deoxyglucose, with areas of high metabolic activity (SUVmax greater than 2.5) appearing hot (or avid) on imaging.
  - Allows for characterization of a known lung nodule as "hot," with a high likelihood of malignancy; up to 96% sensitivity, 88% specificity, 94% accuracy in solitary pulmonary nodules.
  - Allows for characterization of local/regional lymph nodes (hilar, mediastinal, supraclavicular), with avid nodes suspicious for malignant involvement; sensitivity and specificity of approximately 90%.
  - Allows for the evaluation of the entire body distal metastatic disease.
  - Limitations:

    Due to high metabolic activity, the brain is poorly staged with PET scan.

    False positives: infectious and inflammatory disease (granulomatous disease, sarcoidosis).

    False negative: primary cancers with low metabolic activity (adenocarcinoma in situ, carcinoid tumors) and small-sized lung cancers (threshold 8 mm).

    For central tumors, it may be difficult to differentiate activity of primary tumor from hilar/mediastinal node activity.

- MRI brain
  - Recommended for any patients with symptoms and signs on clinical evaluation and for clinical stage II or higher.
  - CT head with and without contrast is an acceptable alternative if there is a contraindication to MRI.
- MRI of primary site
  - For more detailed assessment of suspected invasion into vital structures (T4-brachial plexus, spine, mediastinal structures)
- MRI of distal sites
  - For more detailed assessment of suspected metastatic sites (liver, adrenal, bone)

Invasive Staging Techniques

- Site selection:
  - Select the site of biopsy which will result the highest stage of disease, for example, on a patient with lung mass and a PET-avid liver lesion, biopsy should be directed at the liver rather than the lung.

- Otherwise select the site that is most straightforward/least risk to biopsy.

- Any site suspected of having disease that will alter staging, hence treatment, must be biopsied, for example, PET activity in the contralateral mediastinum (N3) must be proven to be malignant by biopsy prior to deeming patient not a surgical candidate due to advanced disease.
- Consider performing PET/CT scan early in the workup to identify optimal site for biopsy.
- Invasive mediastinal nodal staging:
  - Recommended for central clinical stage IA, or clinical stage IB or higher, with endobronchial ultrasound (EBUS) commonly chosen as the initial technique for biopsy.
  - EBUS with transbronchial needle aspiration (Fig. 5.6a).

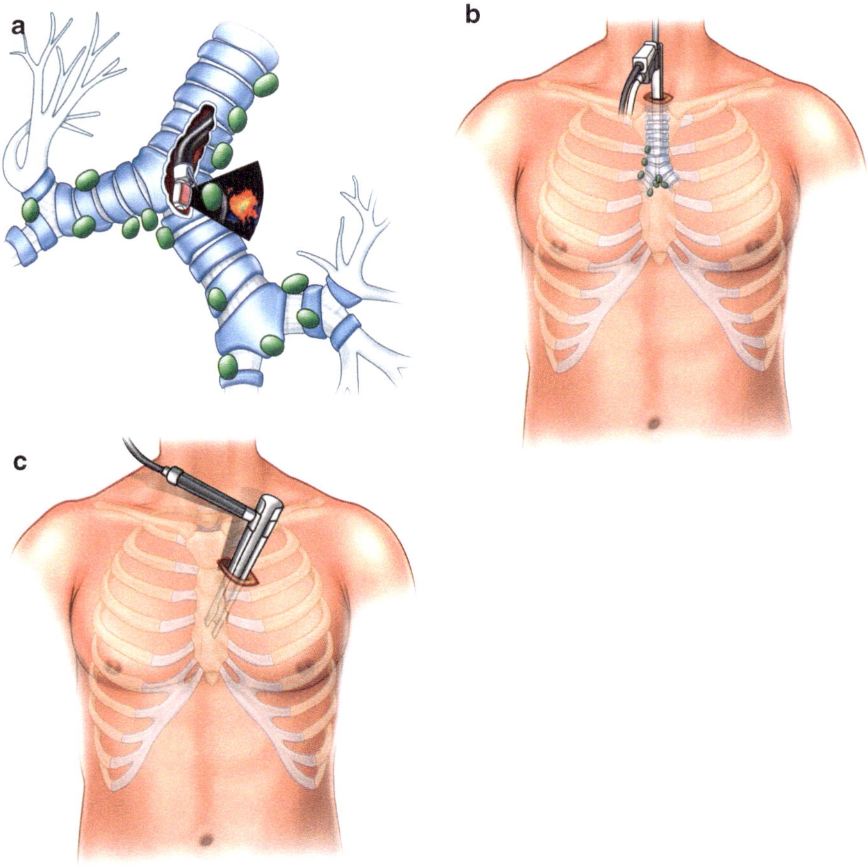

Fig. 5.6 Invasive mediastinal staging technique. (**a**) Endobronchial ultrasound with transbronchial needle aspiration of mediastinal nodes; (**b**) surgical biopsy of mediastinal nodes by cervical mediastinoscopy; (**c**) surgical biopsy of aortopulmonary window and para-aortic nodes by anterior mediastinotomy

Requires general anesthesia.
Less invasive than mediastinoscopy, with similar sensitivity, specificity, and accuracy.
Can access lymph node stations 2, 4, 7, 10, 11, and 12.
Rapid on-site evaluation by cytologist increases diagnostic yield.

- Cervical mediastinoscopy (Fig. 5.6b).

  Surgical biopsy performed under general anesthesia using a mediastinoscope through a neck incision superior to the sternal notch.
  Rare, but risk of massive bleeding from injury to the great vessels, azygos vein, and pulmonary artery; also small risk of injury to the recurrent nerve.
  Risk of mortality is <1%.
  Can access lymph node stations 2, 4, and 7.
  Perform if EBUS is negative or nondiagnostic in a highly suspicious node (large or PET-avid node).
  Can be performed at the same time as the definitive pulmonary resection if mediastinal nodes are found to be negative for malignancy on frozen section pathologic analysis.

- Anterior mediastinotomy (Chamberlain procedure) (Fig. 5.6c).

  Surgical biopsy performed under general anesthesia using a mediastinoscope through a small left parasternal incision in the second intercostal space (historically the second costal cartilage is removed for access, but this is rarely necessary).
  Can stay extrapleural but also can be performed intrapleural with the introduced air evacuated with a catheter at the end of the procedure.
  Can access lymph node stations in the aortopulmonary window (station 5) and periaortic (station 6) lymph nodes.
  Small risk of injury to the great vessels, pulmonary artery, recurrent nerve, and phrenic nerve.

- Endoscopic ultrasound (EUS).

  May require general anesthesia for optimal working conditions.
  Upper endoscopy to perform transesophageal biopsy of mediastinal lymph nodes.
  Can access stations 7, 8, and 9 (nodal stations that neither EBUS nor mediastinoscopy can reach).

- Video-assisted thoracic surgery (VATS).

  Minimally invasive surgical biopsy performed under general anesthesia and one-lung ventilation.
  Most invasive compared to all the above mediastinal staging techniques.
  Can access all ipsilateral mediastinal nodes, stations 2, 3, 4, 5, 6, 7, 8, and 9; thus cannot assess N3 nodes.
  Can also biopsy N1 nodal stations 10, 11, and 12.

- Biopsy of pleural disease:
  - Thoracentesis of pleural effusion for cytology; however, it is not uncommon for malignant effusions to have negative cytology, in which case VATS for direct pleural biopsy is indicated.
- Needle biopsy of distal metastatic site:
  - Commonly with CT or ultrasound image guidance.
  - Biopsy of supraclavicular node, liver, bone, adrenal.

Conclusions

- Components of diagnosis, staging, and treatment of lung cancer are often performed in concert rather than proceeding in a sequential pathway.
- The goals of staging are to determine the extent and spread of disease, which guides treatment selection, and offer prognostic information.
- As vastly different therapies are offered for different cell types and different stages of disease, thus accurate pathologic diagnosis and precise staging for patients with lung cancer are paramount.

Key Reference

- Detterbeck FC, Boffa DJ, Kim AW, Tanoue LT. The eighth edition lung cancer stage classification. Chest. 2017;151(1):193–203.

Further Reading

Detterbeck FC. The eighth edition TNM stage classification for lung cancer: what does it mean on main street? J Thorac Cardiovasc Surg. 2018;155(1):356–9.

Ettinger DS, Wood DE, Aisner DL, Akerley W, Bauman JR, Bharat A, Bruno DS, Chang JY, Chirieac LR, De Camp M, Dilling TJ, Dowell J, Durm GA, Gettinger S, Grotz TE, Gubens MA, Hegde A, Lackner RP, Lanuti M, Lin J, Loo BW, Lovly CM, Maldonado F, Massarelli E, Morgensztern D, Ng T, Otterson GA, Patel SP, Patil T, Polanco PM, Riely GJ, Riess J, Schild SE, Shapiro TA, Singh AP, Stevenson J, Tam A, Tanvetyanon T, Yanagawa J, Yang SC, Yau E, Gregory KM, Hughes M. NCCN guidelines® insights: non-small cell lung cancer, version 2.2023. J Natl Compr Canc Netw. 2023;21(4):340–50.

Goldstraw P, Chansky K, Crowley J, Rami-Porta R, Asamura H, Eberhardt WE, Nicholson AG, Groome P, Mitchell A, Bolejack V; International Association for the Study of Lung Cancer Staging and Prognostic Factors Committee, Advisory Boards, and Participating Institutions; International Association for the Study of Lung Cancer Staging and Prognostic Factors Committee Advisory Boards and Participating Institutions. The IASLC Lung Cancer Staging Project: proposals for revision of the TNM stage groupings in the forthcoming (eighth) edition of the TNM classification for lung cancer. J Thorac Oncol. 2016;11(1):39–51.

Siegel RL, Miller KD, Wagle NS, Jemal A. Cancer statistics, 2023. CA Cancer J Clin. 2023;73(1):17–48.

Travis WD, Asamura H, Bankier AA, Beasley MB, Detterbeck F, Flieder DB, Goo JM, MacMahon H, Naidich D, Nicholson AG, Powell CA, Prokop M, Rami-Porta R, Rusch V, van Schil P, Yatabe Y; International Association for the Study of Lung Cancer Staging and Prognostic Factors Committee and Advisory Board Members. The IASLC Lung Cancer Staging Project: proposals for coding T categories for subsolid nodules and assessment of tumor size in part-solid tumors in the forthcoming eighth edition of the TNM classification of lung cancer. J Thorac Oncol. 2016;11(8):1204–23.

Chapter 6
Early-Stage Non-small Cell Lung Cancer (Stages I and II)

Les James and Amie Kent

Introduction

Lung cancer is the leading cause of cancer deaths worldwide in men and the second leading cause in women. In the United States, lung cancer is the leading cause of cancer deaths. In 2022, an estimated 236,740 new cases of lung and bronchial cancer will be diagnosed, and 130,180 deaths are estimated to occur because of the disease. Lung cancer, generally, has a poor prognosis, with an overall 5-year survival rate of approximately 20%. Lung cancer has one of the lowest 5-year survival rates of all cancers because cases are often diagnosed at later stages, when the disease is less likely to be treatable. Nearly 30% of NSCLC is diagnosed as "early-stage," or disease that is limited to one lung and not involving the mediastinum or more distant sites (stage I or II). Five-year survival for stage I NSCLC is 70–90% and for stage II NSCLC is 53–60%. Unfortunately, patients with early-stage NSCLC are often asymptomatic, highlighting the importance of early and frequent screening for those with significant risk factors. Tobacco smoke is the most well-known risk factor for lung cancer, although numerous other environmental exposures and genetic factors can increase susceptibility for development of NSCLC. The mainstay of therapy for early-stage NSCLC is anatomic surgical resection. Stereotactic body radiation therapy (SBRT) is the treatment of choice for those who are not surgical candidates or refuse surgery.

L. James · A. Kent (✉)
Division of Thoracic Surgery, Department of Cardiothoracic Surgery, New York University Langone Health, New York, NY, USA
e-mail: Leslie.James@nyulangone.org; Amie.Kent@nyulangone.org

T. Ng, T. Geraci (eds.), *Thoracic Surgery Clerkship*, Contemporary Surgical Clerkships, https://doi.org/10.1007/978-3-031-44645-0_6

Clinical Presentation

- The high mortality in lung cancer is largely a consequence of patients presenting late (stage III or IV disease) when the cancer is already locally advanced or has disseminated.
- Detection of early-stage NSCLC, stage I (Fig. 6.1) or stage II (Fig. 6.2) disease, can lead to improved prognosis, although patients can live with lung cancer for years before it becomes apparent.
- Early-stage lung cancer is largely asymptomatic.
- Lung cancer can present with a wide range of nonspecific symptoms, the most common being cough, hemoptysis, chest and shoulder pain, dyspnea, hoarseness, weight loss, anorexia, fever, and weakness.
- Symptoms may be difficult to appreciate in the presence of coexisting respiratory diseases that are prevalent within this patient population, for example, chronic obstructive pulmonary disease (COPD).

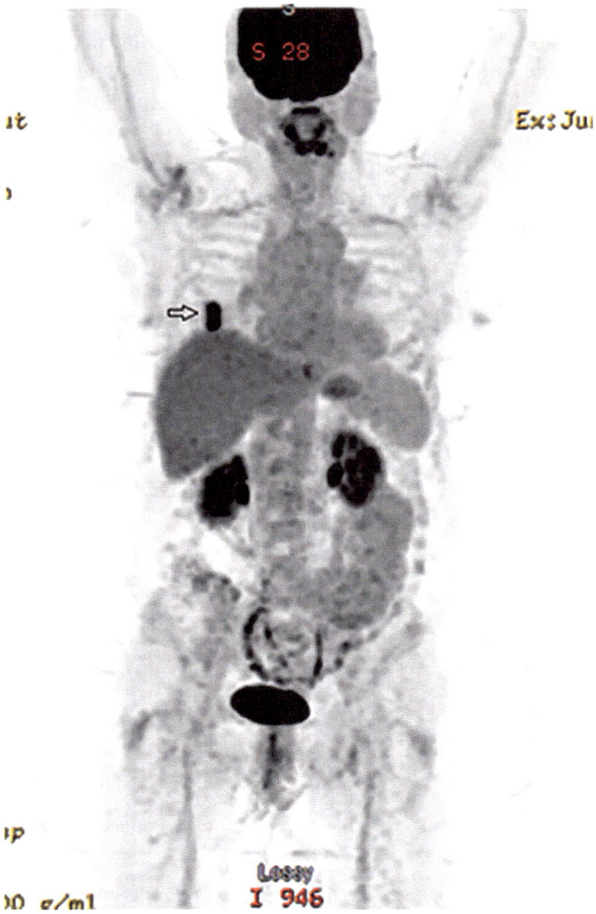

Fig. 6.1 PET scan of a 2 cm avid right lower lobe lung lesion (arrow) without mediastinal or distal activity, clinical stage I (T1bN0) disease

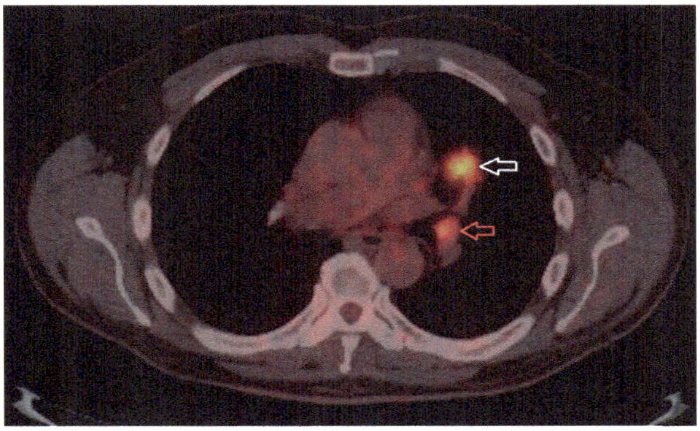

Fig. 6.2 PET/CT scan of a 2.5 cm avid left upper lobe lung lesion (white arrow), with activity in a station 11 lymph node, clinical stage II (T1cN1)

Risk Factors

- Smoking tobacco products (primarily cigarettes) is the most important risk factor for the development of lung cancer; secondhand smoke is also a significant cause of lung cancer:
  - Smoking is estimated to account for about 90% of all lung cancer cases, with a relative risk of lung cancer approximately 20-fold higher than in nonsmokers.
  - Smoking cigars, a pipe, or marijuana is also associated with an increased risk of lung cancer.
  - The effect of electronic cigarettes (e-cigarettes) on the incidence of lung cancer is not well-understood; there may be confounding effects of cigarette smoking among patients who use e-cigarettes.
- Numerous occupational and environmental carcinogens increase the risk of lung cancer, the best known being asbestos and radon.
- Asbestos is a well-established risk factor for lung cancer; patients with asbestos exposure complicated by interstitial fibrosis (asbestosis) are much more likely to develop lung cancer than patients with asbestos exposure alone.
- Radon is a gaseous decay product of uranium-238 and radium-226; it is present in soil, rock, and groundwater and can accumulate in homes:
  - Radon is capable of damaging respiratory epithelium via the emission of alpha particles; exposure to radon and its decay products confers an increased risk of lung cancer, and there is an interactive effect between radon exposure and cigarette smoking.
- Increasing age is also a risk factor for lung cancer; the median age of diagnosis of lung cancer is 70 years.
- Multiple other factors may have an impact on the risk of lung cancer, including radiation therapy, inflammation and benign lung disease, COPD, genetic factors, race/ethnicity, dietary factors, and body mass index (BMI); however, these are relatively less important in contributing to lung cancer burden.

Prevention and Screening

- Prevention is the most effective strategy for reducing the burden of lung cancer in the long term.
- As most lung cancer is attributed to smoking, the promotion of smoking cessation is essential to risk reduction.
- While progress in smoking cessation is demonstrated in the declining lung cancer rates and mortality in men in the United States, the smoking rate remains high and is increasing in many parts of the world.
- A high percentage of lung cancer occurs in former smokers, since the risk for lung cancer does not decline for many years following smoking cessation.
- Lung cancer screening with low-dose CT (LDCT) can reduce death from lung cancer in high-risk smokers.
- National lung cancer screening programs have been implemented in the United States and Korea and are being implemented in Europe and Canada.
- Despite broad recommendations from almost all expert panels, lung cancer screening has been poorly adopted; it is estimated that only approximately 15% of eligible candidates have been screened.
- The National Lung Screening Trial (NLST) was a randomized controlled study involving more than 53,000 current or former heavy smokers that assessed the risks and benefits of low-dose CT scans compared with chest x-rays for detecting lung cancer:
  - The NLST demonstrated that screening individuals with high-risk factors using LDCT decreased the mortality rate from lung cancer by 20%.
  - Individuals with high-risk factors were:

    55–74 years of age
    Current or former smokers with a 30 or more pack-year smoking history (former smokers had quit up to 15 years before enrollment)
    Had no evidence of lung cancer
- In 2021, the United States Preventive Services Task Force (USPSTF) revised its recommendations for annual lung cancer screening with LDCT based on a systematic review on the accuracy of screening and the benefits and harms for screening:
  - Expanded the age range to 50–80 years (previously 55–80 years)
  - Reduced the pack-year history to 20 pack-years of smoking (previously 30 pack-years)

2021 USPSTF Recommendations for Lung Cancer Screening

- Adults aged 50–80 years who have a 20 pack-year smoking history and currently smoke or have quit within the past 15 years.
- Screen for lung cancer with LDCT every year.
- Stop screening once a person has not smoked for 15 years or has a health problem that limits life expectancy or the ability to have lung surgery.

Workup and Staging

- History, physical exam, and chest radiograph are the common evaluations in the initial diagnostic workup for suspected lung cancer.
- National Comprehensive Cancer Network (NCCN) guidelines recommend a CT scan with IV contrast of the chest and upper abdomen (through the adrenals), as it provides the most detailed imaging information needed for a new diagnosis of lung cancer; if available, previous radiographs and CT scans should be reviewed for comparison.
- Tissue diagnosis should be obtained and needs to be tailored to the patient's clinical and radiographic presentation.
- Patients with a strong clinical suspicion of stage I lung cancer based on risk factors and radiologic appearance do not require a biopsy prior to undergoing surgery:
  - Biopsy adds time, costs, and procedural risk and may not be needed for treatment decisions.
  - Preoperative biopsy may be appropriate if an intraoperative diagnosis appears difficult or risky (due to depth and location, the lesion cannot be easily wedge resected for intraoperative frozen section).
  - However if surgical biopsy is to be considered, full staging and pulmonary function workup must be completed prior as anatomic resection may follow under the same anesthesia.
- There are a variety of techniques that can be used to obtain tissue for histologic confirmation of a mass or nodule found on imaging:
  - Percutaneous transthoracic biopsy, bronchoscopic biopsy, navigation bronchoscopy, fine needle aspiration (FNA) using endobronchial ultrasound (EBUS), and FNA using esophageal ultrasound.
  - Endobronchial lesions are most often accessible via standard bronchoscopic biopsy.
  - Lesions adjacent to the central airways may be best accessed by EBUS.
  - More peripheral lesions can be sampled via transthoracic biopsy or navigation bronchoscopy.

- Proper staging requires evaluation of the mediastinum for metastases:
  - In the past, mediastinoscopy was the most common way to stage the mediastinum.
  - Less invasive option, EBUS with transbronchial FNA, has shown similar sensitivity and specificity to mediastinoscopy.
  - Invasive mediastinal staging is indicated for central clinical IA or clinical IB and above tumors.
- Patients with biopsy-proven or suspected early-stage NSCLC should undergo PET/CT:
  - If nodes are clinically positive (>1 cm or avid on PET/CT)

    Mediastinal staging with EBUS and/or mediastinoscopy is warranted.
    If EBUS is performed initially, due to clinical suspicion, mediastinoscopy must follow a negative EBUS.

  - If nodes are clinically negative (≤1 cm and not avid on PET/CT)

    Mediastinal staging with EBUS or mediastinoscopy is performed if lung primary is >3 cm or central in location.

Table 6.1 Definitions for TN descriptors relevant for stage I and stage II lung cancer

T—primary tumor	
Tx	Primary tumor cannot be assessed, or tumor proven by presence of malignant cells in sputum or bronchial washings but not visualized by imaging or bronchoscopy
T0	No evidence of primary tumor
Tis	Carcinoma in situ (squamous or adenocarcinoma, including adenocarcinoma with pure lepidic pattern ≤3 cm)
T1	Tumor ≤3 cm surrounded by lung or visceral pleura, not invading more proximal than lobar bronchus
T1mi	Minimally invasive adenocarcinoma (≤3 cm in size and ≤5 mm invasion)
T1a	Tumor ≤1 cm
T1b	Tumor >1 cm but ≤2 cm
T1c	Tumor <2 cm but ≤3 cm
T2	Tumor >3 cm but ≤5 cm, or tumor with any of the following features: – Involvement of the main bronchus (not the carina) – Invasion of the visceral pleura – Atelectasis or obstructive pneumonitis extending to the hilum
T2a	Tumor >3 cm but ≤4 cm
T2b	Tumor <4 cm but ≤5 cm
T3	Tumor <5 cm but ≤7 cm, or invading the chest wall and pericardium, or satellite nodule in the same lobe
N—regional lymph nodes	
N0	No regional lymph node metastasis
N1	Metastasis in ipsilateral pulmonary or hilar nodes

Table 6.2 Stage I and stage II lung cancer by grouping

T/N	Subcategory	N0	N1
T1	T1a	IA1	IIB
	T1b	IA2	IIB
	T1c	IA3	IIB
T2	T2a	IB	IIB
	T2b	IIA	IIB
T3	T3	IIB	

- Brain MRI is not required for asymptomatic clinical stage I cancers; otherwise it is indicated for all other asymptomatic or symptomatic patients.
- For imaging that is suspicious for lung cancer or lung cancer that is confirmed by tissue, staging is critical to direct treatment and determine prognosis.
- Lung cancer is staged using the TNM classification, outlined in the 8th edition of the AJCC staging manual (Tables 6.1 and 6.2):
  - 8th edition of the AJCC staging manual was adopted in January 2018, and major changes from the 7th edition staging classification relate to the T stage and M stage.

Preoperative Evaluation

- Preoperative evaluation of a patient being considered for surgical resection of lung cancer must assess the risk of resection and weigh them against the benefit of cure:
  - Perioperative risks can be extrapolated from the patient's comorbidities and the tolerability of lung resection (pulmonary parenchymal loss).
- Cardiopulmonary evaluation is necessary to assess perioperative risks, with spirometry being the most commonly used preoperative test (see Chap. 11).
- Spirometry allows measurement of:
  - **Forced expiratory volume in the first second (FEV_1):** the amount of air forced from the lungs in 1 s
  - **Diffusing capacity for carbon monoxide (DLCO):** measurement of conductance of transfer for CO molecules from alveolar gas to the hemoglobin of the red blood cells in the pulmonary circulation
- Predicted postoperative FEV_1 <40% or predicted postoperative DLCO <40% should be considered very high-risk for surgery and prompt consideration of nonoperative treatment strategies.
- Although not performed routinely, cardiopulmonary exercise testing (CPET) and determination of maximum oxygen consumption (VO_2max) can be performed to

assess risk of perioperative complications; VO_2max is considered when predicted postoperative FEV_1 or DLCO are borderline.

- **VO_2max:** the maximum amount of oxygen that an individual can utilize during intense or maximal exercise:
  - Preoperative VO_2max is the most specific predictor of postoperative pulmonary complications.
  - *VO_2max >15 mL/kg/min*—not considered to be at increased risk of pulmonary complications or death.
  - *VO_2max <10 mL/kg/min*—very high risk for postoperative pulmonary complications or death.
- If formal CPET is not available, alternative exercise tests may be used to predict VO_2max (stair climbing, 6-minute walk test):
  - Patients who can climb six to seven flights of stairs correlate with a VO2 max >15 mL/kg/min.

Surgery

- Lobectomy was established as the gold standard for resection by a prospective, multi-institutional randomized trial comparing lobectomy and sub-lobar resection for stage I NSCLC by the Lung Cancer Study Group in 1995, which demonstrated that there is a survival benefit for lobectomy, as well as decreased rates of local recurrence.
- More recently, the randomized studies JCOG 0802 and CALGB 140503 have established, respectively, segmentectomy and sub-lobar resection (segmentectomy and wedge) to be noninferior procedure compared to lobectomy for peripheral clinical stage IA cancers that are less ≤2 cm.
- Thus for peripheral clinical stage IA ≤2 cm, consider segmentectomy if technically feasible, otherwise lobectomy; and for all other stage I and for stage II, lobectomy is recommended.
- Minimally invasive surgery, by thoracoscopy or robotic approach, is preferred over open thoracotomy as studies have found that they decrease morbidity and hospital stay, while not compromising oncologic outcomes, including the recent randomized VIOLET study.
- Patients with suspected NSCLC based on clinical and radiographic findings should undergo wedge resection or core needle biopsy for definitive diagnosis prior to proceeding with definitive anatomic lobectomy.
- Patients with significant comorbidities that preclude standard lobar resection should be considered for segmentectomy or wedge resection:
  - For patients who are not lobectomy candidates, sub-lobar resection with margins equal to or greater than the primary tumor is needed.

- For centrally located tumors, such as those involving the pulmonary artery and/or the bronchus, every attempt should be made to perform a sleeve or bronchoplastic resection rather than pneumonectomy, when a margin-negative resection can be achieved.
- For patients with clinical stage I or II NSCLC, either lymph node sampling or dissection is acceptable; however, the American College of Surgeons Commission on Cancer mandates a minimum of three N2 stations and one hilar be evaluated for accurate pathologic staging:
  - 2022 NCCN guidelines recommend sampling N1 and N2 lymph nodes (Fig. 6.3) at the time of surgical resection; the N2 lymph nodes should be sampled from a minimum of three separate stations:

    N1 lymph nodes: ipsilateral pulmonary or hilar nodes, stations 10, 11, 12, 13, 14
    N2 lymph nodes: ipsilateral mediastinal or subcarinal nodes

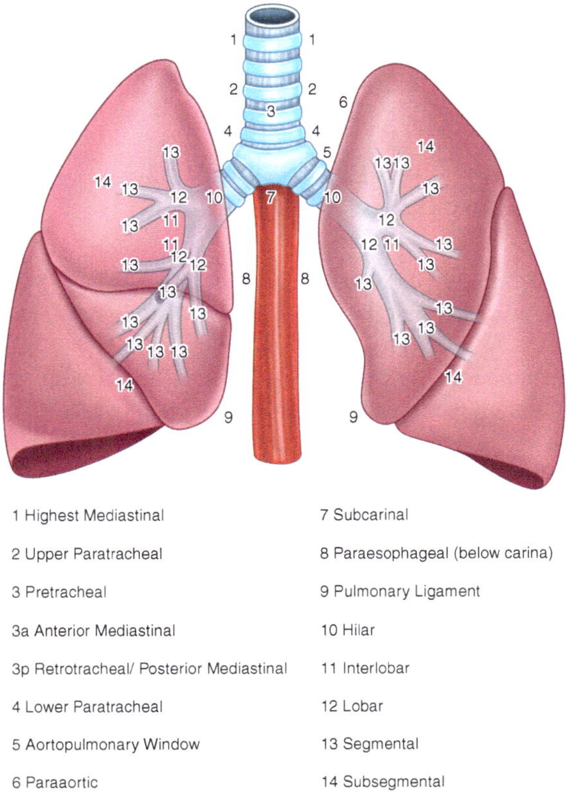

Fig. 6.3 Mediastinal lymph node stations. N2 nodes are the ipsilateral single-digit nodal stations (stations 1–9); N1 nodes are the ipsilateral double-digit stations (stations 10–14)

On the right: stations 2, 4, 7, 8, 9
On the left: stations 5, 6, 7, 8, 9

- Complications after pulmonary resections include postoperative arrhythmias, prolonged air leak, pneumonia, respiratory, and wound infections:
  - Minimally invasive surgical techniques such as video assisted thoracoscopic surgery (VATS) or robotic thoracic surgery have both improved quality of life and significantly decreased postoperative morbidity following pulmonary resection, without oncologic compromise as compared to open.
- Patients with clinical stage I or II (N0) disease who cannot tolerate surgical resection of any extent can benefit from definitive focused radiation therapy, otherwise known as stereotactic body radiation therapy (SBRT), or tumor ablation with microwave or radiofrequency:
  - SBRT involves specialized high-dose radiation delivered directly to the tumor, with a rapid drop-off of the radiation dose delivered to the edge of the target, reducing the exposure of surrounding healthy tissues to radiation.
- Patients with clinical stage II (N1) disease who cannot tolerate surgery will be considered for chemoradiation therapy.

Adjuvant Systemic Therapy, Radiation Postoperative Surveillance

- Based on 2023 NCCN guidelines, patients with stage IA NSCLC who undergo R0 (complete resection/margin negative) resection do not require adjuvant systemic therapy.
- Adjuvant chemotherapy is indicated in select patients with stage IB high-risk features [high-grade neuroendocrine tumors, lymphovascular invasion, visceral pleural invasion, wedge resection, and unknown node status (Nx)] and stage II tumors; first-line chemotherapy is cisplatin-based.
- For R0 resected pathologic stages IB and II, adjuvant targeted therapy for cancers with epidermal growth factor receptor (EGFR) mutation using EGFR-tyrosine kinase inhibitors and immunotherapy for cancers expressing programmed death-ligand (PD-L1) have shown great promise, with improved disease-free survival, but longer follow-up is needed to confirm overall survival benefit of these therapies.
- Patients with stage I or II NSCLC who undergo R0 resection do not benefit from adjuvant radiation; adjuvant radiation may even be harmful in this setting.
- Patients with stage I or II NSCLC who undergo an R1 (microscopic residual disease) or R2 (macroscopic residual disease) resection should ideally undergo re-resection; if this is not possible, adjuvant radiation therapy is indicated.

- Early result of preoperative combined chemotherapy and immunotherapy (in patients without EGFR mutation or ALK translocation) has also shown disease-free survival benefit over preoperative chemotherapy alone; however the role of preoperative targeted therapy and immunotherapy has yet to be precisely defined in the treatment of early-stage lung cancer
- For patients with stage I–II NSCLC who are treated with surgery, surveillance includes:
  - H&P and CT chest ± contrast performed every 6 months for 2–3 years, followed by H&P and low-dose non-contrast CT chest annually thereafter.
  - There is no indication for routine PET/CT surveillance.

Key Reference

- Altorki N, Wang X, Kozono D, Watt C, Landrenau R, Wigle D, Port J, Jones DR, Conti M, Ashrafi AS, Liberman M, Yasufuku K, Yang S, Mitchell JD, Pass H, Keenan R, Bauer T, Miller D, Kohman LJ, Stinchcombe TE, Vokes E. Lobar or sublobar resection for peripheral stage IA non-small-cell lung cancer. N Engl J Med. 2023;388(6):489–98.

Further Reading

Aberle DR, et al. Reduced lung-cancer mortality with low-dose computed tomographic screening. N Engl J Med. 2011;365(5):395–409.

Aberle DR, et al. The national lung screening trial: overview and study design. Radiology. 2011;258(1):243–53.

Aberle DR, et al. Baseline characteristics of participants in the randomized national lung screening trial. J Natl Cancer Inst. 2010;102(23):1771–9.

Altorki N, Wang X, Kozono D, Watt C, Landrenau R, Wigle D, Port J, Jones DR, Conti M, Ashrafi AS, Liberman M, Yasufuku K, Yang S, Mitchell JD, Pass H, Keenan R, Bauer T, Miller D, Kohman LJ, Stinchcombe TE, Vokes E. Lobar or sublobar resection for peripheral stage IA non-small-cell lung cancer. N Engl J Med. 2023;388(6):489–98.

Boffa DJ, Dhamija A, Kosinski AS, Kim AW, Detterbeck FC, Mitchell JD, Onaitis MW, Paul S. Fewer complications result from a video-assisted approach to anatomic resection of clinical stage I lung cancer. J Thorac Cardiovasc Surg. 2014;148(2):637–43.

Burlew JT, Weber C, Banks KP. Anatomy, thorax, mediastinal lymph nodes. In: StatPearls, 2021. Available at https://www.ncbi.nlm.nih.gov/books/NBK532863/.

Burns DM. Primary prevention, smoking, and smoking cessation: implications for future trends in lung cancer prevention. Cancer. 2000;89(11):2506–9.

Darling GE, Allen MS, Decker PA, Ballman K, Malthaner RA, Inculet RI, Jones DR, McKenna RJ, Landreneau RJ, Rusch VW, Putnam JB Jr. Randomized trial of mediastinal lymph node sampling versus complete lymphadenectomy during pulmonary resection in the patient with N0 or N1 (less than hilar) non-small cell carcinoma: results of the American College of Surgery Oncology Group Z0030 Trial. J Thorac Cardiovasc Surg. 2011;141(3):662–70.

Detterbeck FC. The eighth edition TNM stage classification for lung cancer: what does it mean on main street? J Thorac Cardiovasc Surg. 2018;155(1):356–9.

Ettinger DS, Wood DE, Aisner DL, Akerley W, Bauman JR, Bharat A, Bruno DS, Chang JY, Chirieac LR, De Camp M, Dilling TJ, Dowell J, Durm GA, Gettinger S, Grotz TE, Gubens MA, Hegde A, Lackner RP, Lanuti M, Lin J, Loo BW, Lovly CM, Maldonado F, Massarelli E,

Morgensztern D, Ng T, Otterson GA, Patel SP, Patil T, Polanco PM, Riely GJ, Riess J, Schild SE, Shapiro TA, Singh AP, Stevenson J, Tam A, Tanvetyanon T, Yanagawa J, Yang SC, Yau E, Gregory KM, Hughes M. NCCN Guidelines® insights: non-small cell lung cancer, version 2.2023. J Natl Compr Cancer Netw. 2023;21(4):340–50.
Felip E, Altorki N, Zhou C, Csőszi T, Vynnychenko I, Goloborodko O, Luft A, Akopov A, Martinez-Marti A, Kenmotsu H, Chen YM, Chella A, Sugawara S, Voong D, Wu F, Yi J, Deng Y, McCleland M, Bennett E, Gitlitz B, Wakelee H, IMpower010 Investigators. Adjuvant atezolizumab after adjuvant chemotherapy in resected stage IB-IIIA non-small-cell lung cancer (IMpower010): a randomised, multicentre, open-label, phase 3 trial. Lancet. 2021;398(10308):1344–57.
Forde PM, Spicer J, Lu S, Provencio M, Mitsudomi T, Awad MM, Felip E, Broderick SR, Brahmer JR, Swanson SJ, Kerr K, Wang C, Ciuleanu TE, Saylors GB, Tanaka F, Ito H, Chen KN, Liberman M, Vokes EE, Taube JM, Dorange C, Cai J, Fiore J, Jarkowski A, Balli D, Sausen M, Pandya D, Calvet CY, Girard N, CheckMate 816 Investigators. Neoadjuvant nivolumab plus chemotherapy in resectable lung cancer. N Engl J Med. 2022;386(21):1973–85.
Ginsberg RJ, Rubinstein LV. Randomized trial of lobectomy versus limited resection for T1 N0 non-small cell lung cancer. Lung Cancer Study Group. Ann Thorac Surg. 1995;60(3):615–22; discussion 622-3.
Krist AH, et al. Screening for lung cancer: US Preventive Services Task Force Recommendation Statement. JAMA. 2021;325(10):962–70.
Lim E, Batchelor TJP, Dunning J, Shackcloth M, Anikin V, et al. Video-assisted thoracoscopic or open lobectomy in early stage lung cancer. NEJM Evid. 2022;1(3):100016. https://doi.org/10.1056/EVIDoa2100016.
National Cancer Institute. SEER cancer statistics review, 1975-2018, National Cancer Institute. 2021. Available at https://seer.cancer.gov/archive/csr/1975_2018/.
NCCN. Non-small cell lung cancer (version 3.2023). 2023. Available at https://www.nccn.org/professionals/physician_gls/pdf/nscl.pdf.
O'Brien M, Paz-Ares L, Marreaud S, Dafni U, Oselin K, Havel L, Esteban E, Isla D, Martinez-Marti A, Faehling M, Tsuboi M, Lee JS, Nakagawa K, Yang J, Samkari A, Keller SM, Mauer M, Jha N, Stahel R, Besse B, Peters S. EORTC-1416-LCG/ETOP 8-15 PEARLS/KEYNOTE-091 Investigators. Pembrolizumab versus placebo as adjuvant therapy for completely resected stage IB-IIIA non-small-cell lung cancer (PEARLS/KEYNOTE-091): an interim analysis of a randomised, triple-blind, phase 3 trial. Lancet Oncol. 2022;23(10):1274–86.
Pignon JP, Tribodet H, Scagliotti GV, Douillard JY, Shepherd FA, Stephens RJ, Dunant A, Torri V, Rosell R, Seymour L, Spiro SG, Rolland E, Fossati R, Aubert D, Ding K, Waller D, Le Chevalier T, LACE Collaborative Group. Lung adjuvant cisplatin evaluation: a pooled analysis by the LACE Collaborative Group. J Clin Oncol. 2008;26(21):3552–9.
Saji H, Okada M, Tsuboi M, Nakajima R, Suzuki K, Aokage K, Aoki T, Okami J, Yoshino I, Ito H, Okumura N, Yamaguchi M, Ikeda N, Wakabayashi M, Nakamura K, Fukuda H, Nakamura S, Mitsudomi T, Watanabe SI, Asamura H, West Japan Oncology Group and Japan Clinical Oncology Group. Segmentectomy versus lobectomy in small-sized peripheral non-small-cell lung cancer (JCOG0802/WJOG4607L): a multicentre, open-label, phase 3, randomised, controlled, non-inferiority trial. Lancet. 2022;399(10335):1607–17.
Siegel RL, Miller KD, Wagle NS, Jemal A. Cancer statistics, 2023. CA Cancer J Clin. 2023;73(1):17–48.
Wu YL, Tsuboi M, He J, John T, Grohe C, Majem M, Goldman JW, Laktionov K, Kim SW, Kato T, Vu HV, Lu S, Lee KY, Akewanlop C, Yu CJ, de Marinis F, Bonanno L, Domine M, Shepherd FA, Zeng L, Hodge R, Atasoy A, Rukazenkov Y, Herbst RS, ADAURA Investigators. Osimertinib in resected EGFR-mutated non-small-cell lung cancer. N Engl J Med. 2020;383(18):1711–23.
Yang CF, Sun Z, Speicher PJ, Saud SM, Gulack BC, Hartwig MG, Harpole DH Jr, Onaitis MW, Tong BC, D'Amico TA, Berry MF. Use and outcomes of minimally invasive lobectomy for stage I non-small cell lung cancer in the national cancer data base. Ann Thorac Surg. 2016;101(3):1037–42.

Chapter 7
Surgery for Advanced-Stage Non-small Cell Lung Cancer (Stages III and IV)

Nikia T. Toomey and Thomas Ng

Introduction

Surgical resection is considered for selected patients with advanced-stage lung cancer, but often as one arm of a multimodal approach, which may include chemotherapy, radiation, and immunotherapy. A multidisciplinary approach to treatment includes expertise from pulmonology, radiology, medical oncology, and radiation oncology. Surgical resection for advanced-stage lung cancer occurs most commonly in two scenarios, when clinical staging suggests early-stage disease, but final pathology after resection reveals more advanced-stage disease (often with occult mediastinal nodal disease), or when advanced stage is known upfront and multimodality treatment is planned. This chapter focuses on the latter scenario, while the management of the former is also covered in Chaps. 15 and 16.

Advanced-Stage Lung Cancer

- Stages III and IV (see Chap. 6).
- Clinically diagnosed with CT scan, PET scan, and brain MRI; however this clinical stage should be pathologically confirmed with biopsy by either CT-guided

N. T. Toomey
Department of Surgery, University of Tennessee Health Science Center, College of Medicine, Memphis, TN, USA
e-mail: ntoomey1@uthsc.edu

T. Ng (✉)
Division of Thoracic Surgery, University of Tennessee Health Science Center, College of Medicine, Memphis, TN, USA
e-mail: tng4@uthsc.edu

T. Ng, T. Geraci (eds.), *Thoracic Surgery Clerkship*, Contemporary Surgical Clerkships, https://doi.org/10.1007/978-3-031-44645-0_7

percutaneous biopsy, endobronchial ultrasound (EBUS), endoscopic ultrasound (EUS), cervical mediastinoscopy, anterior mediastinotomy, or thoracoscopy (see Chap. 6).

- Advanced stages where surgery may be considered, but as part of multimodality therapeutic approach, include:
  - Stage IIIA: T1-2N2, T3N1, T4N0, T4N1.
  - Stage IIIB: T3N2 (selected T3: satellite nodule, size).
  - Stage IV: T1-3, N0, M1b solitary brain metastasis;
- Curative surgery is not considered for other stage IIIB, stage IIIC and other stage IV.

Stage IIIA: Locally Invasive T3/T4

- Discussed in Chap. 9.

Stage III: N2 Discovered After Surgical Resection (Clinical N0 or N1 with Surprise Pathologic N2)

- Postoperative chemotherapy is indicated.
- Adjuvant targeted therapy for cancers with epidermal growth factor receptor (EGFR) mutation using EGFR-tyrosine kinase inhibitors or immunotherapy for cancers expressing programmed death-ligand (PD-L1).
- Patients with R0 resection do not benefit from adjuvant radiation.

Stage III: N2 Disease Discovered at the Time of Staging

- Approximately 15% of patients with lung cancer present with N2 disease.
- Pathologic confirmation of N2 disease is imperative, as enlarged or PET-avid N2 nodes do not always represent malignant disease (e.g., sarcoidosis or granulomatous disease).
- Invasive mediastinal staging to pathologically confirm N2 nodal disease is often assessed by EBUS; however if enlarged and/or PET-avid N2 nodes are found to be negative after EBUS, surgical evaluation with either mediastinoscopy, anterior mediastinotomy, or thoracoscopy should follow to confirm this finding.
- Selection of patients with N2 disease for surgery as part of their multimodality treatment:
  - Good operative candidate (see Chap. 11)
  - Ideally, single station N2 disease
  - Non-bulky/nonadherent N2 disease (Fig. 7.1)
  - Pneumonectomy not expected

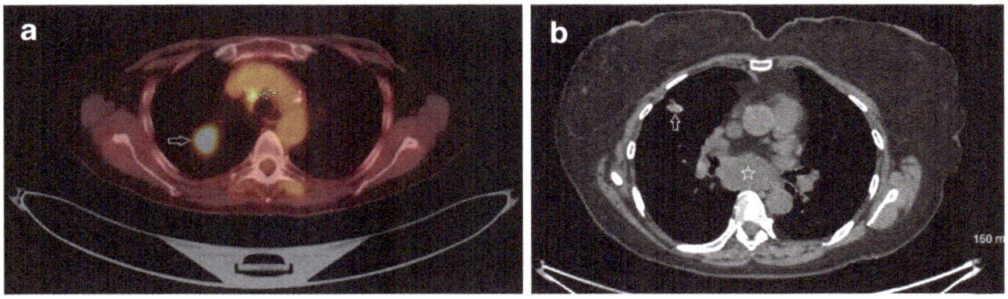

Fig. 7.1 Stage IIIA-N2 disease. (**a**) PET scan showing right upper lobe-avid lung cancer (white arrow) along with an avid right paratracheal lymph node (yellow arrow); this patient with non-bulky N2 disease is a candidate for surgery as a part of a multimodality treatment approach; (**b**) CT scan showing a right middle lobe cancer (arrow) with bulky subcarinal nodal disease (star); this patient with bulky N2 disease would not be a good candidate for surgery

- For patients with N2 disease selected for surgery, multimodality treatment options include:
  - Preoperative chemotherapy and immunotherapy, followed by surgical resection in those without EGFR mutation or ALK translocation
  - Preoperative chemotherapy and radiation, followed by surgical resection
  - Preoperative chemotherapy, followed by surgical resection
- After preoperative therapy (also termed induction or neoadjuvant therapy), restage by CT scan, PET scan, and/or invasive mediastinal evaluation (EBUS, EUS, mediastinoscopy); ideally there is down-staging with absence of N2 disease, but surgical resection can still be considered as long as there is no progression of disease.
- Surgical resection after preoperative therapy:
  - Can be performed by minimally invasive approaches (thoracoscopy or robotic) or by open thoracotomy.
  - For preoperative therapy that includes radiation, surgery is planned approximately 6–10 weeks after therapy (as surgery becomes more difficult after 10 weeks due to radiation fibrosis); surgery may be earlier (4 weeks) if radiation was not given as part of preoperative therapy.
  - Due to possible impaired wound healing from preoperative therapy, especially with radiation, buttressing the bronchial stump with vascularized flap should be considered, with use of muscle flaps, thymic/pericardial fat, or pleural flap.
  - Lobectomy is preferred in good operative candidates.
  - Pneumonectomy, especially right, should be avoided as this procedure carries a high risk for mortality after preoperative chemotherapy and radiation.
  - Full mediastinal lymph node dissection should be performed with a minimum three mediastinal stations and the hilar station, including the station(s) known to be involved with disease.

- Postoperative systemic therapy:
  - Postoperative chemotherapy is indicated.
  - Adjuvant targeted therapy for cancers with epidermal growth factor receptor (EGFR) mutation using EGFR-tyrosine kinase inhibitors or immunotherapy for cancers expressing programmed death-ligand (PD-L1).
- For patients with complete resection (R0), postoperative radiation appears to have no benefit.
- Five-year overall survival for IIIA-N2 disease (including T3N2, per previous 7th edition staging) treated with preoperative chemotherapy and radiation followed by surgical resection is 27%; this increases to 36% if pneumonectomies are excluded; recent trials have shown more promising results with 3-year overall survival of 70–80% but more long-term results are pending.
- Preoperative regimens utilizing combination of chemotherapy and immunotherapy show promise after short-term follow-up, with favorable disease-free survival outcome over preoperative chemotherapy alone; however, long-term results of overall survival have yet to be reported.

Stage IV

- In the rare circumstance, where a patient presents with a solitary brain metastasis (SBM), and no other sites of disease other than the lung primary (T1-3N0M1b), surgical resection as part of multimodality therapy can be considered.
- Treatment sequence should proceed with therapy for the SBM first, followed by pulmonary resection.
- Surgical resection or stereotactic radiosurgery is utilized to treat the SBM, without clear evidence of one modality being superior to the other; combination of surgery and radiation for the SBM is a common treatment regimen.
- For resection of the lung primary, lobectomy is preferred in good surgical candidates.
- As this is stage IV disease, adjuvant systemic therapy is considered; systemic therapy can also be considered prior to thoracic surgery.
- Surgical resection of both the primary lung malignancy and the SBM can achieve a 5-year survival of 20%.

Key Reference

- Forde PM, Spicer J, Lu S, Provencio M, Mitsudomi T, Awad MM, Felip E, Broderick SR, Brahmer JR, Swanson SJ, Kerr K, Wang C, Ciuleanu TE, Saylors GB, Tanaka F, Ito H, Chen KN, Liberman M, Vokes EE, Taube JM, Dorange C, Cai J, Fiore J, Jarkowski A, Balli D, Sausen M, Pandya D, Calvet CY, Girard N; CheckMate 816 Investigators. Neoadjuvant nivolumab plus chemotherapy in resectable lung cancer. N Engl J Med. 2022;386(21):1973-85.

Further Reading

Albain KS, Swann RS, Rusch VW, Turrisi AT 3rd, Shepherd FA, Smith C, Chen Y, Livingston RB, Feins RH, Gandara DR, Fry WA, Darling G, Johnson DH, Green MR, Miller RC, Ley J, Sause WT, Cox JD. Radiotherapy plus chemotherapy with or without surgical resection for stage III non-small-cell lung cancer: a phase III randomised controlled trial. Lancet. 2009;374(9687):379–86.

Billing PS, Miller DL, Allen MS, Deschamps C, Trastek VF, Pairolero PC. Surgical treatment of primary lung cancer with synchronous brain metastases. J Thorac Cardiovasc Surg. 2001;122(3):548–53.

Ettinger DS, Wood DE, Aisner DL, Akerley W, Bauman JR, Bharat A, Bruno DS, Chang JY, Chirieac LR, DeCamp M, Dilling TJ, Dowell J, Durm GA, Gettinger S, Grotz TE, Gubens MA, Hegde A, Lackner RP, Lanuti M, Lin J, Loo BW, Lovly CM, Maldonado F, Massarelli E, Morgensztern D, Ng T, Otterson GA, Patel SP, Patil T, Polanco PM, Riely GJ, Riess J, Schild SE, Shapiro TA, Singh AP, Stevenson J, Tam A, Tanvetyanon T, Yanagawa J, Yang SC, Yau E, Gregory KM, Hughes M. NCCN guidelines® insights: non-small cell lung cancer, version 2.2023. J Natl Compr Canc Netw. 2023;21(4):340–50. https://doi.org/10.6004/jnccn.2023.0020. PMID: 37015337.

Fuentes R, Osorio D, Expósito Hernandez J, Simancas-Racines D, Martinez-Zapata MJ, Bonfill CX. Surgery versus stereotactic radiotherapy for people with single or solitary brain metastasis. Cochrane Database Syst Rev. 2018;8(8):CD012086.

Hui Z, Men Y, Hu C, Kang J, Sun X, Bi N, Zhou Z, Liang J, Lv J, Feng Q, Xiao Z, Chen D, Wang Y, Li J, Wang J, Gao S, Wang L, He J. Effect of postoperative radiotherapy for patients with pIIIA-N2 non-small cell lung cancer after complete resection and adjuvant chemotherapy: the phase 3 PORT-C randomized clinical trial. JAMA Oncol. 2021;7(8):1178–85.

Le Pechoux C, Pourel N, Barlesi F, Lerouge D, Antoni D, Lamezec B, Nestle U, Boisselier P, Dansin E, Paumier A, Peignaux K, Thillays F, Zalcman G, Madelaine J, Pichon E, Larrouy A, Lavole A, Argo-Leignel D, Derollez M, Faivre-Finn C, Hatton MQ, Riesterer O, Bouvier-Morel E, Dunant A, Edwards JG, Thomas PA, Mercier O, Bardet A. Postoperative radiotherapy versus no postoperative radiotherapy in patients with completely resected non-small-cell lung cancer and proven mediastinal N2 involvement (Lung ART): an open-label, randomised, phase 3 trial. Lancet Oncol. 2022;23(1):104–14.

NSCLC Meta-analysis Collaborative Group. Preoperative chemotherapy for non-small-cell lung cancer: a systematic review and meta-analysis of individual participant data. Lancet. 2014;383(9928):1561–71.

Qin H, Wang C, Jiang Y, Zhang X, Zhang Y, Ruan Z. Patients with single brain metastasis from non-small cell lung cancer equally benefit from stereotactic radiosurgery and surgery: a systematic review. Med Sci Monit. 2015;21:144–52.

Chapter 8
Superior Sulcus (Pancoast) Tumors

Brenden P. Sheridan and Thomas Ng

Introduction

- Initially described by radiologist Dr. Henry Pancoast in 1924 within a case series of chest radiographs identifying apical thoracic tumors. Later in 1932, he went on to describe seven cases of "superior sulcus tumors" with a distinct clinical presentation referred to as Pancoast syndrome.
- Dr. José Tobias, also in 1932, similarly described these tumors, but accurately identified their origin as bronchogenic or peripheral lung tumors.
- Definition of Pancoast tumors as provided by the American College of Chest Physicians (ACCP):
  - "A lung cancer arising in the apex of the lung involving the apical chest wall. Invasion of apical chest wall structures is required at the level of the first rib or above, but it is not necessary to have Horner syndrome or pain radiating down the arm. These lesions frequently invade the brachial plexus, subclavian vessels, or spine."
  - Modern literature, however, continues to use Pancoast tumor, Pancoast-Tobias tumor, and superior sulcus tumor interchangeably.

B. P. Sheridan
Department of Surgery, University of Tennessee Health Science Center, College of Medicine, Memphis, TN, USA
e-mail: bsherid2@uthsc.edu

T. Ng (✉)
Division of Thoracic Surgery, University of Tennessee Health Science Center, College of Medicine, Memphis, TN, USA
e-mail: tng4@uthsc.edu

T. Ng, T. Geraci (eds.), *Thoracic Surgery Clerkship*, Contemporary Surgical Clerkships, https://doi.org/10.1007/978-3-031-44645-0_8

Anatomy

- The superior pulmonary sulcus refers to the upper most extent of the costovertebral gutter or the apical recess of the pulmonary sulcus.
- Anatomy of the area affected by Pancoast tumors is defined by the thoracic inlet, subdivided into three compartments (Fig. 8.1):
  - Anterior Compartment: defined by the sternum anteriorly and the anterior scalene muscle posteriorly; includes the sternocleidomastoid and omohyoid muscles, subclavian and jugular veins, and scalene fat pad
  - Middle Compartment: between the anterior and middle scalene muscles; includes the brachial plexus, phrenic nerve (which runs on the anterior scalene), and subclavian artery
  - Posterior Compartment: posterior to the middle scalene muscle; includes the posterior scalene muscle, brachial plexus, nerve roots, stellate ganglion, sympathetic chain, long thoracic and accessory nerves, neural foramina, and vertebral body

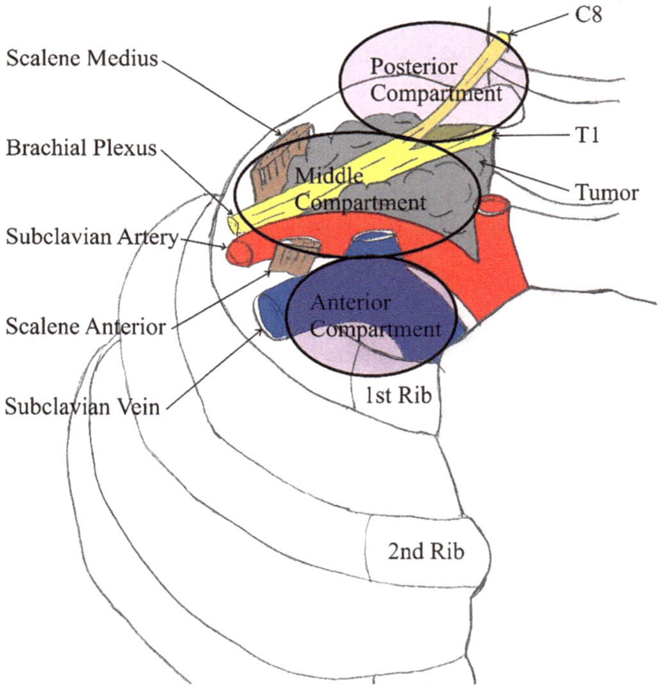

Fig. 8.1 The three compartments of the thoracic inlet, along with the major associated structures

Presentation

- Superior sulcus tumors represent less than 5% of newly diagnosed lung cancers.
- Majority of patients will be symptomatic at presentation due to tumor invasion in the thoracic inlet:
  - The most common symptoms are shoulder pain radiating down the arm, axilla, or scapula.
  - As the tumor invades the thoracic apex from below, the inferior nerve roots of the brachial plexus will be initially involved, T1 and C8, which are the major nerve roots of the ulnar nerve: resulting in pain of the inner arm and forearm and weakness/wasting of the intrinsic muscles of the hand.
  - Approximately 25% present with Horner's syndrome: ptosis, miosis, and anhidrosis.
  - Approximately 10% present with classic Pancoast syndrome: Horner's syndrome, muscle/arm pain, and hand wasting.
- Other associated symptoms: SVC syndrome, shortness of breath, hemoptysis, pneumonia, paraneoplastic syndromes, and weight loss.

Imaging

- Chest radiograph: used for initial evaluation; however as this area may be difficult to image with plain radiograph (Fig. 8.2), CT scan should follow if there is clinical suspicion of a superior sulcus tumor.
- Contrast-enhanced CT scan: establishes diagnosis, evaluates regional lymph node involvement, bony invasion, vascular involvement, and thoracic metastasis.

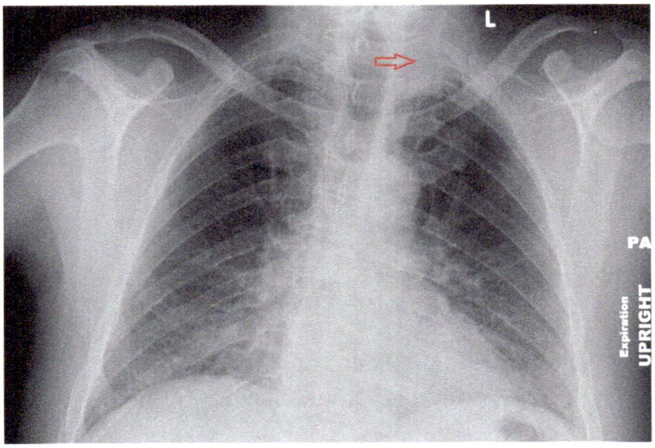

Fig. 8.2 Chest radiograph showing the subtle left apical density (arrow) of a patient with a superior sulcus tumor

- Contrast-enhanced MRI: imaging modality of choice for determining resectability, assesses involvement of the brachial plexus, subclavian vessels, neural foramina, vertebral body, and spinal cord.
- Positron emission tomography (PET)/CT scan for staging.
- Brain MRI assesses for brain metastasis.

Diagnosis and Staging

- Tissue diagnosis is required and can be obtained by image-guided (ultrasound or CT) needle biopsy transthoracic or transcervical, by bronchoscopy, by invasive staging techniques listed below, or by thoracoscopy if necessary:
  - Superior sulcus tumors are most often squamous cell carcinoma or adenocarcinoma, with <5% being small cell lung carcinoma.
  - Differential diagnosis includes metastatic malignancy from other sites, hematologic malignancies, infection (bacterial, fungal, TB), and thoracic outlet syndrome.
- In addition to staging by imaging (CT scan, PET scan, MRI), invasive staging is recommended; this includes EBUS and/or mediastinoscopy and, as indicated, scalene node biopsy and thoracoscopy.
  - Twenty-four percent of patients will have N2 or N3 disease at presentation.
- Staging is per the 8th edition TNM system (see Chap. 6):
  - With the presence of local invasion, superior sulcus tumors are T3 (rib/chest wall) or T4 (adjacent structures: vertebral body, subclavian vessels, brachial plexus).
  - There is controversy whether ipsilateral supraclavicular lymph node should be considered regional N1 rather than N3; this is due to the proximity of this node to the primary tumor.
  - T3N0: Stage IIB
  - T3N1, T4N0, T4N1: Stage IIIA
  - T3N2, T4N2: Stage IIIB
  - T3N3, T4N3: Stage IIIC
  - T3/4Nany Many: Stage IV

Treatment

- Multidisciplinary team: medical oncology, radiation oncology, pulmonology, radiology, pathology, thoracic anesthesia, thoracic surgery, spine surgery, vascular surgery.

- Treatment for curative intent: neoadjuvant (or preoperative) chemotherapy/radiation followed by surgery is offered for stages IIB and IIIA (with resectable T4: <50% vertebral body involvement, no brachial plexus involvement above T1, absent tracheal or absent esophageal involvement) who are operative candidates (see Chap. 11).
  - Neoadjuvant therapy with cisplatin-based chemotherapy, concurrent with 45 Gy radiation, followed by surgical resection has shown to improve survival:
    - Southwest Oncology Group (SWOG) 9416: 44% 5-year overall survival
    - Japan Clinical Oncology Group (JCOG) 9806: 56% 5-year overall survival
- Main goal of surgery is R0 resection along with mediastinal lymph node dissection.
  - Resection of the tumor is often by lobectomy en bloc with:
    - Chest wall, including at least the first rib (Fig. 8.3a)
    - If necessary per tumor involvement:
      - T1 nerve root of the brachial plexus
      - Subclavian artery with reconstruction
      - Subclavian vein with or without reconstruction
      - Sympathetic chain
      - Vertebral body (Fig. 8.3b) with stabilization
  - Contraindications to surgery include stage IIIA with unresectable T4 (>50% vertebral body involvement, brachial plexus involvement above T1, tracheal or esophageal involvement), IIIB, IIIC, and IV disease.
  - Surgical approach is varied and determined by the location of the tumor within the thoracic inlet while adhering to the goals of surgical resection.
  - Tumors located posteriorly (Fig. 8.4a) are approached by high posterolateral thoracotomy (Fig. 8.4b) described by Shaw and Paulson in 1961; a "hook"

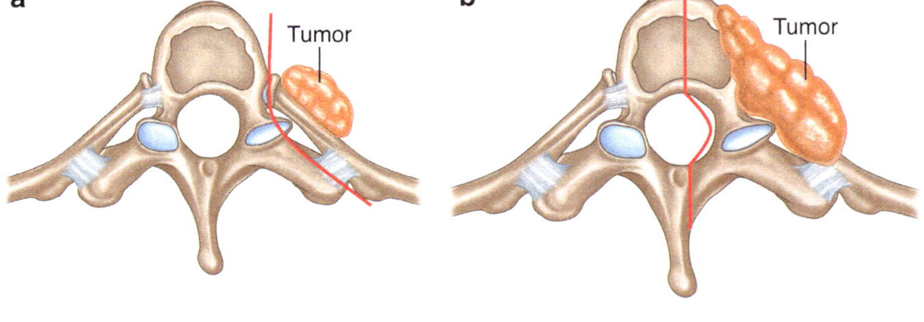

Fig. 8.3 Examples of the extent of resection for superior sulcus tumors. (**a**) Chest wall resection by rib disarticulation (red line); (**b**) rib and vertebral body resection (red line)

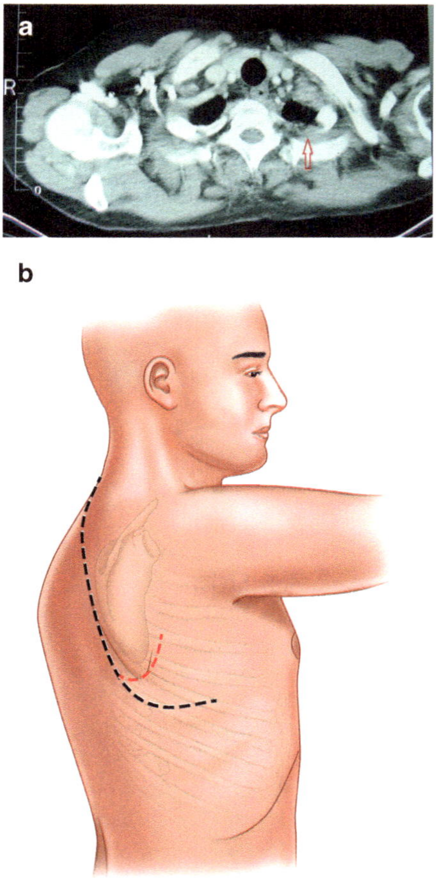

Fig. 8.4 Posterior superior sulcus tumor. (**a**) CT scan of tumor invading posterior aspects of the first and second rib (arrow); (**b**) high posterolateral thoracotomy, with "hook" modification (red line) by extending the incision around the scapula tip toward the axilla to improve subclavian vessel exposure

modification with extension of the incision toward the axilla described by Niwa in 1993 improves exposure of the subclavian vessels.

- Tumors located anteriorly (Fig. 8.5a) are approached by the anterior trans-clavicular approach (Fig. 8.5b) described by Dartevelle in 1993; a modification is the anterior trans-manubrial approach (Fig. 8.5c) described by Grunenwald in 1997 which preserves the clavicle.
- For tumors that span several regions of the thoracic inlet (Fig. 8.6a), the addition of sternotomy such as the Masoka trans-sternal/trap door (Fig. 8.6b) or hemi-clamshell (Fig. 8.6c) incision or utilizing a combination of any of the above incisions may be necessary.
- After en bloc resection by one of the above approaches, lobectomy can then be performed through the posterolateral thoracotomy or sternotomy, if such

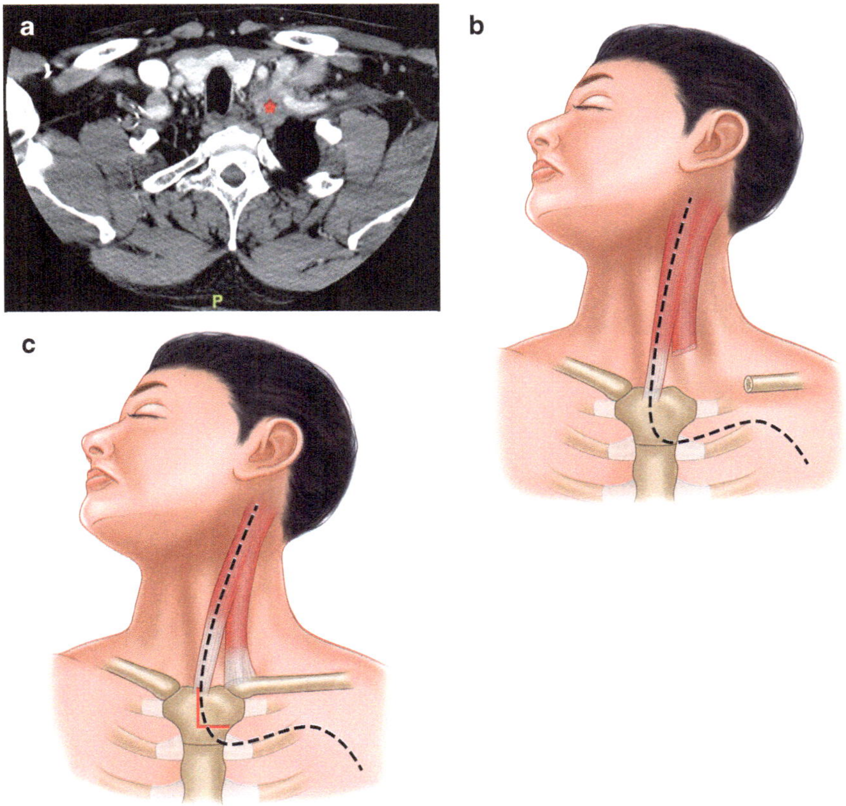

Fig. 8.5 Anterior superior sulcus tumor. (**a**) CT scan of tumor involving the anterior aspect of the first rib and the subclavian artery (star); (**b**) anterior trans-clavicular approach with resection of the medial half of the clavicle for exposure; (**c**) anterior trans-manubrial approach with division of the manubrium (red line), leaving the clavicle intact

incision had been utilized; otherwise (as in the case of anterior trans-clavicular or anterior trans-manubrial approaches) lobectomy can then be performed by minimally invasive thoracoscopic techniques.

- Adjuvant therapy
  - Postoperative chemotherapy is indicated.
  - Adjuvant targeted therapy for cancers with epidermal growth factor receptor (EGFR) mutation using EGFR-tyrosine kinase inhibitors or immunotherapy for cancers expressing programmed death-ligand (PD-L1).

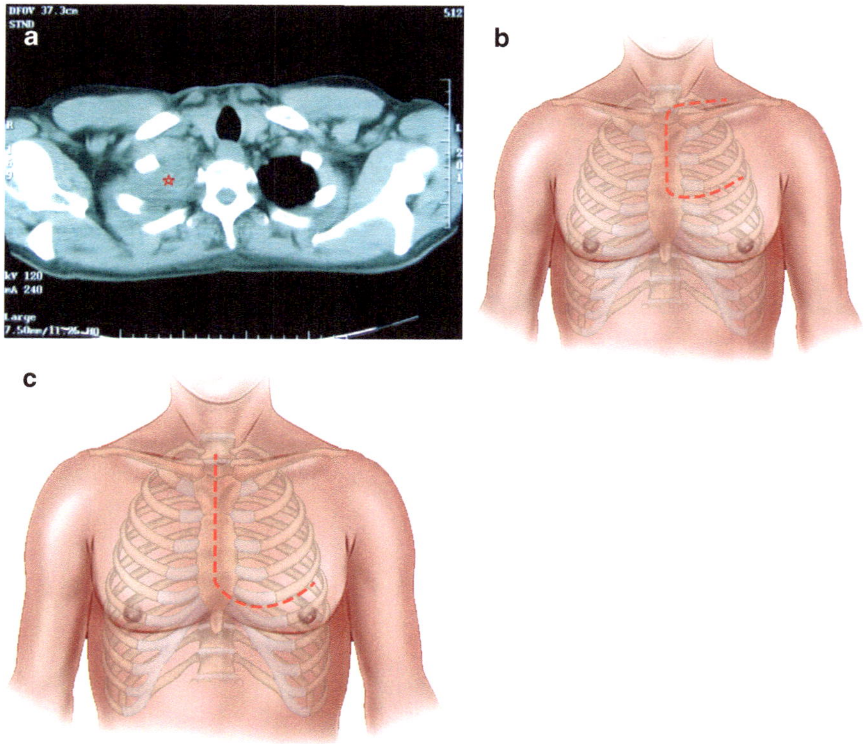

Fig. 8.6 Superior sulcus tumor that involves several regions of the thoracic inlet. (**a**) CT scan showing an extensive apical tumor occupying the entire thoracic inlet (star); (**b**) trans-sternal/trap door incision; (**c**) hemi-clamshell incision

Complications

- Thoracic: prolonged air leak, wound infection, wound dehiscence, bronchopleural fistula, air embolism, hemothorax, empyema, pneumonia, atelectasis, pneumonitis, respiratory failure, ARDS, phrenic nerve injury
- Neurological: hand muscle weakness (claw hand) from T1/C8 nerve root division, Horner's syndrome, peripheral neuropathy, CSF leak, spinal cord injury
- Vascular: subclavian artery injury/thrombosis, subclavian vein thrombosis, edema of the ipsilateral arm, chylothorax
- Postoperative mortality: SWOG 9416 2.3%, JCOG 9806 3%

Clinical Outcomes

- Factors associated with higher tumor recurrence and worse overall survival: higher tumor stage (T4), mediastinal lymph node involvement, invasion into the chest wall or brachial plexus, inability to achieve an R0 resection, patients without a complete pathologic response to induction therapy
- 5-year survival:
  - T3N0: 46%
  - T4N0: 13%
  - N2 disease: 0%

Key Reference

- Kratz JR, Woodard G, Jablons DM. Management of lung cancer invading the superior sulcus. Thorac Surg Clin. 2017;27(2):149–57.

Further Reading

de Perrot M, Rampersaud R. Surgical approaches to apical thoracic malignancies. J Thorac Cardiovasc Surg. 2012;144(1):72–80.

Ettinger DS, Wood DE, Aisner DL, Akerley W, Bauman JR, Bharat A, Bruno DS, Chang JY, Chirieac LR, DeCamp M, Dilling TJ, Dowell J, Durm GA, Gettinger S, Grotz TE, Gubens MA, Hegde A, Lackner RP, Lanuti M, Lin J, Loo BW, Lovly CM, Maldonado F, Massarelli E, Morgensztern D, Ng T, Otterson GA, Patel SP, Patil T, Polanco PM, Riely GJ, Riess J, Schild SE, Shapiro TA, Singh AP, Stevenson J, Tam A, Tanvetyanon T, Yanagawa J, Yang SC, Yau E, Gregory KM, Hughes M. NCCN guidelines® insights: non-small cell lung cancer, version 2.2023. J Natl Compr Cancer Netw. 2023;21(4):340–50.

Kunitoh H, Kato H, Tsuboi M, Shibata T, Asamura H, Ichinose Y, Katakami N, Nagai K, Mitsudomi T, Matsumura A, Nakagawa K, Tada H, Saijo N, Japan Clinical Oncology Group. Phase II trial of preoperative chemoradiotherapy followed by surgical resection in patients with superior sulcus non-small-cell lung cancers: report of Japan Clinical Oncology Group trial 9806. J Clin Oncol. 2008;26(4):644–9.

Marulli G, Battistella L, Mammana M, Calabrese F, Rea F. Superior sulcus tumors (Pancoast tumors). Ann Transl Med. 2016;4(12):239.

Palumbo VD, Fazzotta S, Fatica F, D'Orazio B, Caronia FP, Cajozzo M, Damiano G, Maffongelli A, Cudia BM, Messina M, Lo Monte AI. Pancoast tumour: current therapeutic options. Clin Ter. 2019;170(4):e291–4.

Rusch VW, Giroux DJ, Kraut MJ, Crowley J, Hazuka M, Winton T, Johnson DH, Shulman L, Shepherd F, Deschamps C, Livingston RB, Gandara D. Induction chemoradiation and surgical resection for superior sulcus non-small-cell lung carcinomas: long-term results of Southwest Oncology Group Trial 9416 (Intergroup Trial 0160). J Clin Oncol. 2007;25(3):313–8.

Chapter 9
Neuroendocrine Tumors of the Lung

Nidhi Desai and Thomas Ng

Introduction

The World Health Organization classifies lung neuroendocrine tumors into four different subtypes: typical carcinoids, atypical carcinoids, large cell neuroendocrine tumors, and small cell lung cancer. Neuroendocrine tumors arise from neuroendocrine cells within the gastrointestinal tract (rectum, small bowel) and lungs. The tumors are classified based on their aggressive nature—low grade, intermediate grade, and high grade. In turn, these tumors are more commonly referred to as typical carcinoid, atypical carcinoid, and large/small cell neuroendocrine tumors, respectively.

Typical Carcinoid Lung Cancer (Low Grade)

Epidemiology

- Represent <11% of all lung cancers.
- More common than atypical carcinoid tumors, making up 90% of the well-differentiated neuroendocrine carcinomas.

N. Desai
Department of Surgery, University of Tennessee Health Science Center, College of Medicine, Memphis, TN, USA
e-mail: ndesai4@uthsc.edu

T. Ng (✉)
Division of Thoracic Surgery, University of Tennessee Health Science Center, College of Medicine, Memphis, TN, USA
e-mail: tng4@uthsc.edu

T. Ng, T. Geraci (eds.), *Thoracic Surgery Clerkship*, Contemporary Surgical Clerkships, https://doi.org/10.1007/978-3-031-44645-0_9

- Excellent prognosis, high cure rate with surgical resection.
- Usually more common in patients <60 years of age.
- There is a female predominance.
- Associated with Caucasian race, MEN1 gene, and nonsmokers.

Presentation

- Can be central/endobronchial (Fig. 9.1a, b).
- Symptoms: cough, wheezing, asthma, COPD, chest pain, hemoptysis.
- Carcinoid syndrome and other paraneoplastic syndromes are rare.

Pathologic Diagnosis

- Biopsy will reveal polygonal-shaped cells with round/oval nuclei and salt and pepper chromatin with eosinophilic cytoplasm.
- Neuroendocrine tumor size >5 mm (<5 mm are termed carcinoid "tumorlet").
- Typical carcinoid pathology has <2 mitoses per 2 mm^2.
- Ki-67 is positive in less than 20% of cases.
- Absence of focal necrosis.
- Positive for chromogranin, synaptophysin, CD56, pancytokeratins, Rb.

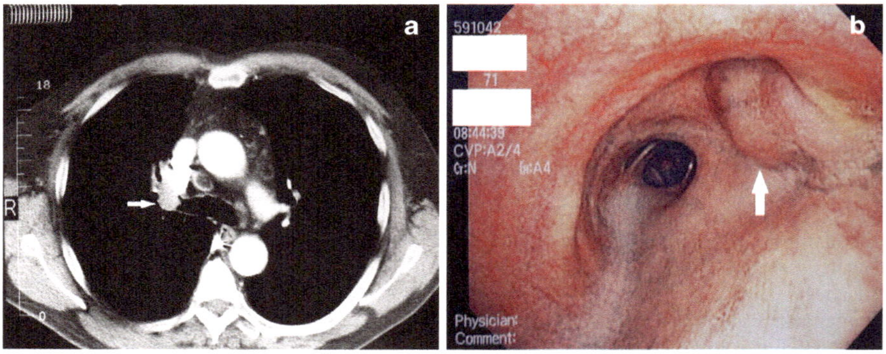

Fig. 9.1 Obstruction endobronchial carcinoid tumor (arrow) of the right upper lobe bronchus. (**a**) CT scan; (**b**) bronchoscopy view

Workup

- History and physical examination
- CT scan of the chest, abdomen, and pelvis with IV contrast
- PET/CT-Ga-DOTATATE scan if there is multifocal disease or suspicion of metastasis
- MRI brain with contrast if symptoms or advanced disease

Staging

- According to AJCC 8th edition staging of lung cancer (see Chap. 6)

Treatment

- Similar to treatment for all other non-small cell lung cancer with some distinctions given below.
- As carcinoid tumors are often less responsive to chemotherapy or radiation, upfront surgery is the mainstay of treatment, even for stage IIIA disease; observation is an option, depending on symptoms and degree of disease progression, balancing with patient comorbidities.
- As carcinoid tumors can be central/endobronchial, sleeve resection is optimal, with the goal of complete resection (negative margins) while preserving lung function (Fig. 9.2).

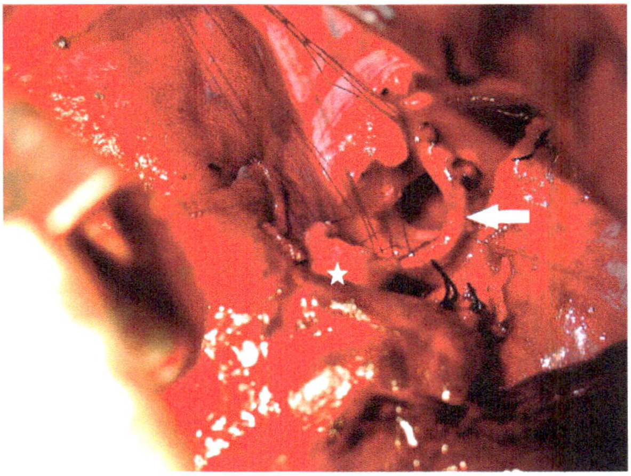

Fig. 9.2 Sleeve right upper lobectomy, after removal of the right upper lobe en bloc with central airway, the right main bronchus (arrow) is being anastomosed to the bronchus intermedius (star), thus preserving right middle and lower lobes

- For advanced disease (locally advanced or metastatic), consider chemotherapy (cisplatin and etoposide or temozolomide ± capecitabine), radiation, octreotide/lanreotide (for somatostatin receptor positive), or everolimus (mTOR inhibitor).

Atypical Carcinoid Lung Cancer (Intermediate Grade)

Epidemiology

- Typically referred to as intermediate-grade neuroendocrine cancer.
- Most are sporadic, but 5–10% can be due to genetic causes (MEN-1, familial pulmonary carcinoid tumors).
- Rare: 2 cases/100,000, less common than typical carcinoids.
- There is a female predominance.
- Most commonly occurs between ages 40 and 60 years.

Presentation

- Can be central/endobronchial causing local symptoms.
- Symptoms: cough, wheezing, asthma, COPD, chest pain, hemoptysis.
- Carcinoid syndrome is present in <5%.
- Can be associated with paraneoplastic syndromes of Cushing syndrome, acromegaly.

Pathologic Diagnosis

- Cells are similar to typical carcinoid tumors, except the cells are looser/more isolated and less uniform, focal necrosis present, mitoses rare but higher than typical carcinoid.
- Atypical pathology has 2–10 mitoses per 2 mm^2.
- Ki-67 is positive in less than 20% of cases.
- Presence of focal necrosis.
- Immunohistochemistry: chromogranin A, synaptophysin, CD 56 positive.

Workup

- History and physical examination
- CT scan of the chest, abdomen, and pelvis with IV contrast
- PET/CT-Ga-DOTATATE scan
- MRI brain with contrast if symptoms or advanced disease

Staging

- According to AJCC 8th edition staging of lung cancer (see Chap. 6)

Treatment

- Similar to treatment for all other non-small cell lung cancer with some distinctions given below.
- As carcinoid tumors are often less responsive to chemotherapy or radiation, upfront surgery is the mainstay of treatment, even for stage IIIA disease, and observation is an option for patients with advanced disease (depending on symptoms and degree of disease progression, balancing with patient comorbidities).
- As carcinoid tumors can be central/endobronchial, in which case sleeve resection is optimal, with the goal of complete resection (negative margins) while preserving lung function.
- For advanced disease (locally advanced or metastatic), consider chemotherapy (cisplatin and etoposide or temozolomide ± capecitabine), radiation, octreotide/lanreotide (for somatostatin receptor positive), or everolimus (mTOR inhibitor).

Large Cell Neuroendocrine Carcinoma (High Grade)

Epidemiology

- Three percent of all lung cancers.
- Associated with heavy smoking.
- There is a male predominance.
- Aggressive neuroendocrine lung carcinoma, comparable to that of small cell neuroendocrine carcinoma.
- Often peripheral more than central.

Pathologic Diagnosis

- Described as "large, polygonal and anaplastic cells growing in sheets or solid nests."
- Neuroendocrine morphology, specifically can have trabeculae, palisading nuclei, organoid nesting, and/or rosettes.
- Tumors have >10 mitoses per 2 mm^2.
- Presence of necrosis.
- High proliferation index Ki-67%.

- Expression of either NCAM/CD56, chromogranin A, or synaptophysin.
- Most sensitive neuroendocrine biomarker is NCAM/CD56.

Presentation

- Presentation can be asymptomatic or with symptoms similar to that of other lung cancers, including bronchopulmonary, extrapulmonary intrathoracic, or metastatic symptoms.
- Paraneoplastic syndromes are not commonly associated with large cell neuroendocrine cancer.

Workup

- History and physical examination
- CT scan of the chest, abdomen, and pelvis with IV contrast
- PET/CT scan
- MRI brain with contrast

Staging

- According to AJCC 8th edition staging of lung cancer (see Chap. 6)

Treatment

- Similar to treatment for all other non-small cell lung cancers with some distinction given below.
- Given high-grade, aggressiveness nature, similar to that of small cell carcinoma:
  - If surgery is planned, preoperative invasive mediastinal lymph node staging is recommended (EBUS or mediastinoscopy).
  - Lobectomy with mediastinal lymph node dissection preferred over sublobar resection.
  - Even for early-stage N0 disease, adjuvant chemotherapy is strongly recommended.

Small Cell Lung Carcinoma (High Grade)

Epidemiology

- Fifteen percent of all lung cancers.
- There is a male predominance.
- High-grade aggressive neuroendocrine lung cancer.
- Risk factors: tobacco, COPD, genetic mutations (EGFR, ALK, TP53, RB1, PTEN).

Pathology

- Cells described as small-sized, round-to-fusiform shape, scant cytoplasm, finely granular nuclear chromatin and absent or inconspicuous nucleoli
- Stains: positive for synaptophysin, chromogranin A, INSM1, CD56

Presentation

- Central location of the tumor, often advanced at presentation with nodal and distal metastatic spread and its associated symptoms (cough, dyspnea, hemoptysis, SVC syndrome, metastatic symptoms)
- Associated with paraneoplastic syndromes like SIADH, Cushing syndrome, Lambert-Eaton
- 10% present with brain metastasis

Workup

- History and physical examination
- CT scan of the chest, abdomen, and pelvis with IV contrast
- PET/CT scan
- MRI brain with contrast

Staging

- Limited stage (stages I–III: T any, N any, M0), disease in the ipsilateral hemithorax that can be safely radiated

  - Includes contralateral mediastinal and ipsilateral supraclavicular lymphadenopathy
  - Earliest stage within this group, T1-2, N0, M0, may be candidates for surgery
- Extensive stage (stage IV: T any, N any, M1a/b/c), disease beyond the ipsilateral hemithorax (includes malignant pleural or pericardial effusion, hematogenous metastasis)
  - Includes contralateral hilar and contralateral supraclavicular lymphadenopathy
  - Includes T4 malignant nodule in the ipsilateral lung but different lobe

Treatment

- Very early-stage small cell lung cancer (T1–T2, N0, M0): rare circumstance, <5%
  - Confirm N0 with mediastinoscopy or EBUS.
  - Surgical resection: lobectomy preferred over sublobar resection, with mediastinal lymph node dissection.
  - Post op systemic therapy/chemotherapy.
  - Post op radiation if N positive on final pathology.
  - Chemotherapy/radiation (consider stereotactic radiation) if medically inoperable.
- Limited-stage small cell lung cancer
  - Chemotherapy (cisplatin-etoposide)/radiation (see Chaps. 15 and 16).
  - Consider prophylactic whole brain radiation if good response.
- Extensive-stage SCLC
  - Chemotherapy + immunotherapy (PD-L1 immune checkpoint inhibitor) (see Chap. 15)
  - Radiation to symptomatic sites

Key Reference

- Soldath P, Petersen RH. The surgical management of lung neuroendocrine neoplasms. Cancers. 2023;15(6):1695.

Further Reading

Beasley MB, Brambilla E, Travis WD. The 2004 World Health Organization classification of lung tumors. Semin Roentgenol. 2005;40(2):90–7.

Fasano M, Della Corte CM, Papaccio F, Ciardiello F, Morgillo F. Pulmonary large-cell neuroendocrine carcinoma: from epidemiology to therapy. J Thorac Oncol. 2015;10:1133–41.

Huang R, et al. Associated links among smoking, chronic obstructive pulmonary disease, and small cell lung cancer: a pooled analysis in the International Lung Cancer Consortium. EBioMedicine. 2015;2:1677–85.

Iyoda A, Hiroshima K, Toyozaki T, Haga Y, Fujisawa T, Ohwada H. Clinical characterization of pulmonary large cell neuroendocrine carcinoma and large cell carcinoma with neuroendocrine morphology. Cancer. 2001;91:1992–2000.

National Comprehensive Cancer Network. 2017 NCCN clinical practice guidelines in oncology: neuroendocrine tumors. Version 3; NCCN: Plymouth meeting, PA, USA, 2017.

Pavel ME, Hainsworth JD, Baudin E, Peeters M, Hörsch D, Winkler RE, Klimovsky J, Lebwohl D, Jehl V, Wolin EM, et al. Everolimus plus octreotide long-acting repeatable for the treatment of advanced neuroendocrine tumours associated with carcinoid syndrome (RADIANT-2): a randomised, placebo-controlled, phase 3 study. Lancet. 2011;378:2005–12.

Rekhtman N. Neuroendocrine tumors of the lung: an update. Arch Pathol Lab Med. 2010;134(11):1628–38.

Rodriguez E, Lilenbaum RC. Small cell lung cancer: past, present, and future. Curr Oncol Rep. 2010;12:327–34.

Rudin CM, Brambilla E, Faivre-Finn C, Sage J. Small-cell lung cancer. Nature reviews. Dis Primers. 2021;7(1):3.

Thandra KC, Barsouk A, Saginala K, Aluru JS, Barsouk A. Epidemiology of lung cancer. Contemp Oncol. 2021;25(1):45–52.

Travis WD, Brambilla E, Burke AP, Marx A, Nicholson AG. WHO classification of tumours of the lung, pleura, thymus and heart. 4th ed. Lyon: IARC Publications; 2015.

Wakeam E, Adibfar A, Stokes S, Leighl NB, Giuliani ME, Varghese TK Jr, Darling GE. Defining the role of adjuvant therapy for early-stage large cell neuroendocrine carcinoma. J Thorac Cardiovasc Surg. 2020;159(5):2043–54.

Chapter 10
Pulmonary Function Testing and Preoperative Assessment

Angel G. Doño, Travis Geraci, and Thomas Ng

Introduction

Lung resection is the best chance for cure in patients with early-stage lung cancer. Pulmonary resection has risks for postoperative complications, including respiratory insufficiency. Lung resection results in loss of pulmonary function, and therefore, surgeons must balance the extent of pulmonary resection aimed at maximizing the chance of cure, with leaving adequate lung volume to survive with an acceptable quality of life. Assessing this balance is a complex process, involving many factors, the most important of which is pulmonary function testing.

Pulmonary Function Testing

Obtaining a detailed history to determine a patient's functional status can provide valuable information regarding candidacy for surgery. However, the cornerstone of objective measure of the adequacy of lung function for pulmonary resection are pulmonary function testing (PFT).

A. G. Doño
Department of Surgery, University of Tennessee Health Science Center, College of Medicine, Memphis, TN, USA
e-mail: adoo@uthsc.edu

T. Geraci
Division of Thoracic Surgery, Department of Cardiothoracic Surgery, New York University Langone Health, New York, NY, USA
e-mail: travis.geraci@nyulangone.org

T. Ng (✉)
Division of Thoracic Surgery, University of Tennessee Health Science Center, College of Medicine, Memphis, TN, USA
e-mail: tng4@uthsc.edu

T. Ng, T. Geraci (eds.), *Thoracic Surgery Clerkship*, Contemporary Surgical Clerkships, https://doi.org/10.1007/978-3-031-44645-0_10

- Most critical measurements of the PFTs are:
  - Percentage of predicted forced expiratory volume in 1 s (FEV1).
  - Percentage of predicted diffusion capacity of the lung for carbon monoxide (DLCO). Arterial blood gas analysis and DLCO reflect the ability of the lung parenchyma to participate in gas exchange.
- Note that the percent predicted values are what is important, not the absolute values, as this accounts for the patient's size.
- If either predicted postoperative % FEV1 (ppo%FEV1) or predicted postoperative % DLCO (ppo%DLCO) is <40% (what remains after resection), then the patient is at high risk, and exercise testing is recommended (see below).
- ppoFEV_1% less than 30% are at very high risk of pulmonary complications.
- Calculation of ppo%FEV1 and ppo%DLCO:
  - Calculation of predicted postoperative values requires knowledge of lung segmental anatomy (Fig. 10.1).
  - ppo%FEV1 = %FEV1 × (1 − # of segments to be resected/# of total segments).
  - ppo%DLCO = %DLCO × (1 − # of segments to be resected/# of total segments).
  - The above formula assumes homogeneous/uniform lung function, thus inaccurate if the tumor has caused atelectasis (Fig. 10.2a), has replaced lung parenchyma (Fig. 10.2b), or is in an area of bullous disease (Fig. 10.2c), in which case nuclear split-lung function may be helpful (see below).
  - Spirometry data should be individualized per each patient as these may vary in its meaning based on age and patient height, weight, and effort. Overall,

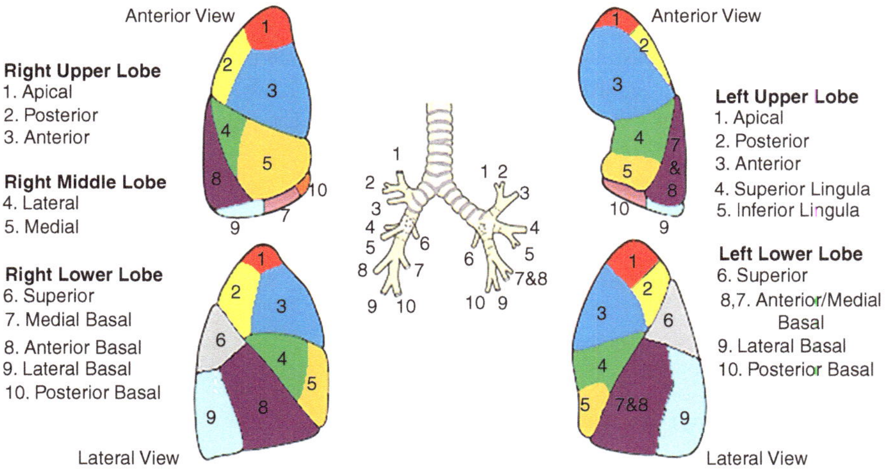

Fig. 10.1 Lung segmental anatomy. The right lung has ten segments. Commonly, the left lung has nine segments, with segments 7 and 8 fused (left lower lobe with four segments). Alternatively, the left lung may be considered to have eight segments, with segments 1 and 2 fused and segments 7 and 8 fused (left upper and lower lobe each having four segments)

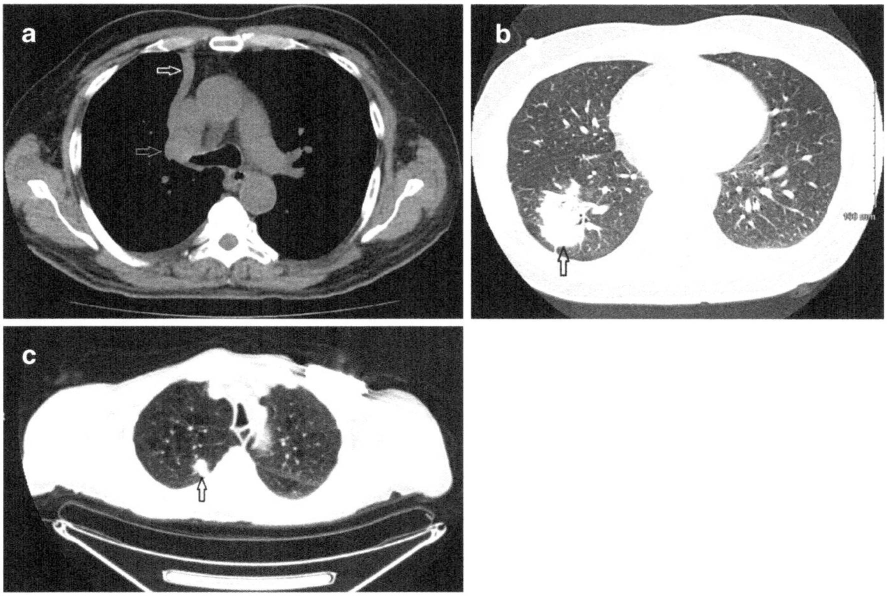

Fig. 10.2 Situations where uniform lung function cannot be assumed when calculating predicted postoperative lung function. (**a**) Centrally located lung cancer obstructing the right upper lobe bronchus (red arrow) resulting in complete right upper lobe atelectasis (white arrow); (**b**) significant amount of lung parenchyma replaced by tumor (arrow); (**c**) tumor located in upper lobe with severe emphysema (arrow)

patients with a ppoFEV1 <40%, while not contraindicated, should have other data input and variables to determine risk of thoracic surgery.

- Example calculation: a patient requiring a right upper lobectomy with FEV1 of 52%:
  - The right upper lobe has three segments for removal (apical, posterior, anterior).
  - ppo%FEV1 = %FEV1 × (1 − # of segments to be resected/# of total segments).
  - ppo%FEV1 = 52 × (1 − 3/19).
  - ppo%FEV1 = 43.8%.
- Flow-volume loops define airflow patterns consistent with specific pathophysiology (Fig. 10.3):
  - Defining between obstructive versus restrictive patterns and response to medications permits preoperative optimization as well as guides perioperative care.

    COPD: emphysema, bronchitis, asthma
    Restriction: parenchymal versus extra-parenchymal diseases
    Airway obstruction: extrathoracic, intrathoracic, fixed, dynamic

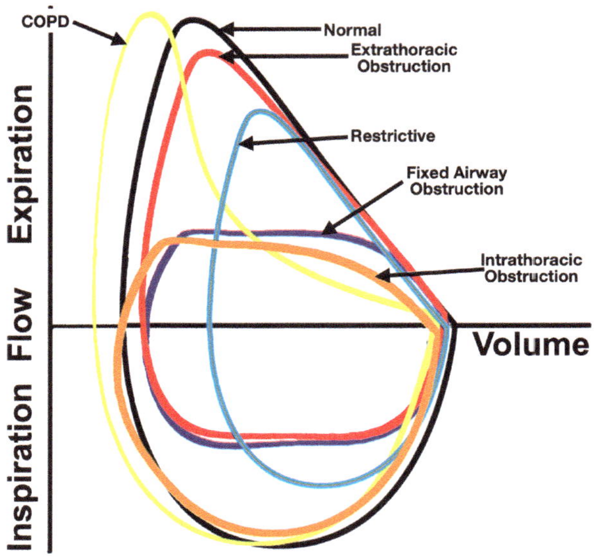

Fig. 10.3 Lung spirometry flow-volume loops

Exercise and Cardiopulmonary Testing

When a patient's ppo%FEV1 or ppo%DLCO is less <40%, exercise testing is indicated to help determine surgical candidacy. Exercise testing is assessed by stair climbing or formal measurement of maximum oxygen consumption (VO_2max).

- Stair climbing
  - Correlates well with VO_2max.
  - Easily performed in the office.
  - Ability to climb a height of 22 m (five flights of stairs) correlates with VO_2max of 15 ml/kg/min, representing low risk for surgery.
  - Patients unable to complete stair climb, then consider VO_2max measurement.
  - Cons: subjective, no standard as to how fast the stair climb should be completed.
- VO_2max measurement
  - Obtained while patient is at maximum exertion on bicycle or treadmill.
  - Measured VO_2max is then used to calculate predicted postoperative VO_2max (ppoVO_2max), utilizing the same formula as for ppo%FEV1 shown above.
  - ppoVO_2max <10 cc/kg/min represents high-risk or inoperable patients and that nonsurgical treatments should be considered such as stereotactic body radiation therapy (see Chap. 16).

Split-Lung Function Perfusion Testing

Split-lung function test is a nuclear test for objectively quantifying the function of specific lung regions by measuring ventilation or perfusion activity of that region and expressing this as a percentage of total lung activity.

- Perfusion is more commonly used than ventilation.
- To calculate ppo%FEV1 utilizing split-lung function test:
  - ppo%FEV1 = %FEV1 × (1 − % of total perfusion of the lung to be resected/100).
  - The same formula is used to calculate ppo%DLCO and ppoVO_2max.
- Split-lung function is most accurate for estimating the function of one entire lung (either side), with preoperative evaluation for pneumonectomy being the specific situation where it is most useful (Fig. 10.4).

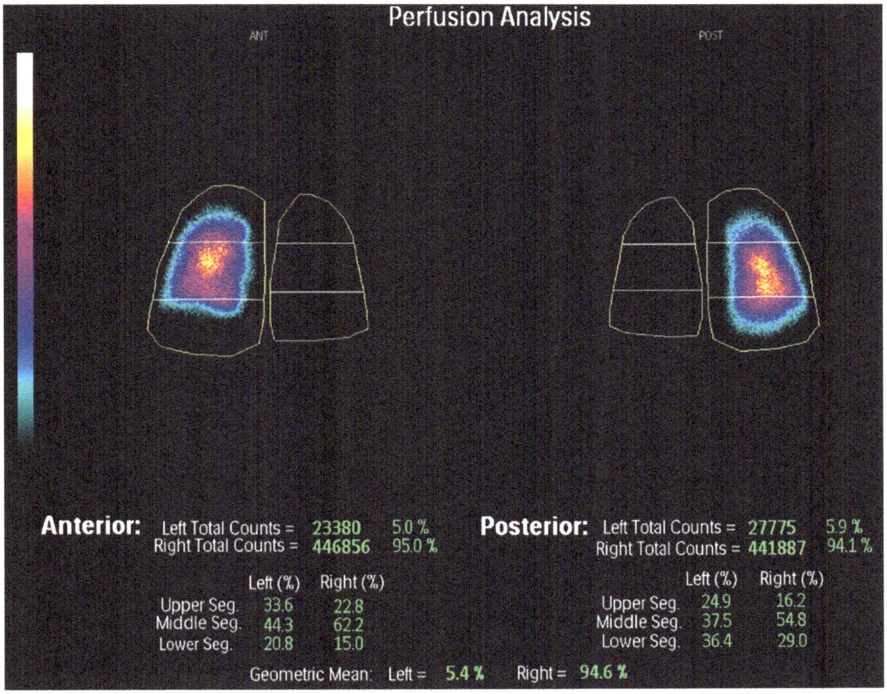

Fig. 10.4 Split-lung function nuclear study of a patient with a large obstructing central left lung cancer, showing very little perfusion activity in the left lung. Although function of each lung is well assessed, note that the function of each lobe of the right side is poorly estimated due to the oblique nature of the major fissure, which results in overlap of lobar activity in the anterior and posterior views

- May be useful when heterogeneous lung function is suspected based on preoperative imaging, such as when the area of lung targeted for resection is atelectatic, replaced by tumor, or has severe emphysema.
- Split-lung function inherently accounts for any lack of function that may exist in both the resected and remaining lung and accounts for any prior resection.
- Limitation of split-lung function testing is its imprecision in estimating lobar function, as the oblique nature of the major fissures results in the overlap of lobar parenchyma in the anterior or posterior views (Fig. 10.4).

Pulmonary Assessment: Special Considerations

- Age and frailty
  - ACCP guidelines state that "age alone is not a contraindication to surgery, and that cardiopulmonary fitness of elderly patients with lung cancer be fully evaluated without any prejudice regarding age."
  - Lung cancer resection in the elderly is feasible, specifically in carefully selected octogenarians.
  - Age may be a surrogate of frailty, but the two are not linearly associated.
  - Although there is limited data in lung cancer, frail patients are at increased risk for postoperative complications.
  - Several assessments, including measurements of sarcopenia, grip strength, and multifaceted clinical scoring systems, are used to determine frailty.
  - For frail patients, preoperative rehabilitation programs are available to optimize functional and nutritional status before surgery.
  - Patients who have undergone 1–4 weeks of prehabilitation before pulmonary resection reported improved postoperative functional status and decreased pulmonary complications.
- Smoking
  - Active smoking increases the risk for postoperative morbidity and mortality and decreases long-term survival.
  - Risk of in-hospital mortality and major pulmonary complications is reduced with smoking cessation for at least 4 weeks before surgery.
  - During the first month after smoking cessation, there are increased mucus burden and disrupted bronchial clearance mechanisms, which can affect clinical recovery after pulmonary resection; thus surgery 4 weeks after smoke cessation is optimal.
  - Smoking cessation programs should be initiated in the preoperative clinic, with the combination of counseling and pharmacotherapy.

- Interstitial lung disease
  - Pulmonary resection in patients with interstitial lung disease (ILD) can result in poor outcomes, with the most feared complication being acute exacerbation of the known ILD.
  - Patients with interstitial pneumonia undergoing pulmonary resection for cancer may have postoperative mortality of 5.5% at 30 days and 12.5% at 90 days.
  - Acute exacerbation of interstitial pneumonia after surgery has an incidence of 9%, with a mortality of 67%.
  - Poor outcomes are reported in ILD patients with low DLCO (associated with pulmonary hypertension) and undergoing lobectomy (versus sublobar resection).
  - Overall, patients with ILD being considered for lung cancer resection need to undergo PFTs and echocardiogram to assess for pulmonary hypertension and are encouraged to stop smoking, and every effort should be made to perform sublobar resection where appropriate.
- Pneumonectomy
  - Pneumonectomy is performed for resection of central tumors otherwise not amenable to lesser resections (sleeve resection, bilobectomy).
  - Pneumonectomy is a morbid procedure, not only with a higher mortality, 5% at 30 days, but also a greater loss of functional capacity and quality of life compared to lesser resections.
  - As oncologic results are equivalent, but morbidity and mortality are higher with pneumonectomy, every effort should be made to resected central tumors by sleeve lobectomy prior to considering pneumonectomy.
  - Preoperative echocardiogram should be added to the preoperative workup, to rule out pulmonary hypertension and/or right ventricular dysfunction.
- Minimally invasive surgery
  - Multiple well-designed propensity-matched studies and more recently, randomized study, have shown minimally invasive approaches (thoracoscopy or robotic) to result in fewer complications, shorter length of stay, and improved physical function as compared to thoracotomy.
  - Studies have also shown that minimally invasive surgery does not compromise oncologic outcomes, with no difference in disease-free survival when compared to thoracotomy.
  - Benefits of minimally invasive surgery may be greatest in patients with compromised pulmonary function.
  - A minimally invasive approach to pulmonary resection should be strongly considered for resection of lung cancer, especially in patients with borderline pulmonary function.

Cardiac Assessment for Pulmonary Resection

- Overall, cardiac complications occur in 3.3% of patients undergoing pulmonary resection.
- The recalibrated thoracic revised cardiac risk index (ThRCRI) assesses cardiac risk, specifically in patients being considered for pulmonary resection.
- ThRCRI comprises of four weighted risk factors:
  - Pneumonectomy = 1.5 points
  - Ischemic heart disease = 1.5 points
  - Cerebrovascular disease = 1.5 points
  - Renal disease (creatinine level >2 mg/dL) = 1 point
- ThRCRI < 2 total points has <1.5% to 5.8% incidence of cardiac complications: low-risk.
- ThRCRI ≥ 2 total points has 19–23% incidence of cardiac complications: high-risk.
- Cardiac evaluation and testing is recommended for ThRCRI ≥ 2, commonly by echocardiogram and stress test.
- Preoperative echocardiogram should be obtained for planned pneumonectomy, patients with borderline PFTs, interstitial lung disease, known cardiac disease, and advanced age (60–70 years; no strict guidelines have been established).

Conclusion

The preoperative evaluation for lung cancer resection mainly focuses on pulmonary function testing, exercise testing, and the ThRCRI; however, other clinical factors also need to be considered when assessing risk (Fig. 10.5). As there are nonsurgical options available for the treatment of early-stage lung cancer, discussion regarding all options, its risks and efficacy, is required. Each patient will be different in their assessment of the level of risk versus the level of cure they are willing to accept. The final determination of treatment should be a shared decision process with the multidisciplinary team.

Key Reference

- Geraci TC, Ng T. When is it safe to operate for lung cancer? Selection of fiscally responsible cardiopulmonary function tests for limited resection (wedge resection and segmentectomy), standard lobectomy, sleeve lobectomy, and pneumonectomy. Thorac Surg Clin. 2021;31(3):255–63.

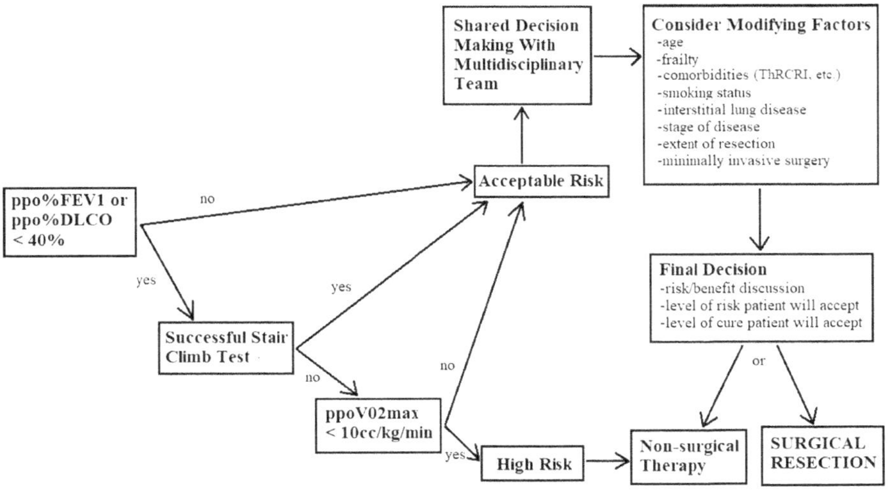

Fig. 10.5 Preoperative assessment for patients being considered for pulmonary resection. *ppo%FEV1* predicted postoperative percent force expiratory volume in 1 s, *ppo%DLCO* predicted postoperative percent diffusion capacity of the lung for carbon monoxide, VO_2max maximum oxygen consumption, *ThRCRI* thoracic revised cardiac risk index

Further Reading

Boffa DJ, Dhamija A, Kosinski AS, Kim AW, Detterbeck FC, Mitchell JD, Onaitis MW, Paul S. Fewer complications result from a video-assisted approach to anatomic resection of clinical stage I lung cancer. J Thorac Cardiovasc Surg. 2014;148(2):637–43.

Brunelli A, Kim AW, Berger KI, Addrizzo-Harris DJ. Physiologic evaluation of the patient with lung cancer being considered for resectional surgery: diagnosis and management of lung cancer, 3rd ed: American College of Chest Physicians evidence-based clinical practice guidelines. Chest. 2013;143(5 Suppl):e166S–90S.

Brunelli A, Varela G, Salati M, Jimenez MF, Pompili C, Novoa N, Sabbatini A. Recalibration of the revised cardiac risk index in lung resection candidates. Ann Thorac Surg. 2010;90(1):199–203. https://doi.org/10.1016/j.athoracsur.2010.03.042. PMID: 20609775.

Burt BM, Kosinski AS, Shrager JB, Onaitis MW, Weigel T. Thoracoscopic lobectomy is associated with acceptable morbidity and mortality in patients with predicted postoperative forced expiratory volume in 1 second or diffusing capacity for carbon monoxide less than 40% of normal. J Thorac Cardiovasc Surg. 2014;148(1):19–28.

Ceppa DP, Kosinski AS, Berry MF, Tong BC, Harpole DH, Mitchell JD, D'Amico TA, Onaitis MW. Thoracoscopic lobectomy has increasing benefit in patients with poor pulmonary function: a Society of Thoracic Surgeons Database analysis. Ann Surg. 2012;256(3):487–93.

Dezube AR, Cooper L, Jaklitsch MT. Prehabilitation of the thoracic surgery patient. Thorac Surg Clin. 2020;30(3):249–58.

Dobson Amato KA, Hyland A, Reed R, Mahoney MC, Marshall J, Giovino G, Bansal-Travers M, Ochs-Balcom HM, Zevon MA, Cummings KM, Nwogu C, Singh AK, Chen H, Warren GW, Reid M. Tobacco cessation may improve lung cancer patient survival. J Thorac Oncol. 2015;10(7):1014–9.

Fernandez FG, Kosinski AS, Burfeind W, Park B, DeCamp MM, Seder C, Marshall B, Magee MJ, Wright CD, Kozower BD. The Society of Thoracic Surgeons Lung cancer resection risk model: higher quality data and superior outcomes. Ann Thorac Surg. 2016;102(2):370–7.

Kuritzky AM, Aswad BI, Jones RN, Ng T. Lobectomy by video-assisted thoracic surgery vs muscle-sparing thoracotomy for stage I lung cancer: a critical evaluation of short- and long-term outcomes. J Am Coll Surg. 2015;220(6):1044–53.

Lim E, Batchelor TJP, Dunning J, Shackcloth M, Anikin V, et al. Video-assisted thoracoscopic or open lobectomy in early stage lung cancer. NEJM Evid. 2022;1:3.

Mason DP, Subramanian S, Nowicki ER, Grab JD, Murthy SC, Rice TW, Blackstone EH. Impact of smoking cessation before resection of lung cancer: a Society of Thoracic Surgeons General Thoracic Surgery Database study. Ann Thorac Surg. 2009;88(2):362–70.

Ohsawa M, Tsutani Y, Fujiwara M, Mimae T, Miyata Y, Okada M. Predicting severe postoperative complication in patients with lung cancer and interstitial pneumonia. Ann Thorac Surg. 2020;109(4):1054–60.

Pagès PB, Mordant P, Renaud S, Brouchet L, Thomas PA, Dahan M, Bernard A, Epithor Project (French Society of Thoracic and Cardiovascular Surgery). Sleeve lobectomy may provide better outcomes than pneumonectomy for non-small cell lung cancer. A decade in a nationwide study. J Thorac Cardiovasc Surg. 2017;153(1):184–95.

Paul S, Isaacs AJ, Treasure T, Altorki NK, Sedrakyan A. Long term survival with thoracoscopic versus open lobectomy: propensity matched comparative analysis using SEER-medicare database. BMJ. 2014;349:g5575.

Rosero ID, Ramírez-Vélez R, Lucia A, Martínez-Velilla N, Santos-Lozano A, Valenzuela PL, Morilla I, Izquierdo M. Systematic review and meta-analysis of randomized, controlled trials on preoperative physical exercise interventions in patients with non-small-cell lung cancer. Cancer. 2019;11(7):944.

Shapiro M, Swanson SJ, Wright CD, Chin C, Sheng S, Wisnivesky J, Weiser TS. Predictors of major morbidity and mortality after pneumonectomy utilizing the Society for Thoracic Surgeons General Thoracic Surgery Database. Ann Thorac Surg. 2010;90(3):927–34.

Shi W, Zhang W, Sun H, Shao Y. Sleeve lobectomy versus pneumonectomy for non-small cell lung cancer: a meta-analysis. World J Surg Oncol. 2012;10:265.

Varela G, Brunelli A, Rocco G, Marasco R, Jiménez MF, Sciarra V, Aranda JL, Gatani T. Predicted versus observed FEV1 in the immediate postoperative period after pulmonary lobectomy. Eur J Cardiothorac Surg. 2006;30(4):644–8.

Wolfenden L, Wiggers J, Knight J, Campbell E, Rissel C, Kerridge R, Spigelman AD, Moore K. A programme for reducing smoking in pre-operative surgical patients: randomised controlled trial. Anaesthesia. 2005;60(2):172–9.

Yang CF, Sun Z, Speicher PJ, Saud SM, Gulack BC, Hartwig MG, Harpole DH Jr, Onaitis MW, Tong BC, D'Amico TA, Berry MF. Use and outcomes of minimally invasive lobectomy for stage I non-small cell lung cancer in the national cancer data base. Ann Thorac Surg. 2016;101(3):1037–42.

Zhou W, Heist RS, Liu G, Park S, Neuberg DS, Asomaning K, Wain JC, Lynch TJ, Christiani DC. Smoking cessation before diagnosis and survival in early stage non-small cell lung cancer patients. Lung Cancer. 2006;53(3):375–80.

Chapter 11
Pulmonary Resection, Approaches and Techniques

Benjamin R. Zambetti and Thomas Ng

Introduction

Pulmonary resection has a variety of indications ranging from benign infectious pathologies to malignant disease. Despite the etiology, the general principles of an anatomic pulmonary resection remain the same, with the division of the corresponding airway, pulmonary vein and pulmonary artery. Pulmonary resection can be performed via thoracotomy, via thoracoscopy, or on a robotic platform. Lung isolation techniques have greatly facilitated the ability to perform pulmonary resection, specifically with minimally invasive approaches.

Indications

- Benign disease: bulla/bleb, lung volume reduction, trauma, interstitial lung disease
- Infectious: bacterial, fungal, tuberculosis
- Congenital: sequestration, cystic malformation
- Vascular: arteriovenous malformation
- Neoplasm: primary malignant or benign lesions of the lung, metastasectomy

B. R. Zambetti
Department of Surgery, University of Tennessee Health Science Center, College of Medicine, Memphis, TN, USA

T. Ng (✉)
Division of Thoracic Surgery, University of Tennessee Health Science Center, College of Medicine, Memphis, TN, USA
e-mail: tng4@uthsc.edu

T. Ng, T. Geraci (eds.), *Thoracic Surgery Clerkship*, Contemporary Surgical Clerkships, https://doi.org/10.1007/978-3-031-44645-0_11

The Approach

Open Approaches

Thoracotomy provides wide exposure that may be necessary for complex thoracic procedures or during thoracic emergencies. The use of rib spreaders is common to all open approaches.

- Posterolateral thoracotomy (Fig. 11.1)
  - Lateral decubitus position.
  - Incision made going around the tip of the scapula.
  - Divide the latissimus dorsi.
  - Serratus anterior can either be mobilized and spared or divided.
  - Chest entry commonly at the fifth interspace as this centers the operative field at the pulmonary hilum, but can vary one space above or below.
  - Small segment of anterior or posterior rib can be removed if needed to improve exposure by allowing wider retraction of the rib space (referred to as "rib shingling").
  - Place rib retractors and begin planned resection; if intercostal muscle flap is to be utilized, harvest during entry into the chest, to avoid damage with retractors.
- Muscle sparing thoracotomy (Fig. 11.2)
  - Lateral decubitus position.
  - Anterior-lateral transverse incision near the level of the nipple.
  - Anterior edge of the latissimus dorsi is mobilized and retracted posteriorly.
  - Serratus anterior is split between its muscle fibers.
  - Chest entry commonly in fifth interspace as this centers the field at the pulmonary hilum, but can vary one space above or below.
  - Place rib retractor.

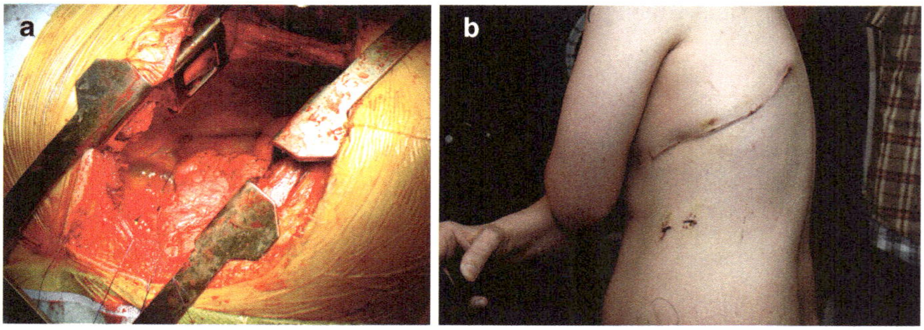

Fig. 11.1 Posterolateral thoracotomy. (**a**) Intraoperative exposure; (**b**) extent of wound

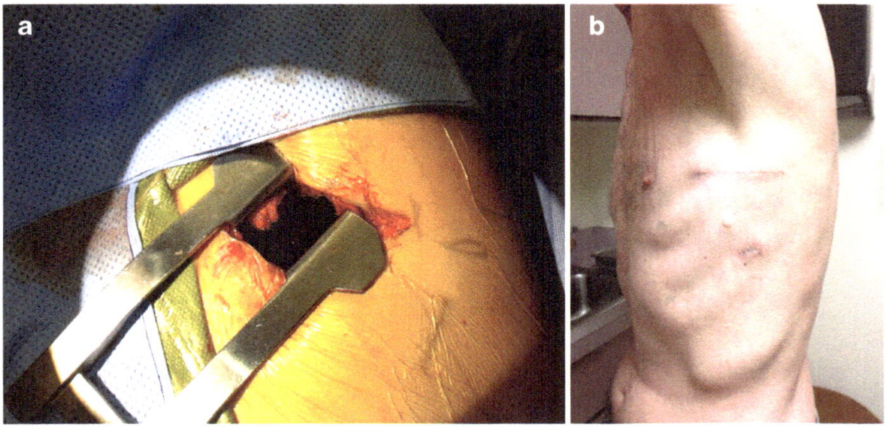

Fig. 11.2 Muscle sparing thoracotomy. (**a**) Intraoperative exposure; (**b**) extent of wound

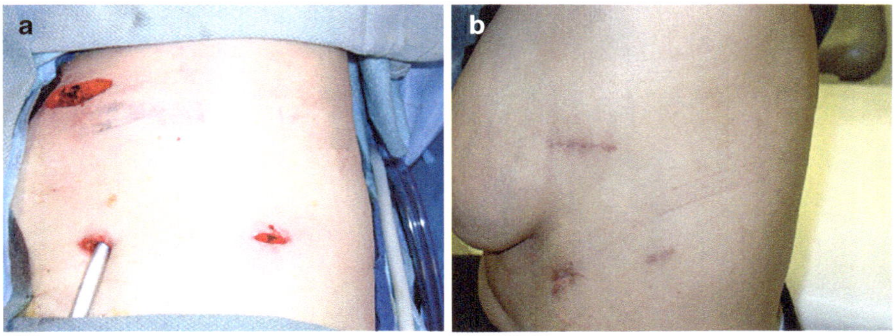

Fig. 11.3 Thoracoscopic approach. (**a**) Three ports for lobectomy; (**b**) extent of wound

Minimally Invasive Approaches

The principles of minimally invasive thoracic surgery are consistent between thoracoscopic and robotic approaches: small incisions, with no division of muscle and no rib spreading, thus reducing incisional pain and morbidity as compared with thoracotomy. Extension of one of these small incisions may be required to extract the specimen with an endoscopic specimen bag.

- Thoracoscopy (Fig. 11.3), also known as video-assisted thoracoscopic surgery (VATS)
  - Lateral decubitus position.
  - Number of ports varies depending on the complexity of the surgery and surgeon preference.
  - Multiple instruments can be passed through a single site by extending the site incision, while still maintaining no rib spreading.

- Can be performed either with all thoracoscopic instruments or in combination with open instruments under thoracoscopic visualization.
- CO_2 insufflation can be utilized to improve visualization but should be set at the lowest pressures required to facilitate the surgery (commonly <10 mmHg), due to risk of hemodynamic instability.

• Robotic (Fig. 11.4)

- Lateral decubitus position.
- Number of trocars or robotic arms varies depending on the complexity of the surgery and surgeon preference.

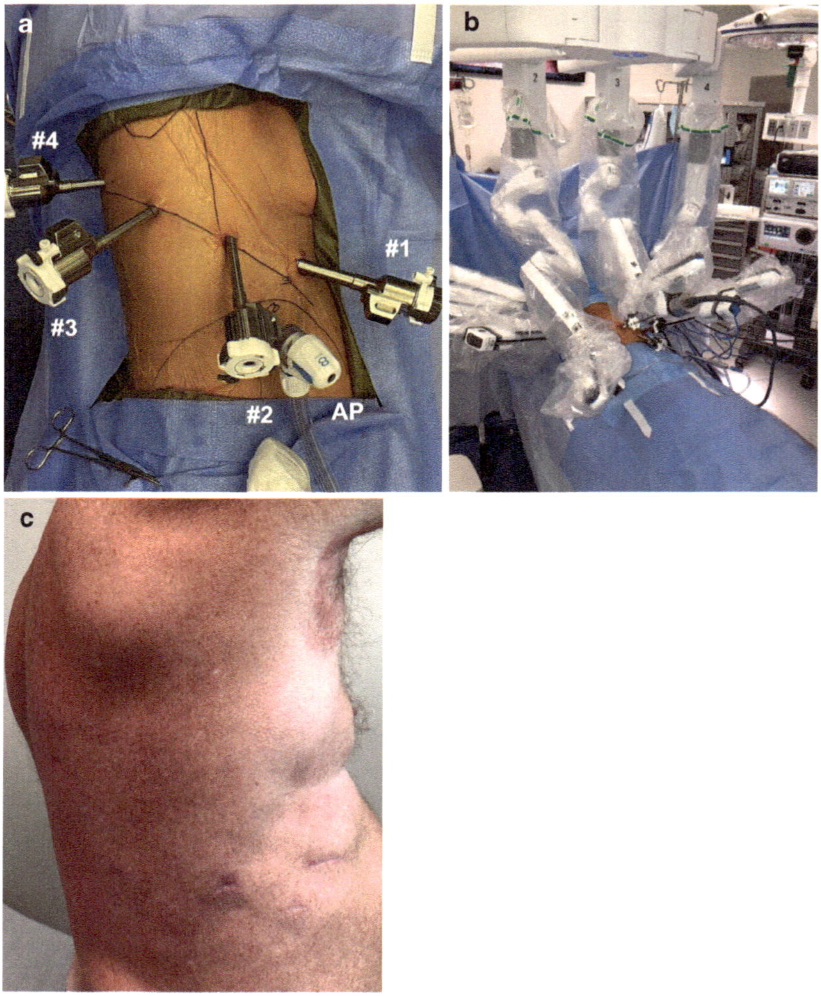

Fig. 11.4 Robotic approach. (**a**) Four robotic ports and one assist port (AP) for lobectomy; (**b**) the four robotic ports docked to the robot; (**c**) extent of wound

- Robotic trocars are placed low (or caudad) on the chest wall and spaced apart (8–10 cm if possible) to optimize mobility of the robotic arms.
- Initial three robotic ports include a camera port placed in mid-axillary line, low on the chest wall to allow for maximum viewing of the entire thoracic cavity; then working robotic ports are placed on either side.
- A fourth robotic port for retraction may be placed, commonly required for anatomical pulmonary resections.
- Additional bedside assistant port (non-robotic), placed even more inferiorly, is commonly required during anatomical pulmonary resections, for suctioning, retrieval of lymph nodes, and exchange of rolled sponges.
- CO_2 insufflation can be utilized to improve visualization but should be set at the lowest pressures required to facilitate the surgery (commonly <10 mmHg), due to risk of hemodynamic instability.

Technical Aspects of Pulmonary Resection

After entering the chest (either via a thoracotomy or minimally invasive approach), a thorough exploration is performed to confirm the targeted pathology, identify presence of any metastatic disease, and identify presence of any other pathologies. At the conclusion of the procedure, most pulmonary resections require intraoperative placement of at least one chest tube (management discussed in Chap. 2).

- Wedge resection
  - Wedge resections are commonly utilized for diagnosis of indeterminate pulmonary nodules, diagnosis of interstitial lung disease, nonneoplastic processes, benign neoplasms, and pulmonary metastases and for selected primary lung cancers (see Chap. 7).
  - Does not require isolation of pulmonary vasculature or bronchi.
  - Parenchymal tissue surrounding the intended lesion is serially divided using a linear cutting stapler.
  - Staple lines should be examined for hemostasis and to evaluate for obvious air leaks.
- Segmentectomy
  - Segmentectomies are performed for select primary lung cancers (peripheral clinical IA, less than 2 cm), nonneoplastic processes, benign neoplasms, and pulmonary metastases that are not amenable to wedge resection, commonly due to size and depth of the pathology.
  - Segmentectomy requires isolation and division of the segmental artery, vein, and bronchus; commonly using linear cutting stapler, however vasculature can also be suture ligated and the bronchus can be sewn closed.
  - There is no definitive order for the division of the segmental structures.
  - The segmental bronchus can be clamped, and with differential inflation/deflation, the segmental plane is identified, allowing for parenchymal division to

separate the segment, commonly using a linear cutting stapler or combination of cautery and blunt dissection. Alternatively, indocyanine green can be administered after division of the vasculature, to define the intersegmental plane.
  - The vascular staple/suture lines should be examined for hemostasis, and the bronchial stump should be tested for air leak with Valsalva maneuver while submerged.

- Lobectomy/bilobectomy
  - Commonly performed for primary lung malignancies; if involving two lobes, then may require upper bilobectomy (right upper and middle) or lower bilobectomy (right lower and middle).
  - Also performed for nonneoplastic processes, benign neoplasms, and pulmonary metastases that are not amenable to sublobar (segmentectomy or wedge) resection, commonly due to the pathology involving the entire lobe.
  - Each lobe should have pulmonary vein and artery branches isolated and divided, commonly with linear cutting stapler or suture ligature; for lower bilobectomy the common arterial trunk to the lower and middle lobe is divided.
  - The lobar bronchus can be isolated and divided commonly with a linear cutting stapler; however sutured closure is also an option; for lower bilobectomy the proximal bronchus intermedius is divided.
  - Division of the lobar fissure can be by cautery if complete; if incomplete, then by linear cutting stapler to minimize air leak from the fissure parenchymal tissue.
  - There is no required order of the division for the pulmonary vein, pulmonary artery, bronchus, or fissure; these structures are divided in whichever order that facilitates safe resection. There is some data that suggests dividing the vein first prevents systemic tumor cell dissemination.
  - The vascular staple/suture lines should be examined for hemostasis, and the bronchial stump should be tested for air leak with Valsalva maneuver while submerged.
  - Orientation of the remaining lobe(s) should be ensured to minimize risk of lobar torsion.

- Sleeve lobectomy
  - Sleeve resections are utilized for central tumors involving the main bronchus, in an effort to avoid pneumonectomy, while maintaining complete or R0 resection.
  - The lobectomy is performed in the same fashion as above, except for the handling of the bronchus.
  - As the tumor is central and involves or is in close proximity of the main bronchus (Fig. 11.5a, b), the main bronchus is divided proximal to the tumor, and the remaining lobar bronchus is divided distal to the tumor, to resect a "sleeve" of the main bronchus en bloc.
  - Frozen section is sent to confirm negative margins on the airway.

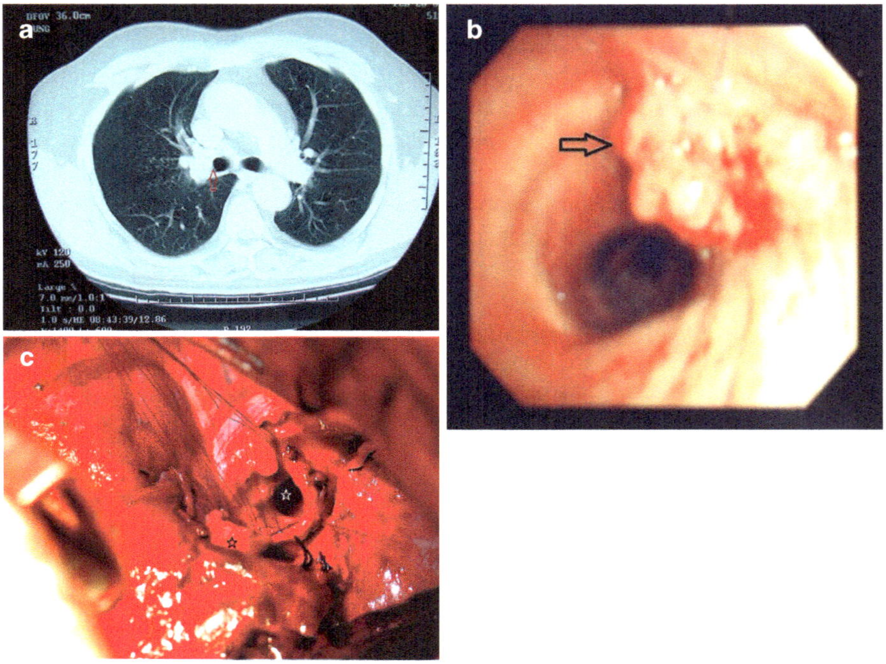

Fig. 11.5 Central right upper lobe tumor involving the main bronchus. (**a**) CT scan of the tumor (arrow); (**b**) bronchoscopic view of the tumor (arrow); (**c**) anastomosis of the right mainstem bronchus (white star) to the bronchus intermedius (black star) after sleeve right upper lobectomy

  - A sutured end-to-end anastomosis of the main bronchus to the bronchus of the remaining lung is performed (Fig. 11.5c).
  - The anastomosis is submerged and tested for air leak with Valsalva maneuver.

- Pneumonectomy
  - Associated with a relatively high morbidity and mortality, therefore should be avoided unless absolutely necessary.
  - Commonly performed for primary lung malignancies that are central, with extensive invasion into the parenchyma of all lobes, main bronchus or main pulmonary artery, that otherwise cannot be completely resected by standard or sleeve lobectomy.
  - Rarely performed for benign or nonneoplastic processes that have resulted in the destruction of the entire lung.
  - The main pulmonary artery and superior and inferior pulmonary veins are isolated and commonly divided with linear cutting stapler, less often suture ligation due to the size of these vessels.
  - If more proximal control of main pulmonary vessels is required, the pericardium is opened, and the intrapericardial aspects of these vessels can then be controlled.

- The mainstem bronchus is isolated and divided, commonly with a linear cutting stapler, less often suture closure.
- Commonly one chest tube is placed, to keep the mediastinum balanced (avoid significant mediastinal shift in the acute postoperative period), with the chest tube placed to waterseal and the drainage system clearly marked to warn against applying suction as this may cause acute dramatic mediastinal shift leading to hemodynamic compromise; this chest tube is removed the next morning to minimize post-pneumonectomy empyema.
- Alternatively no chest tube is placed, but this may require postoperative needle evacuation or introduction of air into the pneumonectomy space, depending on the direction of the excessive mediastinal shift.
- During the intraoperative period and in the postoperative period, excessive intravenous fluids are avoided, as post-pneumonectomy pulmonary edema carries a high risk of mortality.

• Mediastinal lymphadenectomy

- Either mediastinal lymph node sampling or full dissection is acceptable, during resection of early-stage primary lung malignancies.
- For early-stage lung cancer, no difference in complications or long-term survival was found when comparing mediastinal lymph node dissection versus sampling.
- As a measure of quality in lung cancer surgery, the American College of Surgeons Committee on Cancer mandates that a minimum of three mediastinal lymph node stations along with hilar node be sampled or dissected.
- For right-sided tumors, stations 2R (upper paratracheal), 4R (lower paratracheal), 7 (subcarinal), 8 (paraesophageal), 9 (inferior ligament), 10R (hilar), and 11R (interlobar) are commonly sampled or dissected (for details see Chap. 6).
- For left-sided tumors, stations 5 (subaortic), 6 (para-aortic), 7 (subcarinal), 8 (paraesophageal), 9 (inferior ligament), 10L (hilar), and 11L (interlobar) are commonly sampled or dissected (for details see Chap. 6).

• Resection of adjacent structures due to invasion

- For apical tumors see Chap. 9.
- Chest wall:

  Performed en bloc with pulmonary resection (Fig. 11.6a), chest wall resection is usually performed first.

  General rule for reconstruction: anterior defect >5 cm, posterior defect >10 cm; to prevent excessive paradox movement that can impair respiratory mechanics, to prevent lung herniating, and to prevent trapped scapula tip.

  Options for reconstruction include polytetrafluoroethylene (PTFE) (Fig. 11.6b), polypropylene/methyl methacrylate sandwich, and titanium rib bride/strut.

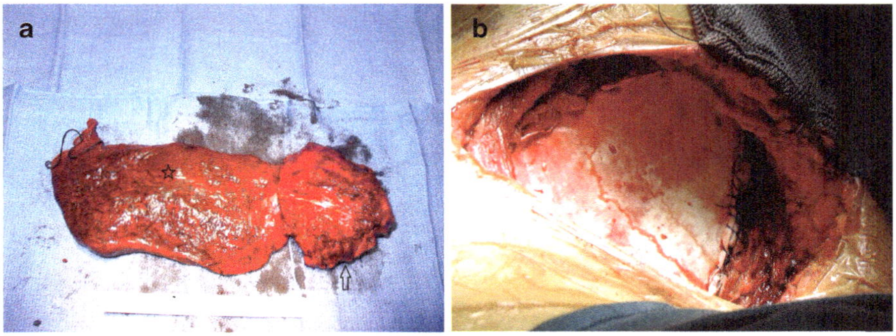

Fig. 11.6 Chest wall resection. (**a**) Pulmonary resection (star) en bloc with chest wall (arrow); (**b**) chest wall reconstruction with 2 mm thick polytetrafluoroethylene (PTFE) patch that is pulled "tight as a drum" to minimize paradoxical motion

- Diaphragm:

  Performed en bloc with pulmonary resection.
  Reconstruction indicated for almost all resections, as any degree of tension with primary repair risks failure of the suture line resulting in herniation of abdominal viscera.
  Reconstruct with PTFE.

Outcomes

- While there is reduced morbidity and length of stay with minimally invasive techniques, complications are generally dependent on the amount of the lung being resected and patient comorbidities.
- Table 11.1 lists the common complications after pulmonary resection, and Table 11.2 lists the morbidity and mortality according to the extent of resection.
- Postoperative outcomes and long-term cancer survival are superior when pulmonary resection is performed at high-volume institutions by experienced thoracic surgeons.

Key Reference

- Wei B, Gleason F. Sublobar resections: indications and approaches. Thorac Surg Clin. 2023;33(2):165–78.

Table 11.1 Complications after pulmonary resection

Complication	% of patients (%)
Tracheostomy	1.0
Reintubation	3.2
Initial ventilatory support >48 h	0.5
Adult respiratory distress syndrome	0.6
Bronchopleural fistula	0.5
Pulmonary embolism	0.5
Pneumonia	4.0
Unexpected return to operating room	3.8
Myocardial infarction	0.3
DVT requiring treatment	0.5
Atrial arrhythmia requiring treatment	10.7
Renal failure	0.8
Sepsis	0.7
Recurrent laryngeal nerve paralysis	0.5
Blood transfusion	
Intraoperative	2.5
Postoperative	5.2
Chylothorax	
Requiring surgical ligation	0.2
Medical treatment only	0.4

Table 11.2 Morbidity and mortality by extent of resection

Procedure	Mortality (%)	Major morbidity (%)	Composite mortality or major morbidity (%)
Wedge	0.8	5.3	5.6
Segmentectomy	0.8	6.5	7.0
Lobectomy	1.3	9.3	9.7
Sleeve lobectomy	1.7	12.1	12.9
Bilobectomy	3.4	15.3	15.7
Pneumonectomy	4.9	16.1	17.5

Further Reading

Altorki N, Wang X, Kozono D, Watt C, Landrenau R, Wigle D, Port J, Jones DR, Conti M, Ashrafi AS, Liberman M, Yasufuku K, Yang S, Mitchell JD, Pass H, Keenan R, Bauer T, Miller D, Kohman LJ, Stinchcombe TE, Vokes E. Lobar or sublobar resection for peripheral stage IA non-small-cell lung cancer. N Engl J Med. 2023;388(6):489–98.

Birkmeyer JD, Siewers AE, Finlayson EV, et al. Hospital volume and surgical mortality in the United States. N Engl J Med. 2002;346(15):1128–37.

Birkmeyer JD, Stukel TA, Siewers AE, Goodney PP, Wennberg DE, Lucas FL. Surgeon volume and operative mortality in the United States. N Engl J Med. 2003;349(22):2117–27.

Birkmeyer JD, Sun Y, Wong SL, Stukel TA. Hospital volume and late survival after cancer surgery. Ann Surg. 2007;245(5):777–83.

Boffa DJ, Allen MS, Grab JD, Gaissert HA, Harpole DH, Wright CD. Data from The Society of Thoracic Surgeons General Thoracic Surgery database: the surgical management of primary lung tumors. J Thorac Cardiovasc Surg. 2008;135(2):247–54.

Boffa DJ, Dhamija A, Kosinski AS, Kim AW, Detterbeck FC, Mitchell JD, Onaitis MW, Paul S. Fewer complications result from a video-assisted approach to anatomic resection of clinical stage I lung cancer. J Thorac Cardiovasc Surg. 2014;148(2):637–43.

Darling GE, Allen MS, Decker PA, Ballman K, Malthaner RA, Inculet RI, Jones DR, McKenna RJ, Landreneau RJ, Rusch VW, Putnam JB Jr. Randomized trial of mediastinal lymph node sampling versus complete lymphadenectomy during pulmonary resection in the patient with N0 or N1 (less than hilar) non-small cell carcinoma: results of the American College of Surgery Oncology Group Z0030 Trial. J Thorac Cardiovasc Surg. 2011;141(3):662–70.

Fernandez FG, Kosinski AS, Burfeind W, Park B, DeCamp MM, Seder C, Marshall B, Magee MJ, Wright CD, Kozower BD. The Society of Thoracic Surgeons lung cancer resection risk model: higher quality data and superior outcomes. Ann Thorac Surg. 2016;102(2):370–7.

Lim E, Batchelor TJP, Dunning J, Shackcloth M, Anikin V, et al. Video-assisted thoracoscopic or open lobectomy in early stage lung cancer. NEJM Evid. 2022;1:3. https://doi.org/10.1056/EVIDoa2100016.

Mansour Z, Kochetkova EA, Santelmo N, et al. Risk factors for early mortality and morbidity after pneumonectomy: a reappraisal. Ann Thorac Surg. 2009;88(6):1737–43.

Pagès PB, Mordant P, Renaud S, Brouchet L, Thomas PA, Dahan M, Bernard A, Epithor Project (French Society of Thoracic and Cardiovascular Surgery). Sleeve lobectomy may provide better outcomes than pneumonectomy for non-small cell lung cancer. A decade in a nationwide study. J Thorac Cardiovasc Surg. 2017;153(1):184–95.

Saji H, Okada M, Tsuboi M, Nakajima R, Suzuki K, Aokage K, Aoki T, Okami J, Yoshino I, Ito H, Okumura N, Yamaguchi M, Ikeda N, Wakabayashi M, Nakamura K, Fukuda H, Nakamura S, Mitsudomi T, Watanabe SI, Asamura H, West Japan Oncology Group and Japan Clinical Oncology Group. Segmentectomy versus lobectomy in small-sized peripheral non-small-cell lung cancer (JCOG0802/WJOG4607L): a multicentre, open-label, phase 3, randomised, controlled, non-inferiority trial. Lancet. 2022;399(10335):1607–17.

Shapiro M, Swanson SJ, Wright CD, et al. Predictors of major morbidity and mortality after pneumonectomy utilizing the Society for Thoracic Surgeons General Thoracic Surgery Database. Ann Thorac Surg. 2010;90(3):927–34; discussion 34-5.

Yang CF, Sun Z, Speicher PJ, Saud SM, Gulack BC, Hartwig MG, Harpole DH Jr, Onaitis MW, Tong BC, D'Amico TA, Berry MF. Use and outcomes of minimally invasive lobectomy for stage I non-small cell lung cancer in the national cancer data base. Ann Thorac Surg. 2016;101(3):1037–42.

Chapter 12
Pulmonary Metastasis and Metastasectomy

Tanvi Subramanian and Jessica Donington

Introduction

Uncontrolled metastatic disease is the most frequent cause of cancer-related death. The lungs are the most common site for cancer metastases. Whereas widespread disease is often not amenable to localized therapy, metastatic spread that is limited to the lungs can often be successfully treated with localized therapy, encompassing both surgical and nonsurgical methods.

Pathophysiology

- Pulmonary tissue has several unique features that make it an ideal site for metastatic seeding:
  - Receives the entire cardiac output every minute
  - Houses the densest capillary bed in the body
  - Acts as a major lymphatic reservoir
- Metastatic spread is therefore easily facilitated by both hematogenous and lymphatic routes, and newly seeded tumor cells have plentiful access to oxygen for survival.

T. Subramanian · J. Donington (✉)
Section of Thoracic Surgery, Department of Surgery, University of Chicago Medicine, Chicago, IL, USA
e-mail: tanvi.subramanian@uchicagomedicine.org; jdonington@bsd.uchicago.edu

T. Ng, T. Geraci (eds.), *Thoracic Surgery Clerkship*, Contemporary Surgical Clerkships, https://doi.org/10.1007/978-3-031-44645-0_12

Presentation

- The majority of pulmonary metastases are asymptomatic and detected radiographically.
- Approximately 15–20% of patients with pulmonary metastases are symptomatic, with cough and hemoptysis being the most common. Patients may also present with chest pain (a possible sign of chest wall invasion) or constitutional symptoms.
  - The presence of symptoms suggests proximity of tumor to larger airways or pleural surface.

Imaging

- Cross-sectional imaging is essential in the evaluation of pulmonary metastases:
  - Computed tomography (CT) is most commonly utilized. Chest CT is accurate, widely available, and associated with a low dose of radiation exposure.
  - FDG-PET (fluorodeoxyglucose-labeled positron emission tomography) enables identification of extrathoracic tumor sites and simultaneously characterizes pulmonary foci of disease metabolically.

    Important in patients who have a short disease-free interval and with high potential for extrathoracic sites of disease

  - Magnetic resonance imaging (MRI) is not a good imaging modality for lung tissue, but can be helpful in demonstrating tumor invasion of the great vessels, heart, chest wall, or nervous structures (spine, brachial plexus) and can be helpful in ruling out synchronous liver metastases.
- Classic radiographic appearance of a pulmonary metastasis: smooth, well-circumscribed, peripheral nodule; a "gumball" or "cannonball" (Fig. 12.1).
- Metastases frequently appear in multiple sites throughout the lungs simultaneously.
- Important to distinguish lesions between infectious processes, primary lung cancer, and metastatic disease.
- In patients with a history of malignancy, the likelihood of pulmonary metastases relative to new primary malignancy is related to the histology of the antecedent cancer, the patient's risk for lung cancers, and the interval from the previous malignancy.

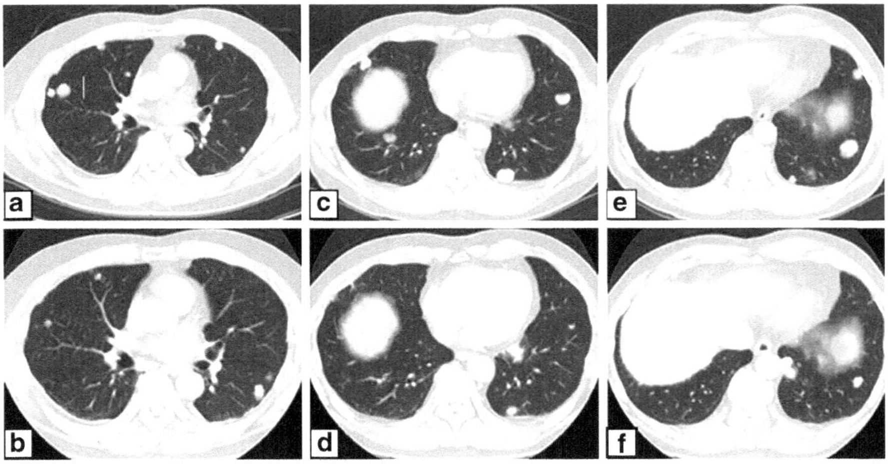

Fig. 12.1 Axial computed tomography images of pulmonary metastases, demonstrating the classical radiologic appearances: circular, well-circumscribed, multiple, and peripheral (**a**–**f**)

Diagnosis

- Histopathologic confirmation is the ultimate determinant of whether a new pulmonary nodule in a patient with a history of cancer is a metastasis.
- If surgical removal will not be pursued, nonoperative biopsy is preferable.
  - Techniques such as image-guided percutaneous biopsy, fluoroscopic-guided transbronchial, endobronchial-ultrasound aided, electromagnetic navigational, or robotic bronchoscopy are all reasonable approaches and should be individualized to the location of the nodule, institutional expertise, and patient-specific concern.
- In patients who cannot be diagnosed by nonoperative means, surgical exploration, and biopsy, preferably by video-assisted thoracoscopic surgery (VATS) is reasonable.

Histologic Subtypes

- Soft tissue and osteogenic sarcoma
  - Both are relatively rare, but have high rates of pulmonary metastases.
  - Failure to control pulmonary metastatic disease is the most frequent cause of death in these patients.

  - Chemotherapy regimens exist, but complete resection of metastatic lesions remains the most effective treatment for long-term survival.
  - Recurrence is common.

- Renal cell carcinoma (RCC)
  - The lung is the most common metastatic site; metastases are frequently present at the time of diagnosis or can develop after nephrectomy.
  - Most patients with systemic disease are treated with systemic immunotherapy or other targeted therapies (tyrosine kinase inhibitors, checkpoint inhibitors, CAR-T cells).
  - Metastasectomy should be considered in patients with few, easily accessible pulmonary metastases with long disease-free interval after nephrectomy or a partial response to targeted therapies.

- Germ cell tumors (testicular cancer)
  - Survival following pulmonary metastasectomy is higher for germ cell tumors than any other histology.

    Multimodal treatment approach combining highly efficacious cisplatin-based chemotherapy and surgery.

- Colorectal cancer (CRC)
  - Lung metastases develop in 5–15% of colorectal cancer (CRC) patients.

    Pulmonary metastasectomy has become an integral part in the multi-modality treatment.

- Head and neck cancers
  - The lung remains the most frequent metastatic site for head and neck cancers (HNC), with origins from oral, pharyngeal, laryngeal, and thyroid primaries.

    Both lung cancer and squamous cell HNC have a common risk factor of smoking, and there is 3–6× increased risk of developing lung cancer in patients with a history of HNC.

  - Metastatic HNC is associated with a notably poor prognosis, with median survival ~10 months after systemic therapy.
  - Treatment commonly involves systemic chemotherapy and immune checkpoint inhibitors; data for pulmonary metastasectomy is still evolving.

- Table 12.1 summarizes outcomes and prognostic factors for the various cancer subtypes.

Table 12.1 Outcomes following surgical metastasectomy for pulmonary metastasis, by tumor histology of primary cancer

Histology	Overall survival at 5 years (%)	Factors associated with improved prognosis
Osteosarcoma	38–43	CSR, small tumor size, long DFI, fewer mets, no progression under chemo, repeat metastasectomy
Soft tissue sarcoma	17–56	CSR, DFI >1 year, age at diagnosis <50, low pathologic grade, tumor subtype
Renal cell carcinoma	44–62	CSR, DFI >32 months, tumor size <2 cm, tumor subtype, fewer/unilateral mets, age <50
Germ cell tumor	73–76	CSR, fewer mets, decreased tumor marker levels
Colorectal cancer	29–48	CSR, fewer mets, tumor size <2 cm, no nodal involvement, CEA level
Head/neck cancer	41–54	DFI >18 months, tumor size <2.5 cm, tumor subtype, no local recurrence before pulmonary mets

CSR complete surgical resection, *DFI* disease-free interval, *mets* metastasis, *CEA* carcinoembryonic antigen

Surgical Metastasectomy

- Criteria for selection of patients for surgical pulmonary metastasectomy:
  - Definitive control of the primary tumor has occurred (or is possible).
  - Absence of (or ability to control) extrathoracic metastatic disease.
  - Lung metastases are amenable to complete resection.
  - Patient can tolerate the planned procedure.
  - There is no better treatment alternative.
- Goal is to identify patients with potential to benefit from metastasectomy from those whose disease has already (or will soon) spread beyond the means of local intervention.
- Open versus minimally invasive surgery (MIS):
  - As thoracoscopic and robotic techniques gain popularity for a wide range of thoracic procedures, surgeons have been keen to apply these to metastasectomy.
  - Benefits to MIS approach: decreased pain, shorter hospital stay, and increased tolerability in patients with poor pulmonary function.
  - Benefit to open approach: improved detection of small metastases afforded by manual palpation of the lung.
  - Recent large European retrospective study demonstrates the advantages of video-assisted thoracoscopic surgery (VATS) combined with improvements in modern CT modalities outweigh the inability to manually detect lesions via open surgery.

- Open approach:
  - Thoracotomy is ideal in the setting of unilateral disease.

    Can proceed with sequential thoracotomy in the setting of bilateral disease, with a 3–6-week interval between operations.

  - Sternotomy may be indicated in the setting of bilateral disease, but affords poor exposure and restricts manual palpation of the posterior aspect of the lower lobes.
  - Clamshell incision offers improved access to both lung fields, but is associated with increased pain and slower postoperative recovery.
- Extent of resection:
  - Goal of metastasectomy is complete removal of all gross tumor.

    A complete (R0) resection is essential for successful metastasectomy, as disease debulking has no clinical benefit.

  - Also important to maintain adequate pulmonary function by removing as little functional lung tissue as possible.

    Metastasectomy is associated with 10–15% decrease in pulmonary function on average.
    This is amplified in patients undergoing bilateral operations and postoperative chemotherapy.
    VATS is associated with a less significant decrease in pulmonary function.

  - Nonanatomic wedge resections are ideal for removal of peripheral nodules.

    Associated with improved postoperative lung function relative to a larger anatomic resection.

  - Lobar and segmental anatomic resections are safe (mortality <1%), but require removal of more functional lung parenchyma.

Nonsurgical Therapies

- Image-guided ablative therapies are frequently used in the lungs and are a popular alternative to surgical metastasectomy.
  - Increasingly used in patients who have undergone numerous previous surgeries and may not tolerate reoperation.
- Stereotactic body radiotherapy (SBRT) or stereotactic ablative body radiotherapy (SABR) is a highly precise and dose-intensive form of external beam radiation therapy frequently used to treat metastases in the thorax.

- Well-tolerated by patients with few respiratory side effects
- Associated with good local control and short-term survival
- Factors associated with positive outcomes: number and pattern of metastases, target volume size, biological effective dose (BED) >90 Gy, absence of previous systemic therapy, no development of new metastases during follow-up, and excellent overall condition.

- Radiofrequency ablation (RFA) is a CT-guided percutaneous ablative technology using coagulative necrosis.
  - Best for tumors <3.5 cm in diameter, located in the middle and outer third of the lung.
  - Large tumors require multiple treatments.
  - Not recommended in areas adjacent to central airways or large blood vessels.
  - Most common complication is pneumothorax.

    Radiographic evidence of fibrosis or cavitation is common, but rarely symptomatic.

  - Other percutaneous therapies include microwave ablation and cryoablation.

Prognosis

- Long-term survival after metastasectomy remains uncommon:
  - Median survival after complete metastasectomy is ~35 months.
  - This likely reflects the fact that resected disease does not represent the entirety of their metastatic burden in most patients.
- Large international retrospective analysis (International Registry of Lung Metastasis) demonstrated improved survival in patients who underwent complete (R0) surgical resection, disease-free interval >36 months, and single metastasis:
  - Patients with favorable risk in these three categories had ~50% 5-year survival, compared to <15% in patients with unfavorable risk in all three categories.
  - Repeat metastasectomy associated with favorable 5-year survival.

Key Reference

- Gerull WD, Puri V, Kozower BD. The epidemiology and biology of pulmonary metastases. J Thorac Dis. 2021;13(4):2585-2589.

Further Reading

Bong CY, Smithers BM, Chua TC. Pulmonary metastasectomy in the era of targeted therapy and immunotherapy. J Thorac Dis. 2021;13(4):2618–27.

Ceppa DP, Kosinski AS, Berry MF, et al. Thoracoscopic lobectomy has increasing benefit in patients with poor pulmonary function: a Society of Thoracic Surgeons Database analysis. Ann Surg. 2012;256(3):487–93.

Gonzalez M, Brunelli A, Szanto Z, Passani S, Falcoz PE. Report from the European Society of Thoracic Surgeons database 2019: current surgical practice and perioperative outcomes of pulmonary metastasectomy. Eur J Cardiothorac Surg. 2021;59(5):996–1003.

Herrera LJ, Fernando HC, Perry Y, et al. Radiofrequency ablation of pulmonary malignant tumors in nonsurgical candidates. J Thorac Cardiovasc Surg. 2003;125(4):929–37.

Kesler KA, Kruter LE, Perkins SM, et al. Survival after resection for metastatic testicular nonseminomatous germ cell cancer to the lung or mediastinum. Ann Thorac Surg. 2011;91(4):1085–93. discussion 1093

Kessel KA, Grosser RCE, Kraus KM, Hoffmann H, Oechsner M, Combs SE. Stereotactic body radiotherapy (SBRT) in patients with lung metastases - prognostic factors and long-term survival using patient self-reported outcome (PRO). BMC Cancer. 2020;20(1):442.

Molnar TF, Gebitekin C, Turna A. What are the considerations in the surgical approach in pulmonary metastasectomy? J Thorac Oncol. 2010;5(6 Suppl 2):S140–4.

Palma DA, Olson R, Harrow S, Gaede S, Louie AV, Haasbeek C, Mulroy L, Lock M, Rodrigues GB, Yaremko BP, Schellenberg D, Ahmad B, Senthi S, Swaminath A, Kopek N, Liu M, Moore K, Currie S, Schlijper R, Bauman GS, Laba J, Qu XM, Warner A, Senan S. Stereotactic ablative radiotherapy for the comprehensive treatment of oligometastatic cancers: long-term results of the SABR-COMET phase II randomized trial. J Clin Oncol. 2020;38(25):2830–8.

Pastorino U, Buyse M, Friedel G, et al. Long-term results of lung metastasectomy: prognostic analyses based on 5206 cases. The International Registry of Lung Metastases. J Thorac Cardiovasc Surg. 1997;113(1):37–49.

Saricam M. Factors affecting long-term survival following pulmonary metastasectomy of renal cell carcinoma. Urol J. 2020;17(5):492–6. https://doi.org/10.22037/uj.v16i7.5927. PMID: 32869257.

Stamenovic D, Hohenberger P, Roessner E. Pulmonary metastasectomy in soft tissue sarcomas: a systematic review. J Thorac Dis. 2021;13(4):2649–60.

Treasure T, Farewell V, Macbeth F, Monson K, Williams NR, Brew-Graves C, Lees B, Grigg O, Fallowfield L, PulMiCC Trial Group. Pulmonary metastasectomy versus continued active monitoring in colorectal cancer (PulMiCC): a multicentre randomised clinical trial. Trials. 2019;20(1):718.

Welter S, Cheufou D, Ketscher C, et al. Risk factors for impaired lung function after pulmonary metastasectomy: a prospective observational study of 117 cases. Eur J Cardiothorac Surg. 2012;42(2):22–7.

Chapter 13
Mesothelioma and Solitary Fibrous Tumor of the Pleura

David Chen and Harvey Pass

Introduction

Mesotheliomas are neoplasms that arise from the surface serosal cells that line the cavity of the pleura, peritoneum, and pericardium. They are classified into benign and malignant subtypes. Here, we focus on malignant mesotheliomas of the pleura. The management of solitary fibrous tumor of the pleural, a rare, favorably behaving tumor, is also discussed.

Malignant Pleural Mesothelioma

Pathogenesis

- Malignant pleural mesotheliomas (MPM) are highly aggressive neoplasms of the cells lining the pleural cavity that are associated most commonly with asbestos exposure and classically exhibit a long latency period from the time of asbestos exposure to the onset of disease.
  - Multiple somatic genetic events lead to malignant transformation over time. Additionally, there is a familial inherited genetic syndrome that predisposes to malignant mesothelioma.

D. Chen (✉) · H. Pass
Division of Thoracic Surgery, Department of Cardiothoracic Surgery, New York University Langone Health, New York, NY, USA
e-mail: harvey.pass@nyulangone.org

T. Ng, T. Geraci (eds.), *Thoracic Surgery Clerkship*, Contemporary Surgical Clerkships, https://doi.org/10.1007/978-3-031-44645-0_13

- Asbestos mineral fibers contribute to chronic inflammation that ultimately leads to carcinogenesis.

- There are three major histopathological subtypes: epithelioid (60%, most favorable prognosis), sarcomatoid (10%, least favorable prognosis), and biphasic or mixed (30%, display features of both epithelioid and sarcomatoid).
- Association with loss of tumor suppressor genes: BAP1, TP53.

Epidemiology

- Rare disease: in the United States (US), the incidence is 3000 cases/year with an equal mortality rate of 3000 deaths/year.
- Male/female ratio = 4:1. Age of diagnosis in males: 50–70 years old. 20–40 years latency period.
- Association with industrial exposure: miners, shipyard workers, construction workers, plumbers.
- BAP1 cancer syndrome: familial heterozygous inheritance of germline mutations of BAP1 (tumor suppressor) gene, resulting in multiple malignancies: malignant mesothelioma, uveal melanoma, and, less frequently, cutaneous malignancies, clear cell renal cell carcinoma, breast carcinoma, cholangiocarcinoma, sarcoma, and various brain tumors. 200 families harboring the BAP1 cancer syndrome have been described in the USA, Europe, Australia, and Asia. Distinguished from somatic BAP1 mutations.
- Prognosis poor: 5-year overall survival for all stages: 10%.

Clinical Presentation

- Dyspnea (50–70%) and nonpleuritic chest pain (60%).
- Protracted course of symptoms occurs over many months (25% report >6 months of symptoms).
- Physical exam notable for evidence of pleural effusion and cachexia in late-stage disease.

Diagnosis and Staging

- Imaging:
  - Chest X-ray and CT scan (Fig. 13.1): pleural thickening/nodularity and effusion, mediastinal lymphadenopathy.
  - PET scan: metabolic activity may be increased in areas of locoregional and metastatic disease; however, not a highly sensitive or specific modality.
- Biopsy:
  - Pleural fluid cytology via thoracentesis may yield diagnosis, but its sensitivity is only 80%.
  - Often requires en bloc tissue evaluation with pleural biopsy (VATS or limited thoracotomy) showing evidence of stromal invasion.
- Immunohistochemical analysis:
  - Diagnosis with positive stain for WT1, pankeratin, keratin 5/6, calretinin. Differentiation between reactive mesothelial hyperplasia and malignant mesothelioma determined by combination of IHC staining indicating loss of BAP1 + MTAP, along with overexpression of EZH2.
- Staging. AJCC 8th edition TNM (tumor, node, metastasis) classification (Table 13.1). Imaging with CT and PET can only identify macroscopic disease and has limitations. Tissue diagnosis remains the most reliable method for determining stage.

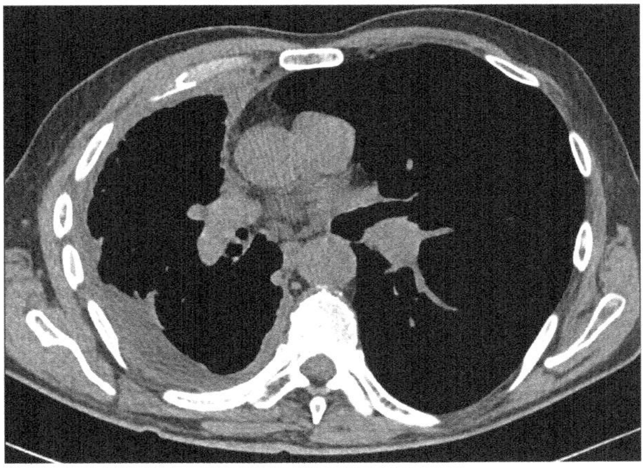

Fig. 13.1 CT chest of a 77-year-old man with right-sided MPM; there is nodular pleural thickening of the right pleura with shifting of the mediastinum toward the diseased side

Table 13.1 AJCC 8th edition TNM classification

Primary tumor site (T)	
Tx	Primary tumor not assessable
T0	No evidence of a primary tumor
T1	Tumor involving the ipsilateral parietal pleura (including mediastinal and diaphragmatic pleura) with or without involvement of the visceral pleura
T2	Tumor involving each of the ipsilateral pleural surfaces (parietal, mediastinal, diaphragmatic, and visceral pleura) with at least one of the following features: Confluent visceral pleural tumor (including fissures) Involvement of diaphragmatic muscle Invasion of the lung parenchyma
T3	Tumor involving all of the ipsilateral pleural surfaces (parietal, mediastinal, diaphragmatic, and visceral pleura) with at least one of the following features: Invasion of the endothoracic fascia Extension into the mediastinal fat Solitary, completely resectable focus invading soft tissues of the chest wall Non-transmittal involvement of the pericardium
T4	Tumor involving all of the ipsilateral pleural surfaces with at least one of the following features: Diffuse or multifocal invasion of soft tissues of the chest wall Any rib involvement Invasion of the peritoneum through the diaphragm Invasion of any mediastinal organ Direct extension to the contralateral pleura Invasions of the spine or brachial plexus Transmural invasion of the pericardium (with or without pericardial effusion or myocardium invasion)
Nodule metastases (N)	
Nx	Regional lymph nodes not assessable
N0	No regional lymph node metastases
N1	Metastasis in the ipsilateral bronchopulmonary, hilar, or mediastinal lymph nodes (including the internal mammary, peridiaphragmatic, pericardial fat pad, or intercostal lymph nodes)
N2	Metastasis in the contralateral bronchopulmonary, hilar, or mediastinal lymph nodes or ipsilateral or contralateral supraclavicular lymph nodes
Distant metastases (M)	
Mx	Presence of distant metastases not assessable
M0	No evidence of distant metastases
M1	Evidence of distant metastases

Staging			
Stage	T	N	M
IA IB	T1 T2-T3	N0 N0	M0 M0
II	T1-T2	N1	M0
IIIA IIIB	T3 T1-T3 T4	N1 N2 Any N	M0 M0 M0
IV	Any T	Any N	M1

Treatment

Surgery

The goal of surgery should be macroscopic cytoreduction with the safest operation.
Consensus nomenclature for mesothelioma operations (IASLC + IMIG 2011):

- Pleurectomy/decortication (PD): parietal and visceral pleurectomy without resection of the diaphragm or pericardium
- Extrapleural pneumonectomy (EPP): en bloc resection of the parietal and visceral pleura + ipsilateral lung, pericardium, and diaphragm
- Partial pleurectomy: partial removal of the parietal and/or visceral pleura for diagnostics or palliation, leaving gross tumor unresected
- Extended pleurectomy/decortication: PD + resection of the pericardium or diaphragm (Fig. 13.2)

There are no randomized controlled trials evaluating surgical approaches, and benefits of PD and EPP are controversial. A recent 20-year single-institution retrospective analysis at MD Anderson Cancer Center evaluated 187 and 95 patients that underwent EPP (66%) and PD (34%), respectively. Perioperative mortality was higher for EPP versus PD (11% versus 0%, $p = 0.031$); median overall survival was lower for EPP versus PD (15 months versus 22 months, $p = 0.276$).

Fig. 13.2 Left-sided extended PD. GoreTex reconstruction of the diaphragm (top) and pericardium (right)

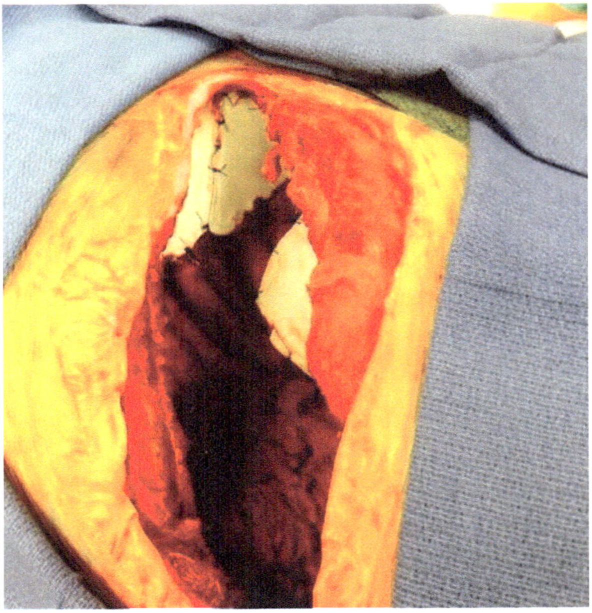

Radiation (RT)

- IASLC 2019 expert consensus. Radiation should be indicated primarily in three settings:
  - Post-PD
  - Post-EPP
  - Palliation
- Dose: 45–54 Gy (up to 60 Gy for R1 or R2 resection)

Chemotherapy

- Platinum-based therapy has shown overall survival benefit in adjuvant setting (cisplatin + pemetrexed).
- The following neoadjuvant trials are notable:
  - Krug et al., J Clin Oncol 2009, phase II trial evaluating treatment of stages I–III with neoadjuvant cisplatin + pemetrexed, followed by EPP + radiation therapy: 77 patients received chemotherapy, 54 patients completed EPP, and 40 patients completed RT—median overall survival for the entire cohort was 16.8 months, and patients who completed all therapy had median overall survival of 29 months and 2-year overall survival of 61%.
  - MARS trial: Treasure et al., Lancet 2011, multicenter randomized controlled feasibility study evaluating induction platinum-based chemotherapy ± EPP/RT: the primary endpoint of enrolling 50 patients in 1 year was not met as they randomized 50 patients over 3 years; of 24 assigned to EPP/RT, 16 completed EPP, and 8 completed RT; EPP was associated with a high 18% operative mortality; the results of this trial are uninterpretable given the inadequate power, patient crossover, and insufficient proportion of patients completing the regimen in the treatment arm.
  - EORTC phase II feasibility study evaluating neoadjuvant chemotherapy, EPP, RT, Van Schil et al., Eur Resp J 2010: EPP was associated with a 6.5% 90-day mortality, and of 55 patients, only 24 successfully completed the treatment; thus the primary endpoint of feasibility was not reached.
  - Weder et al., J Clin Oncol 2004, pilot study evaluating neoadjuvant chemotherapy + EPP: 19 patients enrolled, 16 patients underwent EPP without perioperative mortality, and 13 patients received RT with a median overall survival of 23 months.
- Neoadjuvant therapy continues to be evaluated going forward. EORTC 1205 is a phase II randomized trial evaluating neoadjuvant chemotherapy + surgery versus surgery + adjuvant chemotherapy (both arms utilizing cisplatin + pemetrexed, three cycles; extended PD for surgery). Primary endpoint is successful completion of multimodality treatment in 20 weeks:

- Immunotherapy

    FDA approval in 2020 based on the CheckMate 743 randomized controlled trial for use of nivolumab (anti-PD-1) + ipilimumab (anti-CTLA-4) vs chemotherapy in patients with unresectable disease. Improved median overall survival compared to chemotherapy (18 months versus 14 months)

        First approval in 16 years for MPM. Second FDA-approved systemic therapy for MPM

- Principles

    Evidence so far has not demonstrated a clearly superior approach to treatment and consensus is generally lacking. MPM are relatively radiosensitive. Chemotherapy has limited efficacy and, used alone, is not curative.
    Treatment is best performed at high-volume centers for this rare disease.
    Locoregional disease is treated with multimodal therapy. Surgical resection is often inadequate to remove all microscopic disease (R0 resection).
    Adjuvant radiation and systemic therapy (chemotherapy classically) are used; studies evaluating neoadjuvant and adjuvant therapy are ongoing.
    Metastatic disease is generally treated with radiation and systemic therapy.
    Palliation can employ surgery, radiation, or systemic therapy.

Prognosis

- Prognostic variables have been determined: clinical stage, histology, sex, age, platelet count, hemoglobin, white blood cell count, treatment intent, adjuvant treatment, tumor volume, and metabolic activity.
- BAP1 inherited germline mutation favorable, associated with sevenfold improvement in overall survival.
- Investigational treatments, particularly immunotherapy, may soon alter the paradigm and prognosis for this disease.

Solitary Fibrous Tumor of the Pleura

Presentation

- Rare tumor originating from the sub-mesothelial mesenchymal cells of the pleura.
- Mean age of presentation: fifth–sixth decades of life.
- Slightly more common in males than in females.
- Slow-growing tumors (Fig. 13.3a, b), can never be deemed benign as they have malignant potential.
- Symptoms:

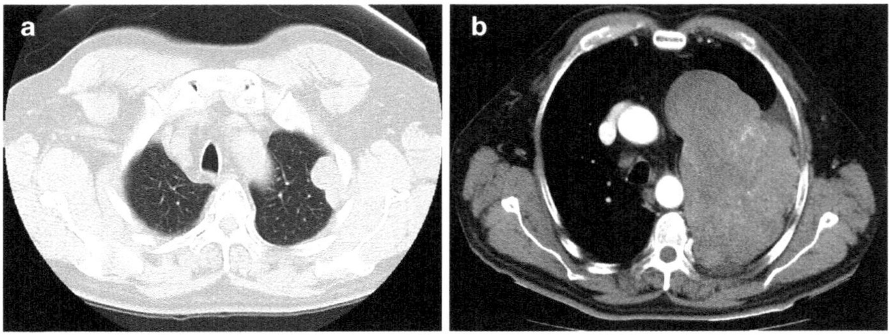

Fig. 13.3 CT image showing growth of a solitary fibrous tumor of the pleural over 7 years of time. (**a**) Initial scan of a lobulated, well-defined lesion abutting the pleura; (**b**) scan 7 years later showing a large left thoracic mass with compression on the ipsilateral lung and mediastinal shift to the right

- Dyspnea
- Chest pain
- Cough
- Paraneoplastic (5–10%)

  Doege-Potter: hypoglycemia from insulin-like growth factor II

  Pierre-Marie Bamberg: bone surface and soft tissue calcification (hypertrophic osteoarthropathy) leading to digital clubbing and arthritis

Imaging (Chest Radiograph or CT Scan)

- Shows a lobulated, well-defined, homogenous mass that abuts the pleura.
- May be difficult to determine if it arises from the visceral (Fig. 13.4a, b) or parietal pleural (Fig. 13.5a, b).
- Compress adjacent structures if large (Fig. 13.3b).

Pathology

- Majority arise from the visceral pleura.
- Spindle cells arranged in short intersecting fascicles with collagenous stroma.
- Stain positive for CD-34, Bcl-2, and CD-99; negative for keratin and S-100.
- Malignant features:
  - Atypia
  - Necrosis
  - Mitosis

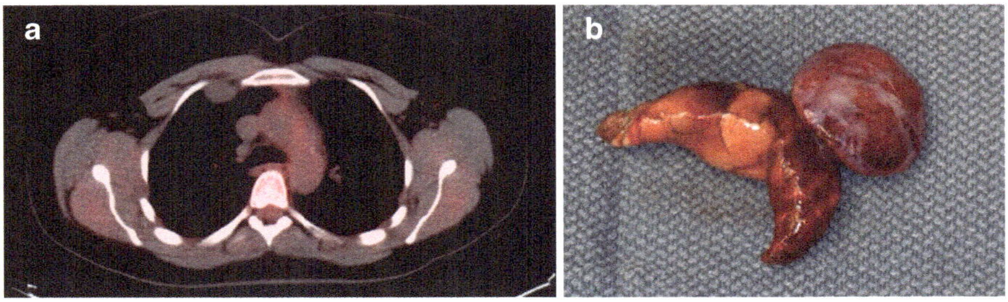

Fig. 13.4 Solitary fibrous tumor of the pleura arising from the visceral pleura of the right upper lobe lung. (**a**) PET/CT scan showing a well-circumscribed lesion abutting the pleura (unclear visceral or parietal by imaging) without avidity; (**b**) resected specimen by en bloc wedge resection of the right upper lobe, with the lesion attached to the visceral pleural by a "stalk"

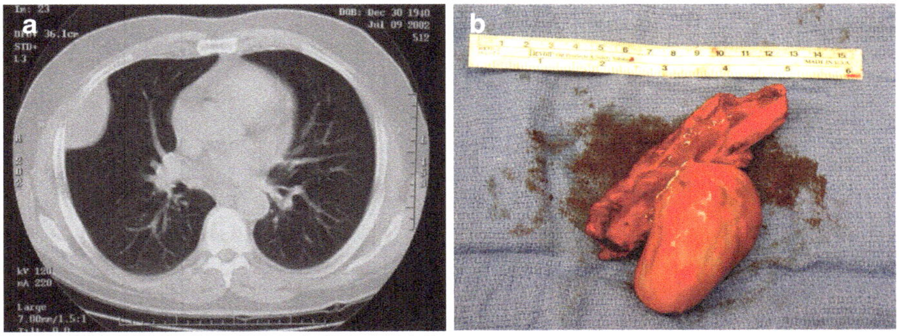

Fig. 13.5 Solitary fibrous tumor of the pleura arising from the parietal pleura. (**a**) CT scan showing a well-circumscribed lesion abutting the pleura (unclear visceral or parietal by imaging); (**b**) resected specimen by en bloc resection of the parietal pleura/rib segment, with the lesion attached to the parietal pleural by a "stalk"

  - Parietal pleural
  - Large size

Treatment

- Mainstay of treatment is complete surgical resection (R0).
  - Surgery should be considered upon diagnosis.
  - If arise from visceral pleural: en bloc pulmonary resection: wedge, segmentectomy, lobectomy, and pneumonectomy.
  - If arise from parietal pleural: en bloc parietal pleura/chest wall resection.
  - Often can be performed by minimally invasive techniques (thoracoscopic or robotic approaches).
  - Role of neoadjuvant and adjuvant therapy has yet to be defined.

- Chemotherapy (ifosfamide and Adriamycin) and radiation
  - Incomplete resection
  - Unresectable disease
  - Metastatic disease

Prognosis

- Benign features, 90–95% 10-year survival; malignant features, 45–60% 10-year survival
- Poor prognostic features
  - Size ≥15–10 cm
  - Age ≥55
  - ≥4 mitosis per 10 high-power field
  - Hypercellularity
  - Necrosis
  - Parietal pleura (vs visceral pleural)
  - Sessile (vs pedunculated)

Key Reference

- Zhou N, Rice DC, Tsao AS, Lee PP, Haymaker CL, Corsini EM, Antonoff MB, Hofstetter WL, Rajaram R, Roth JA, Swisher SG, Vaporciyan AA, Walsh GL, Mehran RJ, Sepesi B. Extrapleural pneumonectomy versus pleurectomy/decortication for malignant pleural mesothelioma. Ann Thorac Surg 2022;113(1):200–8.

Further Reading

Baas P, Scherpereel A, Nowak AK, Fujimoto N, Peters S, Tsao AS, Mansfield AS, Popat S, Jahan T, Antonia S, Oulkhouir Y, Bautista Y, Cornelissen R, Greillier L, Grossi F, Kowalski D, Rodríguez-Cid J, Aanur P, Oukessou A, Baudelet C, Zalcman G. First-line nivolumab plus ipilimumab in unresectable malignant pleural mesothelioma (CheckMate 743): a multicentre, randomised, open-label, phase 3 trial. Lancet. 2021;397(10272):375–86.

Billé A, Krug LM, Woo KM, Rusch VW, Zauderer MG. Contemporary analysis of prognostic factors in patients with unresectable malignant pleural mesothelioma. J Thorac Oncol. 2016;11(2):249–55.

Carbone M, Adusumilli PS, Alexander HR Jr, Baas P, Bardelli F, Bononi A, Bueno R, Felley-Bosco E, Galateau-Salle F, Jablons D, Mansfield AS, Minaai M, de Perrot M, Pesavento P, Rusch V, Severson DT, Taioli E, Tsao A, Woodard G, Yang H, Pass HI. Mesothelioma: scientific clues for prevention, diagnosis, and therapy. CA Cancer J Clin. 2019;69(5):402–29.

Cardillo G, Carbone L, Carleo F, Masala N, Graziano P, Bray A, Martelli M. Solitary fibrous tumors of the pleura: an analysis of 110 patients treated in a single institution. Ann Thorac Surg. 2009;88(5):1632–7.

de Perrot M, Fischer S, Bründler MA, Sekine Y, Keshavjee S. Solitary fibrous tumors of the pleura. Ann Thorac Surg. 2002;74(1):285–93.

Demicco EG, Park MS, Araujo DM, Fox PS, Bassett RL, Pollock RE, Lazar AJ, Wang WL. Solitary fibrous tumor: a clinicopathological study of 110 cases and proposed risk assessment model. Mod Pathol. 2012;25(9):1298–306.

DeVita VT Jr, Lawrence TS, Rosenberg SA. Devita, Hellman, and Rosenberg's cancer: principles & practice of oncology. 11th ed. Philadelphia: Wolters Kluwer; 2018. p. 1863–83.

England DM, Hochholzer L, McCarthy MJ. Localized benign and malignant fibrous tumors of the pleura. A clinicopathologic review of 223 cases. Am J Surg Pathol. 1989;13(8):640–58. Erratum in: Am J Surg Pathol 1991;15(8):818.

Flores RM, Pass HI, Seshan VE, Dycoco J, Zakowski M, Carbone M, Bains MS, Rusch VW. Extrapleural pneumonectomy versus pleurectomy/decortication in the surgical management of malignant pleural mesothelioma: results in 663 patients. J Thorac Cardiovasc Surg. 2008;135(3):620–6.

Gomez DR, Rimner A, Simone CB, Cho BCJ, de Perrot M, Adjei AA, Bueno R, Gill RR, Harpole DH, Hesdorffer M, Hirsch FR, Jackson AA, Pass HI, Rice DC, Rusch VW, Tsao AS, Yorke E, Rosenzweig K. The use of radiation therapy for the treatment of malignant pleural mesothelioma: expert opinion from the National Cancer Institute Thoracic Malignancy Steering Committee, International Association for the Study of Lung Cancer, and Mesothelioma Applied Research Foundation. J Thorac Oncol. 2019;14(7):1172–83.

Krug LM, Pass HI, Rusch VW, Kindler HL, Sugarbaker DJ, Rosenzweig KE, Flores R, Friedberg JS, Pisters K, Monberg M, Obasaju CK, Vogelzang NJ. Multicenter phase II trial of neoadjuvant pemetrexed plus cisplatin followed by extrapleural pneumonectomy and radiation for malignant pleural mesothelioma. J Clin Oncol. 2009;27(18):3007–13.

Lahon B, Mercier O, Fadel E, Ghigna MR, Petkova B, Mussot S, Fabre D, Le Chevalier T, Dartevelle P. Solitary fibrous tumor of the pleura: outcomes of 157 complete resections in a single center. Ann Thorac Surg. 2012;94(2):394–400.

Pass HI, Giroux D, Kennedy C, Ruffini E, Cangir AK, Rice D, Asamura H, Waller D, Edwards J, Weder W, Hoffmann H, van Meerbeeck JP, Rusch VW, IASLC Staging Committee and Participating Institutions. Supplementary prognostic variables for pleural mesothelioma: a report from the IASLC staging committee. J Thorac Oncol. 2014;9(6):856–64.

Rice D, Rusch V, Pass H, Asamura H, Nakano T, Edwards J, Giroux DJ, Hasegawa S, Kernstine KH, Waller D, Rami-Porta R, International Association for the Study of Lung Cancer International Staging Committee and the International Mesothelioma Interest Group. Recommendations for uniform definitions of surgical techniques for malignant pleural mesothelioma: a consensus report of the international association for the study of lung cancer international staging committee and the international mesothelioma interest group. J Thorac Oncol. 2011;6:1304–12.

Rusch VW, Chansky K, Kindler HL, Nowak AK, Pass HI, Rice DC, Shemanski L, Galateau-Sallé F, McCaughan BC, Nakano T, Ruffini E, van Meerbeeck JP, Yoshimura M, IASLC Staging and Prognostic Factors Committee. The IASLC mesothelioma staging project: proposals for the M descriptors and for revision of the TNM stage groupings in the forthcoming (Eighth) edition of the TNM classification for mesothelioma. J Thorac Oncol. 2016;11(12):2112–9.

Sauter JL, Dacic S, Galateau-Salle F, Attanoos RL, Butnor KJ, Churg A, Husain AN, Kadota K, Khoor A, Nicholson AG, Roggli V, Schmitt F, Tsao MS, Travis WD. The 2021 WHO classification of tumors of the pleura: advances since the 2015 classification. J Thorac Oncol. 2022;17(5):608–22.

Scrimgeour LA, Grada Z, Aswad BI, Ng T. Lessons learned from an untreated "benign" thoracic tumor. Ann Thorac Surg. 2017;103(2):e135–7.

Tapias LF, Mino-Kenudson M, Lee H, Wright C, Gaissert HA, Wain JC, Mathisen DJ, Lanuti M. Risk factor analysis for the recurrence of resected solitary fibrous tumours of the pleura: a 33-year experience and proposal for a scoring system. Eur J Cardiothorac Surg. 2013;44(1):111–7.

Treasure T, Lang-Lazdunski L, Waller D, Bliss JM, Tan C, Entwisle J, Snee M, O'Brien M, Thomas G, Senan S, O'Byrne K, Kilburn LS, Spicer J, Landau D, Edwards J, Coombes G, Darlison L, Peto J, MARS trialists. Extra-pleural pneumonectomy versus no extra-pleural pneumonectomy

for patients with malignant pleural mesothelioma: clinical outcomes of the Mesothelioma and Radical Surgery (MARS) randomised feasibility study. Lancet Oncol. 2011;12(8):763–72.
Van Schil PE, Baas P, Gaafar R, Maat AP, Van de Pol M, Hasan B, Klomp HM, Abdelrahman AM, Welch J, van Meerbeeck JP, European Organisation for Research and Treatment of Cancer (EORTC) Lung Cancer Group. Trimodality therapy for malignant pleural mesothelioma: results from an EORTC phase II multicentre trial. Eur Respir J. 2010;36(6):1362–9.
Weder W, Kestenholz P, Taverna C, Bodis S, Lardinois D, Jerman M, Stahel RA. Neoadjuvant chemotherapy followed by extrapleural pneumonectomy in malignant pleural mesothelioma. J Clin Oncol. 2004;22(17):3451–7.

Chapter 14
Thoracic Oncology

Christopher G. Azzoli

Introduction

The practice of thoracic oncology (or thoracic medical oncology) requires multidisciplinary care coordination and the prescription of drugs to increase survival time and quality of life in patients with cancers of the chest (lung cancer, thymoma, and mesothelioma). Historically, these cancers were treated with surgery or radiation alone, and thoracic oncology emerged as a solid tumor subspecialty in the 1990s to support thoracic surgeons in their work.

The first high-level evidence of clinical benefit of traditional chemotherapy was observed when it was delivered prior to surgery, or radiation, in patients with stage III non-small cell lung cancers (NSCLC). At that time, prognosis for patients with stage IV lung cancer was dismal, with or without drug therapy, and it was reasonable to manage them with supportive care only. Since 2005, major advances in anticancer drug therapy have increased overall survival of patients with stage IV NSCLC by two- to fivefold and doubled the survival proportion of patients with stage III disease.

Types of Lung Cancer

Small Cell Lung Cancer

- All solid organs in the body generate small cell cancers.

C. G. Azzoli (✉)
Department of Oncology, Warren Alpert Medical School of Brown University, Providence, RI, USA
e-mail: cazzoli@lifespan.org

T. Ng, T. Geraci (eds.), *Thoracic Surgery Clerkship*, Contemporary Surgical Clerkships, https://doi.org/10.1007/978-3-031-44645-0_14

- By microscopic exam and hematoxylin and eosin (H&E) staining, the cancer cells are undifferentiated, small, round, blue, and with scant cytoplasm, nuclear molding without nucleoli, smudging of cells with crush artifact, and high mitotic rate and express proteins of neuroendocrine differentiation such as synaptophysin and chromogranin A.
- On a molecular level, small cell cancers are notable for loss of function of key tumor suppressor genes, such as TP53 and RB1.
- While all organs generate small cell cancers, the tobacco cigarette has caused a century-long epidemic of small cell lung cancer (SCLC), which represents 12–15% of all lung cancers. There are over 30,000 Americans per year diagnosed with SCLC.
- The incidence of SCLC is declining as fewer people smoke tobacco cigarettes.
- Small cell lung cancers grow rapidly, with a doubling time of 30 days. They are highly likely to spread (metastasize) around the body, typically to the bone, brain, liver, lymph nodes, and adrenal glands.
- All patients with SCLC require chemotherapy as part of their care, regardless of the stage of disease, including chemotherapy with radiation or after surgery for limited-stage disease and chemotherapy alone for extensive-stage disease.
- Due to SCLC proclivity to spread to the brain, even prophylactic cranial irradiation (PCI) can be beneficial in selected patients.

Non-Small Cell Lung Cancer

- All other types of lung cancer are histopathologically distinct from small cell lung cancer and are lumped together by the historical term, non-small cell lung cancer (NSCLC). These cancers can be distinguished by their unique appearance under the microscope and patterns of protein expression which can be measured by immunohistochemistry (Fig. 14.1).
- Large cell neuroendocrine cancer (LCNEC) overlaps with small cell lung cancer in terms of appearance and the types of proteins expressed, but is treated more like NSCLC. Stage for stage, LCNEC carries a worse prognosis than NSCLC and is less responsive to available drug therapies.
- With discoveries in cancer biology, important subgroups have emerged such that the term NSCLC should not be used if a more specific term, which better represents that subgroup of lung cancer, is available (Fig. 14.2).
- Cancers with activating/sensitizing mutations in EGFR are best referred to as "EGFR-mutant lung cancers." Cancers with activating/sensitizing gene rearrangements driving ALK are best referred to as "ALK-positive lung cancer," and so on, and so forth.

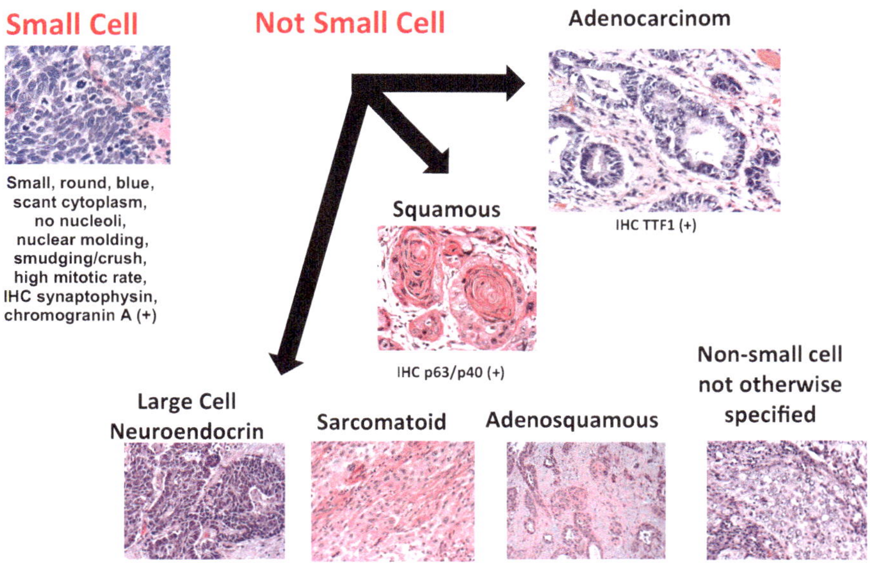

Fig. 14.1 Lung cancer subtypes based on histopathology

Fig. 14.2 Clinically relevant histopathologically or genomically defined subgroups of NSCLC. *UMD* unknown mitogenic driver, *LCNEC* large cell neuroendocrine carcinoma

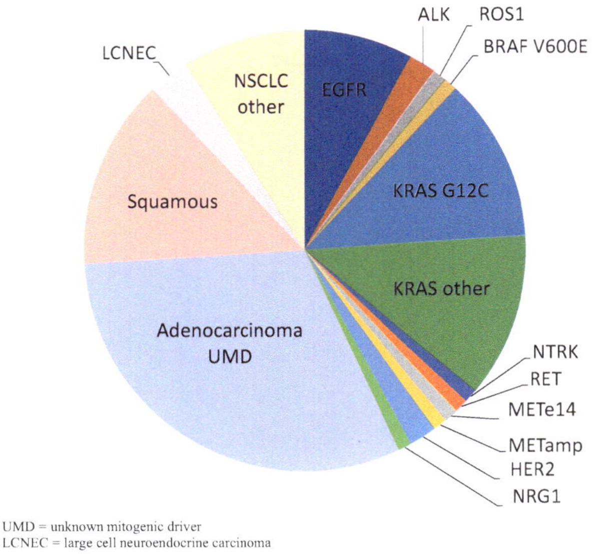

Molecular Pathology of Lung Cancer

- NSCLC (primarily adenocarcinomas) are driven by activating mutations in oncogenes which result in expression of mutant oncoproteins, which are typically signaling molecules (receptor tyrosine kinases).
- The pro-growth signal of these so-called activating mutations can sometimes be blocked by drugs designed to prevent the molecular signal (tyrosine kinase inhibitors).
- The discovery of oncogene mutations which are both activating to growth and sensitizing to a specific drug treatment has revolutionized the diagnosis and treatment of lung cancer.
- Figure 14.2 shows the current (as of 2022) clinically relevant histopathologically or genetically defined subgroups of NSCLC based on the detection of a driver mutation for which there is a specific drug therapy.
- Table 14.1 lists the current pharmacopoeia of molecularly targeted drugs.

Palliative Drug Therapy

- The natural history of lung cancer is to grow and spread around the body, causing debility and death in a matter of months.
- New drugs can control the growth or spread of lung cancer for many months or even years.

Table 14.1 Selected oncogene-targeted drugs which are commercially available in 2022

EGFR: Osimertinib, gefitinib, erlotinib, afatinib, dacomitinib
ALK: Alectinib, lorlatinib, brigatinib, ceritinib, crizotinib
ROS1: Crizotinib, entrectinib, lorlatinib, ceritinib
BRAF V600E: Trametinib + dabrafenib
NTRK 1,2,3: Larotrectinib, entrectinib
RET: Pralsetinib, selpercatinib
MET ex14: Capmatinib, tepotinib, crizotinib
MET amp: Crizotinib, capmatinib
HER2: Trastuzumab deruxtecan
EGFR exon 20: Amivantamab, mobocertinib
KRAS G12C: Sotorasib, adagrasib
NRG1: Afatinib

- Durable disease control is not the same as cure. Treatment is ongoing and indefinite. When the goal is control and not cure, the therapy is often referred to as *palliative*.
- *Palliative care* is a subspecialty of medicine which focuses on relief of pain, symptoms, and stress caused by serious illnesses. Early palliative care has been shown to improve quality of life and overall survival time in patients with advanced lung cancer.

Chemotherapy

- Drugs which interfere with DNA replication and cell division are traditionally called chemotherapy.
- These drugs also damage normal cells which grow and divide as part of their normal function. This results in lowering of blood counts, mouth sores, diarrhea, and, for some drugs, hair loss.
- Chemotherapy drugs are also more likely to cause nausea or vomiting.
- Platinum salts (cisplatin, carboplatin) combined with one other chemotherapy drug (a so-called platinum doublet) is the most effective chemotherapy for lung cancer. Platinum salts bind to DNA, causing DNA double-strand breaks, which result in programmed cell death.
- Taxanes (paclitaxel, docetaxel, albumin-bound paclitaxel) and vinca alkaloids (vinorelbine) bind to microtubules and block cell division which results in programmed cell death.
- Antimetabolites like pemetrexed block the enzymes that make purines and pyrimidines for DNA synthesis, and gemcitabine blocks DNA synthesis, which results in programmed cell death.
- Etoposide blocks DNA synthesis by forming a complex with topoisomerase II and DNA which both induce DNA double-strand breaks and prevent repair. Etoposide is particularly effective in the treatment of SCLC.
- Historically, platinum doublets alone provide median survival times of 10–12 months for patients with metastatic NSCLC or SCLC.

Oncogene-Targeted Drugs

- A comprehensive oncogene target and drug list is in Table 14.1.
- These mutations are primarily found in lung adenocarcinoma, but any NSCLC or lung cancer with mixed histology may harbor them so it is important to test all histologies of NSCLC, especially in small biopsy specimens where histopathology may be uncertain.
- Diagnosis of these genetic changes requires extraction of DNA from biopsy tissue or circulating tumor DNA in the blood. Some of the changes are gene muta-

tions, and others are gene rearrangements, such that you can either find them one at a time using older techniques or all at once using next-generation sequencing (NGS) techniques.

- NGS is also called massively parallel sequencing. The technique involves breaking DNA, or RNA, into pieces and adding adapters to allow the pieces to be amplified and sequenced, and then a computer reassembles the data to figure out the overall sequence.
- Once a patient has been diagnosed with an oncogene-driven, stage IV (metastatic) lung cancer, drug therapy can be initiated to control or shrink the cancer.
- Randomized trials have shown that EGFR tyrosine kinase inhibitors (TKIs), and ALK TKIs, are more effective than chemotherapy for patients with advanced lung cancer and their respective targets.
- Other targeted drugs have not been tested in randomized studies, but in single-arm studies, they result in response rates and progression-free survival times which rival chemotherapy.
- While not as dangerous as chemotherapy, these drugs also have difficult side effects which require close monitoring and supportive care. Common side effects are listed in Table 14.2.

Table 14.2 Selected side effects of oncogene-targeted drugs

Osimertinib (EGFR): mild skin rash, mild diarrhea, paronychia
Mobocertinib, afatinib (EGFR): moderate to severe rash or diarrhea
Alectinib (ALK): body aches, fatigue, hepatitis, increased CPK
Lorlatinib (ALK, ROS1): cognitive impairment, edema, high cholesterol
Trametinib + dabrafenib (MEK, BRAF): fever, rash, fatigue, blurred vision
Entrectinib (NTRK, ROS1): fatigue, vision changes, confusion, anorexia
Larotrectinib (NTRK): cognitive effects, mood effects, edema, anorexia
Selpercatinib, pralsetinib (RET): cytopenias, hypertension, edema
Capmatinib, tepotinib (MET): hepatitis, peripheral edema
Trastuzumab deruxtecan (HER2): pneumonitis, cytopenias, heart injury
Amivantamab (EGFR, MET): transfusion-related reactions, rash
Sotorasib, adagrasib (KRAS G12C): hepatitis, nausea, anorexia, diarrhea

Table 14.3 NSCLC survival based on stage, subtype, and type of drug therapy

Disease state, type of treatment	Rate of radiologic response	Median survival (months)	2-year survival	5-year survival
Stage IV NSCLC, supportive care only	0	6	1%	0%
Stage IV NSCLC, **platinum doublet** chemotherapy	25%	10	20%	1%
Stage IV NSCLC, no EGFR/ALK, **chemo + ipilimumab + nivolumab**	38%	16	38%	–
Stage IV NSCLC, no EGFR/ALK, PDL1 ≥ 1%, **ipilimumab + nivolumab**	36%	17	40%	–
Stage IV NSCLC, no EGFR/ALK, **chemotherapy + pembrolizumab**	48%	22	45%	–
Stage IV NSCLC, no EGFR/ALK, PDL1 ≥ 50%, **pembrolizumab**	45%	24	51%	–
Stage IIIA/N2 NSCLC, neoadjuvant chemoradiation, then surgery	N/A	24	50%	25%
Stage III NSCLC, chemoradiation, then **durvalumab**	N/A	48	66%	43%
Stage IV NSCLC, EGFR mutation on **osimertinib**	80 + %	39	75%	–
Stage IV NSCLC, ALK fusion on **alectinib**	80 + %	N/A	75%	62%
Stage II–III NSCLC, PDL1 ≥ 1%, resected, adjuvant **atezolizumab**	N/A	Improved disease-free survival		
Stage II–III NSCLC, neoadjuvant **chemo + nivolumab**, then surgery	54%	Improved disease-free survival		

- The discovery of oncogene-targeted therapy has improved overall survival two- to fivefold compared to chemotherapy alone (Table 14.3).

Acquired Resistance to Oncogene-Targeted Drugs

- For stage IV disease, targeted drug therapy is palliative in intent, and eventually the cancer becomes resistant to the targeted drug.
- Repeat biopsy of lung cancers with acquired resistance to targeted therapy, or serial blood tests to isolate circulating tumor DNA, can reveal a molecular mechanism of acquired resistance which can be targeted by a different drug.
- Prominent mutations which cause drug resistance include EGFR T790M which causes resistance to gefitinib or erlotinib; EGFR C797S causes resistance to osimertinib; ALK G1202R causes resistance to alectinib.
- On-target mutations which are sensitizing to a different drug are rare (5% or less). Similarly, the development of a different activating/sensitizing genetic change (called *bypass tract activation*, such as MET amplification) is also rare.

- While intensive research is ongoing, most patients with acquired resistance to oncogene-targeted drug therapy must move on to traditional chemotherapy.
- Studies combining chemotherapy and targeted drug therapy are ongoing.

Immune Checkpoint Blockade

- Cancers grow and spread by actively evading the immune system.
- The innate and adaptive immune system is constantly searching for dangerous, nonself targets, like environmental pathogens, virally infected cells, and cancer cells, to eliminate effector cells and antibodies.
- T cells are the major effector cells for the adaptive immune system and are controlled by co-inhibitory and co-stimulatory receptors which help block or foster immune attack (Fig. 14.3).
- Antibodies have been engineered to block co-inhibitory receptors, which unleash immune cells to attack the target. These so-called immune checkpoint inhibitors (ICPIs) block the ability of the cancer cells to evade the immune system and are a powerful anticancer drug therapy.

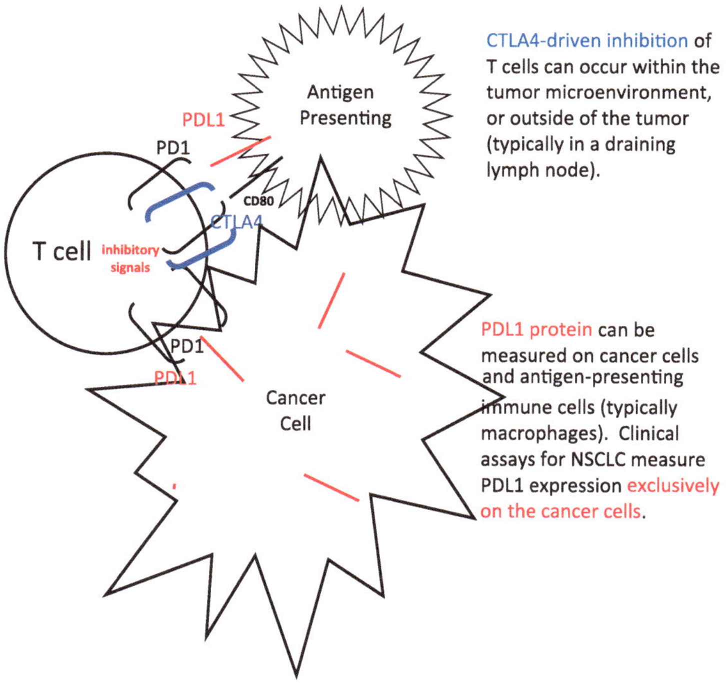

Fig. 14.3 Co-inhibitory immune checkpoint molecules

- Antibodies to the PD1/PDL1 co-inhibitory receptor interaction have single-agent activity, especially in patients with cancer with high PDL1 protein expression (as measured by immunohistochemistry).
- It is a standard practice to measure PDL1 expression in all NSCLC to determine if there is an option for single-agent drug therapy (pembrolizumab, atezolizumab, cemiplimab-rwlc).
- Combinations of chemotherapy and PD1/PDL1 checkpoint blockade are more effective than chemotherapy alone, even in patients with low PDL1 score.
- Another immune checkpoint, CTLA4, can be blocked with an antibody (ipilimumab), and combination of CTLA4 + PD1 checkpoint blockade is an approved first-line regimen, with or without chemotherapy.
- Regular use of immune checkpoint inhibitors has doubled median overall survival time in patients with advanced NSCLC up to 2 years.
- Immune checkpoint inhibitors improve overall survival in patients with extensive-stage small cell lung cancer. The benefit is not as large as it is for NSCLC.
- The side effects of immune checkpoint blockade are unwanted, autoimmune inflammation, typically skin rash, diarrhea, or thyroiditis which causes hypothyroidism. Autoimmune inflammatory damage of vital organs (lung, liver, kidneys, and rarely heart or brain) can be life-threatening and requires urgent immunosuppression, typically with corticosteroids.

Oligo-Metastatic Disease States

- The Greek work *oligos* means few or scanty.
- Traditionally, oligo-metastatic NSCLC referred to a patient with a solitary brain or adrenal metastasis, in which case up to 20% of patients could be cured with aggressive local treatment of the primary tumor and metastasis, typically surgery.
- Attempts at curative surgery for oligo-metastatic NSCLC predated drug therapy and failed to cure most patients.
- Now that there are lifesaving drugs available, these same patients are treated with drug therapy with palliative intent, but also offered treatment of the primary tumor and metastasis with curative intent.
- In the modern era, with drug responses improving, the definition of oligo-metastatic lung cancer has evolved to include multiple metastases, but typically fewer than three metastatic locations.
- For oligo-metastatic patients, after a response to drug therapy, they may be offered local consolidative radiation therapy to all sites of disease based on the results of early, randomized studies. Confirmatory studies are in progress.

Pre-/Postoperative Drug Therapy

- Since 2005, four cycles of a cisplatin doublet have been used after surgical resection to decrease the risk of death from high-risk, completely resected NSCLC. This is called postoperative or adjuvant chemotherapy.
- The benefit of adjuvant chemotherapy is to reduce the risk of death by 5% at 5 years (absolute risk reduction) for all patients. There is greater benefit for higher stages and less benefit for lower stages. Chemotherapy is more harmful than helpful for stage IA.
- As better drugs are being developed for stage IV NSCLC, they are being applied in the adjuvant setting with clear benefit in preventing lung cancer recurrence. High-risk, resected NSCLC (stages II–III) should be tested for PDL1 by IHC and at least EGFR and ALK genetic changes to determine optimal postoperative therapy.
- For resected lung cancers with EGFR activating/sensitizing mutations, it is now standard of care to offer 3 years of the oral, EGFR tyrosine kinase inhibitor, osimertinib.
- Anti-PD1/PDL1 immune checkpoint inhibitors may be offered for 1 year for patients with stage II–III, PDL1-positive NSCLC.
- Delivering immune therapy prior to surgery (to allow immune interaction with the cancer) may be more effective than delivering it after the cancer has been removed. Preoperative drug therapy is also called *neoadjuvant therapy*.
- A groundbreaking study published in 2022 demonstrated that neoadjuvant chemotherapy combined with PD1 checkpoint blockade for resectable NSCLC (tested negative for EGFR and ALK genetic changes) resulted in a pathologic complete response in 25% of patients and improved disease-free survival compared to neoadjuvant chemotherapy alone.
- The availability of preoperative chemotherapy + nivolumab as a lifesaving treatment requires genomic testing of NSCLC *prior to surgery* in patients who might be considered for neoadjuvant therapy.

Radiation Sensitization and Immune Therapy for Stage III NSCLC

- One of the first studies to demonstrate the benefit of drug therapy in the treatment of NSCLC treated patients with locally advanced stage III NSCLC with cisplatin-based combination chemotherapy prior to chest radiation.
- Subsequent studies have shown that chemotherapy is most effective when it is delivered at the same time as radiation therapy, so-called *concurrent* chemoradiation.
- The value of concurrent chemoradiation comes from the cancer-killing synergy between chemotherapy and radiation. In the studies that established concurrent

chemotherapy as standard of care, most of the benefit came in the form of improved local control.
- Concurrent chemoradiation is standard of care for unresectable stage III NSCLC, with a variety of chemotherapy options available, typically carboplatin + paclitaxel, but also cisplatin + etoposide, or cisplatin + pemetrexed.
- Chemotherapy can only be given with radiation at a low dose per fraction. When high doses of radiation are applied to a small tumor (stereotactic radiosurgery), local control is achieved with radiation alone, and adding chemotherapy may be too dangerous.
- One year of anti-PDL1 immune checkpoint blockade following chemoradiation (so-called consolidation therapy) doubles overall survival in patients with stage III NSCLC treated with concurrent chemoradiation.

Thymoma and Thymic Carcinoma

- Cancers of the thymus are rare tumors of the anterior mediastinum derived from thymic epithelium.
- Because the thymus also interacts with the immune system, thymic cancers are associated with autoimmune disorders, and 30% of thymoma patients have coincident myasthenia gravis.
- Surgical resection is the key to cure.
- Recurrence is typically limited to the anterior mediastinum or lining of the chest (pleura), and repeat surgeries may provide long disease-free intervals.
- For thymic malignancy, the grade of the cancer is as important as the stage in determining prognosis.
- Low-grade thymomas are types A, AB, B1, and B2. High-grade thymic malignancies are well-differentiated (B3) or overt thymic carcinoma (C).
- Postoperative radiation is commonly given if the thymic malignancy invades structures in the mediastinum (lung, pleura/pericardium, blood vessels) which make it stage III.
- Radiation alone may be used if the cancer is unresectable but amenable to radiation.
- There is no reliable postoperative drug therapy for resected thymic malignancy. Traditional combination chemotherapy can be given prior to surgery for thymic malignancies of higher stage or higher risk.
- Because thymic malignancy is so rare, there is no comparative efficacy data to guide best practices for palliative drug therapy. Supportive care only is reasonable for low-grade, slow-growing, metastatic thymoma. There is a long list of active drugs for higher-grade thymoma which includes chemotherapy, as well as angiokinase inhibitors for thymic carcinoma.

Mesothelioma

- Malignant pleural mesothelioma is a rare cancer of the lining of the lung, often associated with a remote history of asbestos exposure.
- It must be distinguished from lung cancer based on unique, epithelioid histopathology and protein expression (calretinin, WT1). There are also sarcomatoid or mixed variants of mesothelioma with a worse prognosis.
- Radical surgeries, like extrapleural pneumonectomy, have fallen out of favor due to accumulated evidence of patient harm.
- Pleurectomy, or stripping of the pleura to remove the mesothelioma, is safer but is always incomplete.
- The best survival is seen when patients receive surgery, as well as chemotherapy (cisplatin or carboplatin, with pemetrexed) delivered before or after surgery.
- Surgically unresectable mesothelioma may be treated effectively with either chemotherapy or immune checkpoint blockade.
- Immune checkpoint blockade (ipilimumab + nivolumab) is particularly effective against the sarcomatoid variant, which is a major breakthrough.

Key Reference

- Spigel DR, Faivre-Finn C, Gray JE, et al. Five-year survival outcomes from the PACIFIC trial: durvalumab after chemoradiotherapy in stage III non–small-cell lung cancer. J Clin Oncol. 2022;40(12):1301–11.

Further Reading

Baas P, Scherpereel A, Nowak AK, et al. First-line nivolumab plus ipilimumab in unresectable malignant pleural mesothelioma (CheckMate 743): a multicentre, randomised, open-label, phase 3 trial. Lancet. 2021;397(10272):375–86.

Dillman RO, Seagren SL, Propert KJ, et al. A randomized trial of induction chemotherapy plus high-dose radiation versus radiation alone in stage III non-small-cell lung cancer. N Engl J Med. 1990;323(14):940–5.

Felip E, Altorki N, Zhou C, Csőszi T, Vynnychenko I, Goloborodko O, Luft A, Akopov A, Martinez-Marti A, Kenmotsu H, Chen YM, Chella A, Sugawara S, Voong D, Wu F, Yi J, Deng Y, McCleland M, Bennett E, Gitlitz B, Wakelee H, IMpower010 Investigators. Adjuvant atezolizumab after adjuvant chemotherapy in resected stage IB-IIIA non-small-cell lung cancer (IMpower010): a randomised, multicentre, open-label, phase 3 trial. Lancet. 2021;398(10308):1344–57. https://doi.org/10.1016/S0140-6736(21)02098-5. Epub 2021 Sep 20. Erratum in: Lancet. 2021 Sep 23.

Forde PM, Spicer J, Lu S, et al. Neoadjuvant nivolumab plus chemotherapy in resectable lung cancer. N Engl J Med. 2022;386:1973–85.

Gandhi L, Rodríguez-Abreu D, Gadgeel S, et al. Pembrolizumab plus chemotherapy in metastatic non-small-cell lung cancer. N Engl J Med. 2018;378(22):2078–92.

Gomez DR, Tang C, Zhang J, et al. Local consolidative therapy vs. maintenance therapy or observation for patients with oligometastatic non-small-cell lung cancer: long-term results of a multi-institutional, phase II, randomized study. J Clin Oncol. 2019;37(18):1558–65.

Hellmann MD, Paz-Ares L, Bernabe Caro R, et al. Nivolumab plus ipilimumab in advanced non-small-cell lung cancer. N Engl J Med. 2019;381(21):2020–31.

Mok TS, Wu YL, Thongprasert S, et al. Gefitinib or carboplatin-paclitaxel in pulmonary adenocarcinoma. N Engl J Med. 2009;361(10):947–57.

O'Brien M, Paz-Ares L, Marreaud S, Dafni U, Oselin K, Havel L, Esteban E, Isla D, Martinez-Marti A, Faehling M, Tsuboi M, Lee JS, Nakagawa K, Yang J, Samkari A, Keller SM, Mauer M, Jha N, Stahel R, Besse B, Peters S, EORTC-1416-LCG/ETOP 8-15—PEARLS/KEYNOTE-091 Investigators. Pembrolizumab versus placebo as adjuvant therapy for completely resected stage IB-IIIA non-small-cell lung cancer (PEARLS/KEYNOTE-091): an interim analysis of a randomised, triple-blind, phase 3 trial. Lancet Oncol. 2022;23(10):1274–86.

Reck M, Rodríguez-Abreu D, Robinson AG, et al. Pembrolizumab versus chemotherapy for PD-L1-positive non-small-cell lung cancer. N Engl J Med. 2016;375(19):1823–33.

Roth JA, Fossella F, Komaki R, et al. A randomized trial comparing perioperative chemotherapy and surgery with surgery alone in resectable stage IIIA non-small-cell lung cancer. J Natl Cancer Inst. 1994;86(9):673–80.

Winton T, Livingston R, Johnson D, et al. Vinorelbine plus cisplatin vs. observation in resected non-small-cell lung cancer. N Engl J Med. 2005;352:2589–97.

Wu YL, Tsuboi M, He J, John T, Grohe C, Majem M, Goldman JW, Laktionov K, Kim SW, Kato T, Vu HV, Lu S, Lee KY, Akewanlop C, Yu CJ, de Marinis F, Bonanno L, Domine M, Shepherd FA, Zeng L, Hodge R, Atasoy A, Rukazenkov Y, Herbst RS, ADAURA Investigators. Osimertinib in resected EGFR-mutated non-small-cell lung cancer. N Engl J Med. 2020;383(18):1711–23. https://doi.org/10.1056/NEJMoa2027071. Epub 2020 Sep 19. PMID: 32955177.

Chapter 15
Radiotherapy for Primary and Metastatic Lung Cancer

David L. Schwartz and Stephen G. Chun

Radiation Treatment Modalities

- Three-dimensional conformal radiation therapy (3D-CRT): Since the 1990s, radiation has been delivered with fixed beams which were shaped to exclude as much normal lung, mediastinum, and abdomen as possible. Moderate to severe esophagitis and pneumonitis were common, up to 30% in cooperative group trials testing chemoradiotherapy.
- Intensity-modulated radiation treatment (IMRT): Treatment transitioned to this automated, computer-controlled technology in the early 2000s–2010s, permitting personalized treatment carved away from the central mediastinum, lung, and spine (Fig. 15.1). Treatment is given under CT, MRI, PET, and/or virtual video CT imaging to correct for breathing motion and to limit target sizes only to PET-avid disease. This modality has become more routine as prospective data has suggested reduced toxicity to bystander organs previously difficult to spare, such as the heart and lungs.
- Stereotactic body radiation treatment (SBRT): This extremely precise treatment can deliver ablative treatment in one to five large doses over 1 or 2 weeks. Almost no normal tissues are included in the treatment target (Fig. 15.2); however, careful technique is required to limit excess intermediate-risk radiation doses to the

D. L. Schwartz (✉)
Department of Radiation Oncology, University of Tennessee Health Science Center, Memphis, TN, USA
e-mail: dschwar4@uthsc.edu

S. G. Chun
Department of Radiation Oncology, University of Texas M.D. Anderson Cancer Center, Houston, TX, USA
e-mail: SGChun@mdanderson.org

T. Ng, T. Geraci (eds.), *Thoracic Surgery Clerkship*, Contemporary Surgical Clerkships, https://doi.org/10.1007/978-3-031-44645-0_15

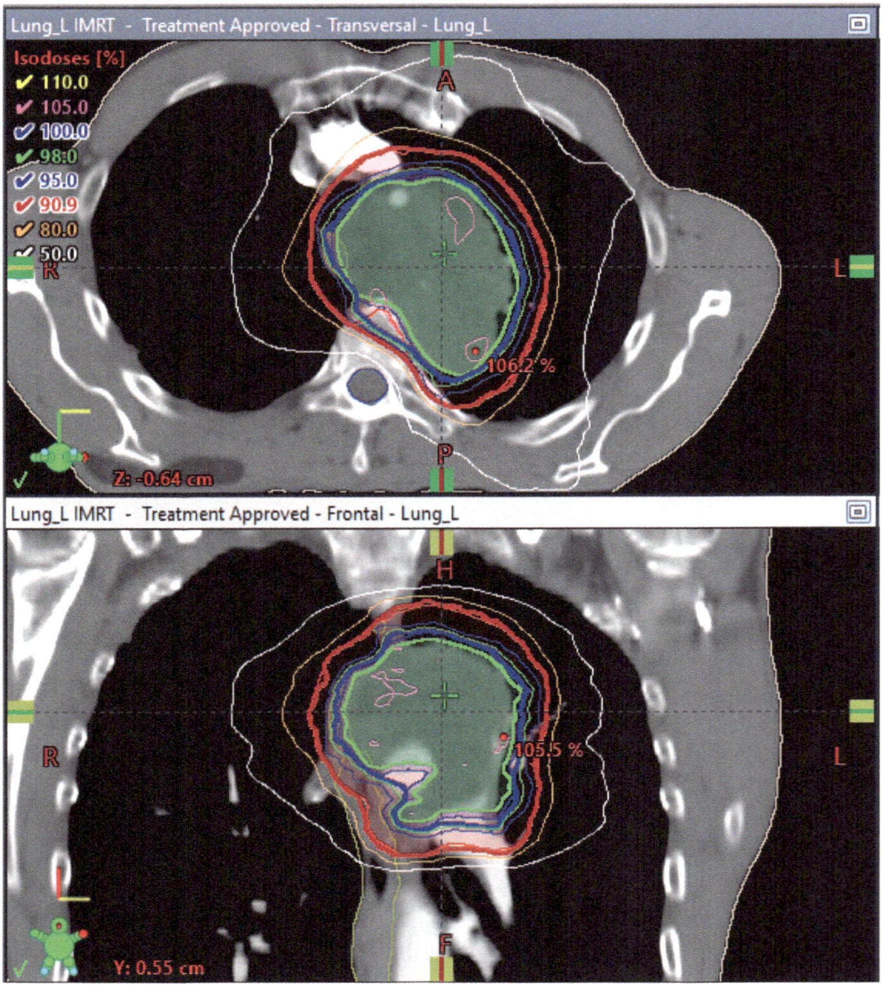

Fig. 15.1 IMRT treatment plan for a T4N0 centralized NSCLC of the left upper lobe. Treatment spares dose to the spinal cord and normal lung

normal lung. SBRT has been tested prospectively since the early 2000s and has been shown to provide survival outcomes for early-stage NSCLC equivalent to historical surgical results (see below). Moderate-severe side effects are uncommon.

- Particle radiation treatment (PRT): In the United States, this consists of proton radiotherapy, available at specialized referral centers (Fig. 15.3). Although institutional data suggest PRT can improve upon therapeutic ratio of standard IMRT

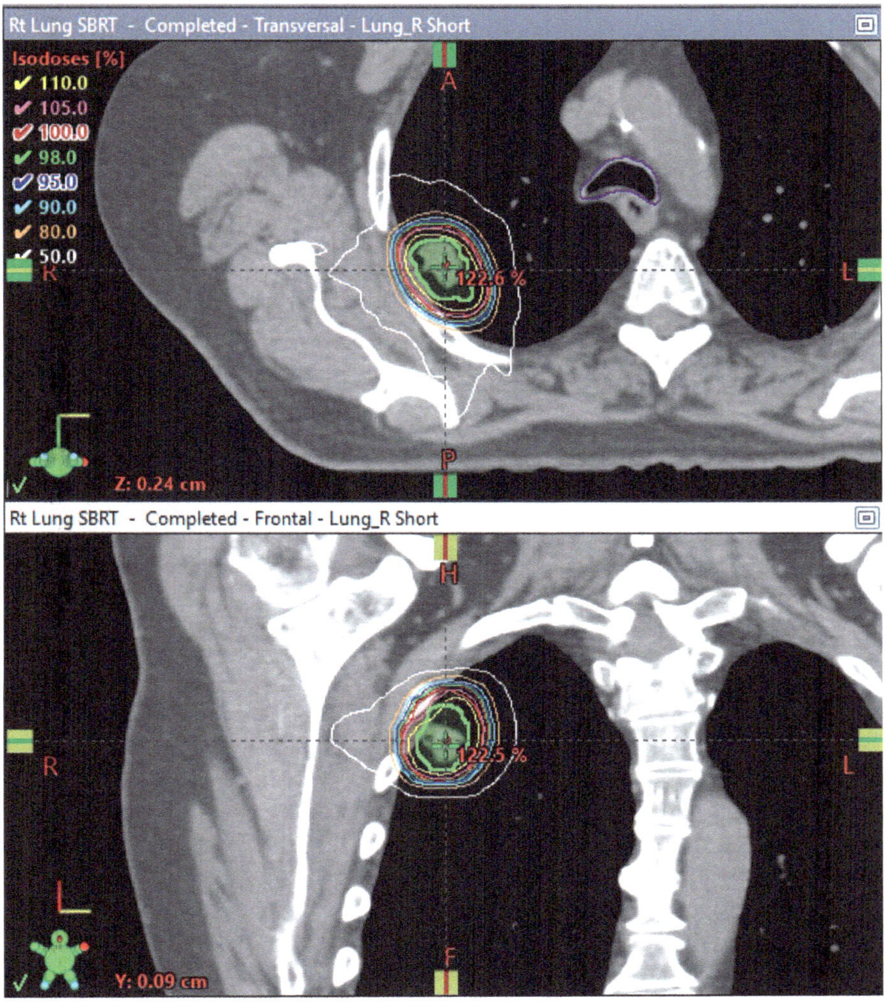

Fig. 15.2 SBRT treatment plan for a T1N0 peripherally located NSCLC of the right upper lobe. Treatment corrects for tumor motion throughout the respiratory cycle and spares dose to the adjacent rib and chest wall. However, note that neighboring normal lung tissue still receives some scattered radiation dose

in selected patients, a single-institution Bayesian adaptive phase II trial comparing IMRT with proton therapy showed promising results, which led to the ongoing national cooperative group phase III randomized trial NRG Oncology-RTOG 1308 which is directly comparing PRT to IMRT for unresectable stage II–III NSCLC.

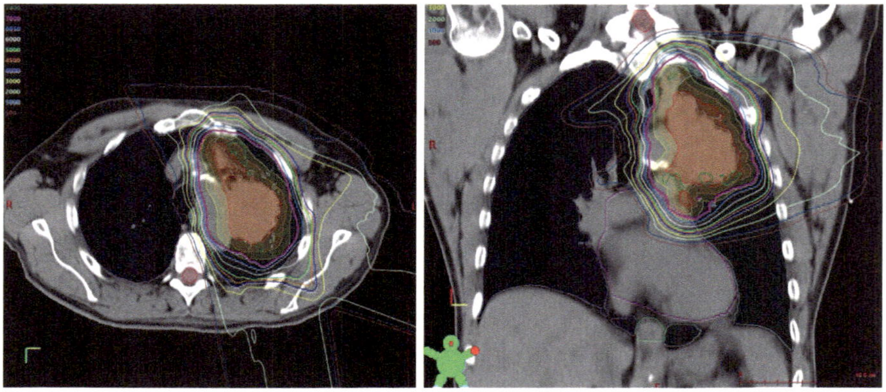

Fig. 15.3 Proton treatment plan for a T4N0 centralized NSCLC of the left upper lobe. Use of protons instead of standard photon IMRT permits coverage of gross disease with improved protection of neighboring normal lung and mediastinum from scattered radiation dose

Early-Stage NSCLC

- SBRT: Successive cooperative group trials (RTOG 0236, 0618, 0813, 0915) have consistently confirmed 82–96% in-field disease control of T1-2 disease with 1–5 fraction regimens. Gr 2 or greater toxicity is <10% for peripheral disease separate from the chest wall. However, the risk for severe damage to the proximal airway, esophagus, and great vessels increases for central disease located <2 cm away from mediastinal structures, necessitating incrementally lower doses. The impact of such dose deintensification is being studied.
- Stage T3 or multiple T1–T2 primaries: Although these disease presentations increase the amount of the normal lung exposed to scattered radiation from SBRT, growing institutional data suggests the safety of careful lung dose constraints or modestly deaccelerated schedules, such as ten treatment fractions over 2 weeks.
- Combined SBRT and PD-L1-directed immunotherapy: Concurrent and/or adjuvant administration of immune checkpoint inhibitors (nivolumab, durvalumab, avelumab, atezolizumab, or pembrolizumab) with SBRT remains unproven, but is being tested in phase II–III trials.

Advanced-Stage NSCLC

- Concurrent Chemoradiotherapy (CRT): Chemoradiotherapy represents preferred first-line treatment for patients with unresectable stage IIIA–IIIB disease. Phase III cooperative group trials have consistently demonstrated improved survival outcomes using CRT vs. radiation alone, with a median progression-free survival of 8–10 months. IMRT can reduce the lung and cardiac toxicity of CRT compared to traditional 3DRT. However, CRT does not improve distant disease spread, and the addition of induction or consolidative cytotoxic chemotherapy has not corrected this shortfall.

- Adjuvant Immunotherapy: PACIFIC was a landmark phase III trial which randomized unresectable, good-performance stage III NSCLC CRT patients to consolidative durvalumab or placebo. The durvalumab arm outperformed placebo at every time point, demonstrating unprecedented 83% 12-month and 66% 36-month overall survival rates. These results have been confirmed at 5 years (43% overall survival vs. 33% for placebo); 1 year of consolidative durvalumab after CRT is now standard of care for this indication.
- Postoperative Radiotherapy: This approach is typically reserved for use in carefully selected cases of mediastinal adenopathy and/or positive surgical margins at an airway reanastomosis or adjoining chest wall. No proven survival benefit has been shown in advanced-stage populations either by clinical trial or meta-analysis.

Limited-Stage Small Cell Lung Cancer (SCLC)

- Concurrent Chemoradiotherapy: For patients who present with disease confined to one hemithorax with or without ipsilateral supraclavicular nodal involvement, twice-daily treatment delivering 45 Gy during platinum-based chemotherapy has been standard of care since publication of the Intergroup 0096 trial. Two recent phase III trials have confirmed equivalence of this approach to once-daily CRT to 66–70 Gy. RT dose escalation via intensified hyperfractionation or moderate hypofractionation (higher dose per treatment) is currently a promising avenue for phase III testing, as is consolidative immunotherapy. An early start to RT by the second cycle of chemotherapy is favored. Since bulky mediastinal disease is common, use of advanced IMRT planning with strict lung constraints and motion correction is frequently desirable. Currently, NRG Oncology-LU005 is a randomized phase III trial evaluating CRT +/− atezolizumab for limited-stage SCLC.
- Prophylactic Cranial Irradiation (PCI): Treatment of the brain to low prophylactic doses (25 Gy over ten fractions) immediately following CRT has been standard of care since the 1990s, significantly reducing intracranial failure. Hippocampal-sparing IMRT, SBRT, and MRI staging/surveillance alone are currently being investigated as alternative approaches to reduce risk for PCI-associated neurocognitive decline. The n-methyl-d-aspartate (NMDA) inhibitor memantine is now routinely used in cooperative group trials with PCI to prevent neurocognitive decline.
- Extensive-Stage SCLC: Initial platinum and etoposide chemotherapy with PD-L1-directed immunotherapy (durvalumab or atezolizumab) followed by maintenance PD-L1-directed immunotherapy is the new standard of care for extensive-stage SCLC. The vast majority of patients respond to first-line sys-

temic therapy and are candidates for consolidative thoracic RT, which has been shown to have an overall survival benefit in multiple trials. At least 30 Gy in ten fractions is recommended, with treatment up to 45–54 Gy in selected favorable cases. Similar to limited-stage disease, PCI or MRI surveillance of the brain can be offered following good response.

Metastatic Disease and Palliation

- Oligometastatic Disease: Patients in otherwise good health, limited metastatic burden (one to five sites), and stable primary disease are candidates for site-directed ablative treatment with SBRT following upfront chemotherapy. Three randomized phase II trials all suggested excellent in-field disease control, improved progression-free and/or overall survival, and limited side effects following SBRT to one to five metastases. There is currently very active investigation to validate these findings via larger multi-institutional trials and to broaden the application of this approach to patients with ≥4 metastases or with limited (one to five) sites of metastatic progression.
- Symptomatic Advanced Disease: Debilitated patients with active or impending disease progression at thoracic or distant sites can frequently be palliated with short-course RT over one to five fractions. Local pain, bleeding, and mass effect with secondary compression (impacting critical structures such as the spinal cord, brain, airway, or great vessels) are presentations most likely to be improved by RT.

Key Reference

- Timmerman RD, Hu C, Michalski JM, Bradley JC, Galvin J, Johnstone DW, Choy H. Long-term results of stereotactic body radiation therapy in medically inoperable stage I non-small cell lung cancer. JAMA Oncol. 2018;4(9):1287–88.

Further Reading

Auperin A, Arriagada R, Pignon JP, et al. Prophylactic cranial irradiation for patients with small-cell lung cancer in complete remission. Prophylactic cranial irradiation overview collaborative group. N Engl J Med. 1999;341(7):476–84.

Bogart JA, Wang X, Masters GA, et al. Short communication: interim toxicity analysis for patients with limited stage small cell lung cancer (LSCLC) treated on CALGB 30610 (Alliance)/RTOG 0538. Lung Cancer. 2021;156:68–71.

Bogart JA, Waqar SN, Mix MD. Radiation and systemic therapy for limited-stage small-cell lung cancer. J Clin Oncol. 2022;40(6):661–70.

Bradley JD, Bae K, Graham MV, et al. Primary analysis of the phase II component of a phase I/II dose intensification study using three-dimensional conformal radiation therapy and concurrent chemotherapy for patients with inoperable non-small-cell lung cancer: RTOG 0117. J Clin Oncol. 2010;28(14):2475–80.

Bradley JD, Paulus R, Komaki R, et al. Standard-dose versus high-dose conformal radiotherapy with concurrent and consolidation carboplatin plus paclitaxel with or without cetuximab for patients with stage IIIA or IIIB non-small-cell lung cancer (RTOG 0617): a randomised, two-by-two factorial phase 3 study. Lancet Oncol. 2015;16(2):187–99. https://doi.org/10.1016/S1470-2045(14)71207-0.

Brown PD, Pugh S, Laack NN, et al. Memantine for the prevention of cognitive dysfunction in patients receiving whole-brain radiotherapy: a randomized, double-blind, placebo-controlled trial. Neuro-Oncology. 2013;15(10):1429–37.

Chang JY, Verma V, Li M, et al. Proton beam radiotherapy and concurrent chemotherapy for unresectable stage III non-small cell lung cancer: final results of a phase 2 study. JAMA Oncol. 2017;3(8):e172032.

Chun SG, Hu C, Choy H, et al. Impact of intensity-modulated radiation therapy technique for locally advanced non-small-cell lung cancer: a secondary analysis of the NRG oncology RTOG 0617 randomized clinical trial. J Clin Oncol. 2017;35(1):56–62.

Daly ME, Ismaila N, Decker RH, et al. Radiation therapy for small-cell lung cancer: ASCO guideline endorsement of an ASTRO guideline. J Clin Oncol. 2021;39(8):931–9.

Faivre-Finn C, Snee M, Ashcroft L, et al. Concurrent once-daily versus twice-daily chemoradiotherapy in patients with limited-stage small-cell lung cancer (CONVERT): an open-label, phase 3, randomised, superiority trial. Lancet Oncol. 2017;18(8):1116–25.

Gomez DR, Tang C, Zhang J, et al. Local consolidative therapy vs. maintenance therapy or observation for patients with oligometastatic non-small-cell lung cancer: long-term results of a multi-institutional, phase II, randomized study. J Clin Oncol. 2019;37(18):1558–65.

Gore EM, Hu C, Sun AY, et al. Randomized phase II study comparing prophylactic cranial irradiation alone to prophylactic cranial irradiation and consolidative extracranial irradiation for extensive-disease small cell lung cancer (ED SCLC): NRG oncology RTOG 0937. J Thorac Oncol. 2017;12(10):1561–70.

Higgins KA, Puri S, Gray JE. Systemic and radiation therapy approaches for locally advanced non-small-cell lung cancer. J Clin Oncol. 2022;40(6):576–85.

Horn L, Mansfield AS, Szczesna A, et al. First-line atezolizumab plus chemotherapy in extensive-stage small-cell lung cancer. N Engl J Med. 2018;379(23):2220–9. https://doi.org/10.1056/NEJMoa1809064.

Iyengar P, Wardak Z, Gerber DE, et al. Consolidative radiotherapy for limited metastatic non-small-cell lung cancer: a phase 2 randomized clinical trial. JAMA Oncol. 2018;4(1):e173501.

Jeremic B, Shibamoto Y, Nikolic N, et al. Role of radiation therapy in the combined-modality treatment of patients with extensive disease small-cell lung cancer: a randomized study. J Clin Oncol. 1999;17(7):2092–9.

Le Pechoux C, Pourel N, Barlesi F, et al. Postoperative radiotherapy versus no postoperative radiotherapy in patients with completely resected non-small-cell lung cancer and proven mediastinal N2 involvement (lung ART): an open-label, randomised, phase 3 trial. Lancet Oncol. 2022;23(1):104–14.

Levy A, Mercier O, Le Pechoux C. Indications and parameters around postoperative radiation therapy for lung cancer. J Clin Oncol. 2022;40(6):556–66.

Li Q, Swanick CW, Allen PK, et al. Stereotactic ablative radiotherapy (SABR) using 70 Gy in 10 fractions for non-small cell lung cancer: exploration of clinical indications. Radiother Oncol. 2014;112(2):256–61.

Liao Z, Lee JJ, Komaki R, et al. Bayesian adaptive randomization trial of passive scattering proton therapy and intensity-modulated photon radiotherapy for locally advanced non-small-cell lung cancer. J Clin Oncol. 2018;36(18):1813–22.

Palma DA, Olson R, Harrow S, et al. Stereotactic ablative radiotherapy for the comprehensive treatment of oligometastatic cancers: long-term results of the SABR-COMET phase II randomized trial. J Clin Oncol. 2020;38(25):2830–8.

Paz-Ares L, Dvorkin M, Chen Y, et al. Durvalumab plus platinum-etoposide versus platinum-etoposide in first-line treatment of extensive-stage small-cell lung cancer (CASPIAN): a randomised, controlled, open-label, phase 3 trial. Lancet. 2019;394(10212):1929–39. https://doi.org/10.1016/S0140-6736(19)32222-6.

Robinson C, Kruser TJ, Owen D, Salama J, Daly ME. Fast and furious: new data examining accelerated radiation therapy for limited-stage small cell lung cancer. Int J Radiat Oncol Biol Phys. 2022;112(5):1067–70.

Ryckman JM, Baine M, Carmicheal J, et al. Correction to: correlation of dosimetric factors with the development of symptomatic radiation pneumonitis in stereotactic body radiotherapy. Radiat Oncol. 2021;16(1):67.

Schild SE, Sio TT, Daniels TB, Chun SG, Rades D. Prophylactic cranial irradiation for extensive small-cell lung cancer. J Oncol Pract. 2017;13(11):732–8.

Slotman BJ, van Tinteren H, Praag JO, et al. Use of thoracic radiotherapy for extensive stage small-cell lung cancer: a phase 3 randomised controlled trial. Lancet. 2015;385(9962):36–42.

Spigel DR, Faivre-Finn C, Gray JE, et al. Five-year survival outcomes from the PACIFIC trial: durvalumab after chemoradiotherapy in stage III non-small-cell lung cancer. J Clin Oncol. 2022;40(12):1301–11.

Takahashi T, Yamanaka T, Seto T, et al. Prophylactic cranial irradiation versus observation in patients with extensive-disease small-cell lung cancer: a multicentre, randomised, open-label, phase 3 trial. Lancet Oncol. 2017;18(5):663–71.

Turrisi AT 3rd, Kim K, Blum R, et al. Twice-daily compared with once-daily thoracic radiotherapy in limited small-cell lung cancer treated concurrently with cisplatin and etoposide. N Engl J Med. 1999;340(4):265–71.

Curran WJ Jr, Paulus R, Langer CJ, et al. Sequential vs. concurrent chemoradiation for stage III non-small cell lung cancer: randomized phase III trial RTOG 9410. J Natl Cancer Inst. 2011;103(19):1452–60.

Chapter 16
Massive Hemoptysis

Joseph R. Slaughter and Thomas Ng

Introduction

Massive hemoptysis is quantitatively defined as blood loss from the lungs >500 mL per 24 h or > 100 mL per hour. However, quantifying the exact amount of hemoptysis is not accurate, and clinicians must keep in mind that even small amounts of hemoptysis can be life threatening. Up to 15% of hemoptysis presentations are life threatening, with mortality as high as 38%. Prompt action is essential in the successful treatment of patients with massive hemoptysis, to quickly diagnose, clear blood clot from the airway, and protect the normal lung. Control of the bleeding source can be obtained by endoluminal methods or vascular embolization, most often a bronchial artery. Once the patient has recovered from bleeding, definitive surgical treatment of the inciting pathology, if necessary, can be electively planned.

J. R. Slaughter
Department of Surgery, University of Tennessee Health Science Center, College of Medicine, Memphis, TN, USA
e-mail: jslaugh4@uthsc.edu

T. Ng (✉)
Division of Thoracic Surgery, University of Tennessee Health Science Center, College of Medicine, Memphis, TN, USA
e-mail: tng4@uthsc.edu

T. Ng, T. Geraci (eds.), *Thoracic Surgery Clerkship*, Contemporary Surgical Clerkships, https://doi.org/10.1007/978-3-031-44645-0_16

Anatomy

Source of Bleeding

- Systemic circulation.
  - Bronchial artery source in 90%.

    Commonly arise from descending aorta T4–6.
    Typically there are two major arteries on the left and one on the right (but this is highly variable).
    Anomalous bronchial arteries can arise from the aortic arch, subclavian artery, innominate artery, intercostal arteries, thyrocervical trunk, internal mammary artery, inferior phrenic artery, and the coronary arteries, with prevalence as high as 35%.

  - Systemic collaterals.

    Arise from descending thoracic aorta, subclavian, intercostal, innominate, axillary, and internal mammary arteries.

- Pulmonary artery circulation.
  - Less common source than systemic circulation.
  - Can arise from a lung abscess eroding into the pulmonary artery, such as Rasmussen aneurysm from tuberculosis.
  - May be iatrogenically injured during Swan-Ganz catheter placement.

Etiologies

The cause of hemoptysis varies from infectious and inflammatory to neoplastic, traumatic, iatrogenic, cardiovascular, vascular, and coagulopathic diseases (Table 16.1). Tuberculosis remains the most common cause of hemoptysis worldwide, while malignancy is most prevalent among developed nations.

Table 16.1 Etiologies of massive hemoptysis, common causes are in bold

Iatrogenic Bronchoscopy **Lung biopsy** Radiotherapy **Pulmonary artery catheterization** Transtracheal aspiration Endobronchial brachytherapy Erosion of airway stent	*Pulmonary* **Bronchiectasis** Cystic fibrosis Lymphangioleiomyomatosis Diffuse alveolar hemorrhage Bronchogenic cyst Granulomatous tracheobronchitis (ulcerative colitis, Crohn disease, Wegener granulomatosis)
Infectious **Tuberculosis** **Fungal infection** (aspergillosis, mucormycosis, coccidioidomycosis, histoplasmosis, maduromycosis) Bronchitis **Necrotizing pneumonia** (*Staphylococcus aureus*, *Legionella*, *Actinomyces*, gram-negative aerobes) **Mycetoma** **Lung abscess** Parasitic infection (amebiasis, ascariasis, clonorchiasis, echinococcosis, hookworm, strongyloidiasis, trichinosis, paragonimiasis, schistosomiasis) Septic emboli	*Cardiovascular and Vasculitis* Pulmonary embolism/infarction Pulmonary artery aneurysms **Bronchial arterial fistula** Congenital heart disease Congestive heart failure Mitral stenosis Systemic lupus erythematosus Antiphospholipid syndrome Henoch-Schonlein purpura Cryoglobulinemia Hughes-Stovin syndrome Arteriovenous malformations Osler-Weber-Rendu syndrome Takayasu arteritis Aortic aneurysms Trachea–innominate artery fistulas Dieulafoy disease of the bronchus Hemangioma (sclerosing, cavernous, tracheal)
Neoplastic **Lung cancer** Bronchial adenoma Pulmonary metastases Sarcoma Metastatic disease	*Interstitial lung disease* Lymphangioleiomyomatosis Sarcoidosis Tuberous sclerosis Pneumoconiosis Langerhans cell granulomatosis
Drugs Bevacizumab Anticoagulants/antiplatelet Volatile solvent Trimellitic anhydride Cocaine Nitrofurantoin	*Traumatic* Blunt chest trauma Penetrating injury Ruptured bronchus Traumatic pseudoaneurysms
Miscellaneous Idiopathic/cryptogenic Amyloidosis Thoracic endometriosis Foreign body aspiration Organophosphate aspiration Chronic pancreatitis	*Hematologic* Platelet disease TTP Coagulopathies

Initial Management

Establish Airway and Breathing

- The priority of management involves rapid initiation of lifesaving interventions that are aimed at establishing the patient's airway and breathing.
- Again, death from asphyxiation due to blood occluding the airway is the immediate risk, this ensuing well before hypovolemia from bleeding, as it does not take much volume of blood to occlude one's airway.
- Blood and blood clots must be cleared from the non-diseased lung so that ventilation and oxygenation can at least be re-established in this one lung.
- Figure 16.1 illustrates the initial management, with the following important points to stress:
  - Other sources of bleeding, such as the nose, mouth, throat, and gastrointestinal tract, can be aspirated and mistaken for hemoptysis. Bronchoscopy, flexible or rigid, and, if necessary, upper endoscopy and ENT evaluation can confirm the source of bleeding.
  - The classic teaching of placing the patient in lateral decubitus position, with the diseased lung down, may be appropriate for submassive hemoptysis and if

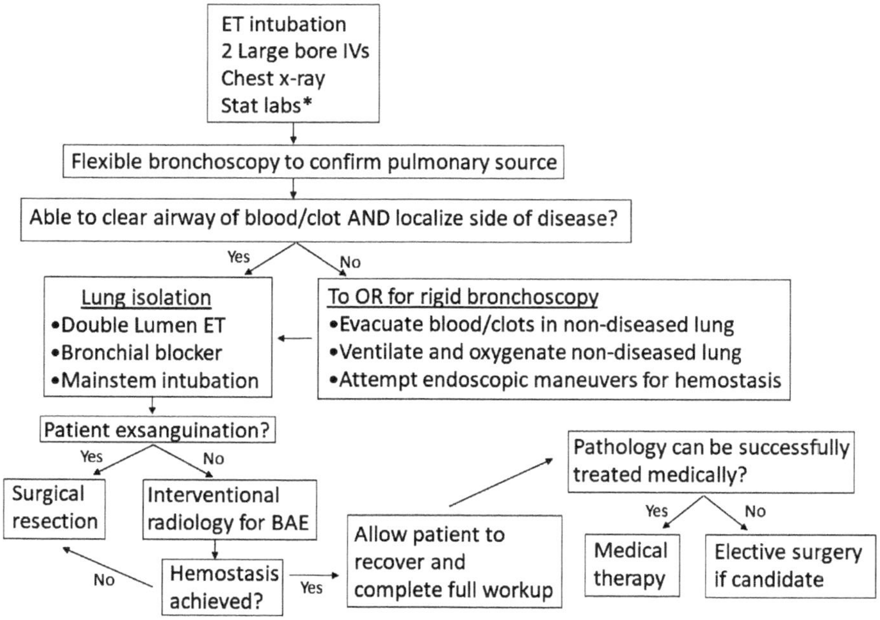

Fig. 16.1 Management algorithm for massive hemoptysis. *ET* endotracheal tube, *IV* intravenous, *BAE* bronchial artery embolization, *blood work (artery blood gas, type and crossmatch blood, coagulation parameters, etc.)

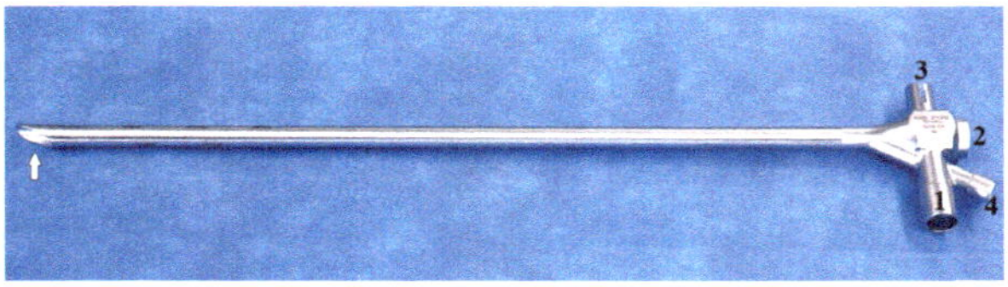

Fig. 16.2 Rigid bronchoscope with large bore lumen (arrow) ideal for suctioning blood clots; (1) ventilation port; (2) visualization port by scope or with the eye; (3) light source port; (4) utility port

the laterality of the pathology is known. However, in cases of true massive hemoptysis, this maneuver is not practical nor helpful as the volume of blood will quickly overwhelm the patient, leading to an unstable airway and a patient in extremis from asphyxiation.

- Unlike upper airway obstruction, oral endotracheal intubation does not secure the patient's airway or breathing as the source of the obstruction is due to bleeding from below.
- Note that if flexible bronchoscopy is not able to rapidly clear the airway due to excessive blood and blood clots, then rigid bronchoscopy (Fig. 16.2) should be performed without delay. One must not persist with flexible bronchoscopy but have a very low threshold for rigid bronchoscopy as this is a much more effective method for clearing large clots.
- Note that CT scan is not listed in the initial management outline in Fig. 16.1. In cases of true massive hemoptysis, this will delay lifesaving interventions. However, in a stable patient who has successfully achieved lung isolation, CT scan can be considered for diagnosis and to guide treatment.

Lung Isolation

After clearing blood from the good lung, it is vital to secure this lung for ventilation and protect it from further filling with blood by one of three lung isolation techniques (also see Chap. 3).

- Double-lumen endotracheal tube (Fig. 16.3).
  - Most secure isolation technique, thus preferred approach if amenable.
  - Left-sided preferred (Fig. 16.3a), as right-sided tube is more difficult to place and maintain due to the short right mainstem and the need to ensure that the bronchial side channel is facing the right upper lobe bronchus for ventilation (Fig. 16.3b).
  - Can access the diseased lung: monitor bleeding, suction, and ventilate as needed.

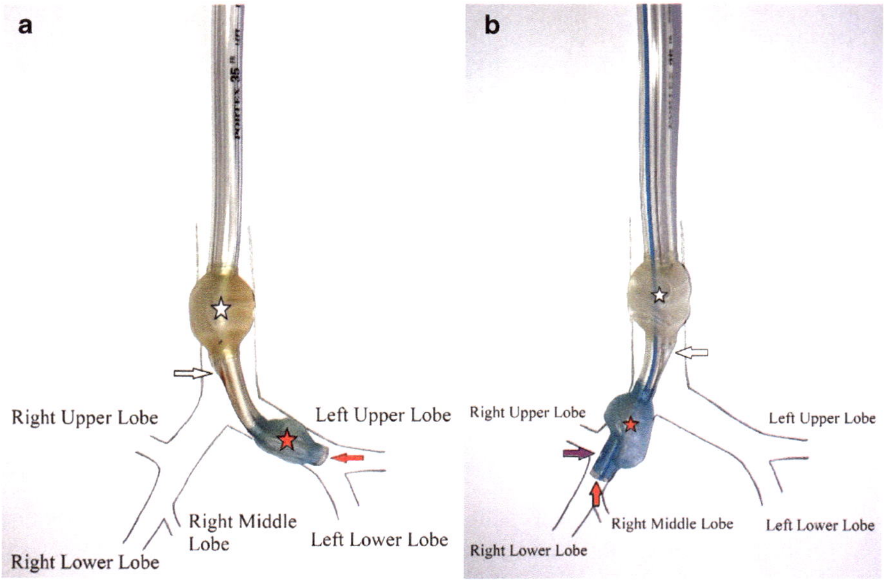

Fig. 16.3 Lung isolation by double-lumen tube with tracheal cuff (white star) and bronchial cuff (red star). (**a**) Left-sided double-lumen tube with bronchial channel (red arrow) to ventilate/suction the left lung and tracheal channel (white arrow) to ventilate/suction the right lung; (**b**) right-sided double lumen with bronchial channel to ventilate/suction the right lung and tracheal channel (white arrow) to ventilate/suction the left lung; note bronchial channel has two openings, one for the right upper lobe (purple arrow) and one for the right middle and lower lobes (red arrow), thus making right-sided harder to position than left-sided double-lumen tube

- Bronchial blocker (Fig. 16.4).
  - Can isolate one lung, but also can isolate specific lobes and segments.
  - Unable to access the diseased lung while the balloon is inflated.
  - Expertise needed to place, often more difficult to place than double lumen.
- Mainstem intubation (Fig. 16.5).
  - Quickest technique for lung isolation.
  - Not ideal for right mainstem isolation as the right upper lobe is often not ventilated.
  - No access to the diseased lung.

Stop the Bleeding

- Rigid bronchoscopy.

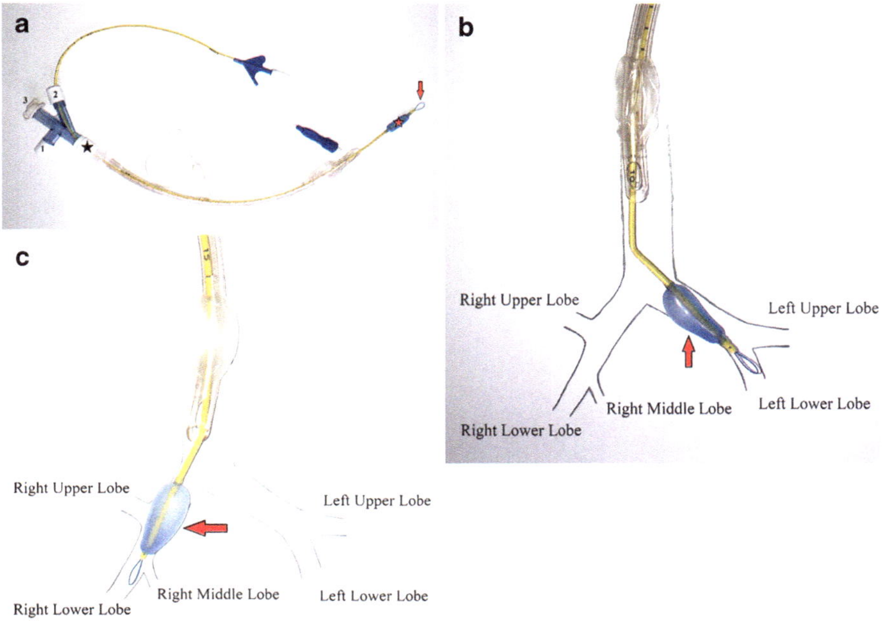

Fig. 16.4 Lung isolation by bronchial blocker placed through a standard single-lumen endotracheal tube. (**a**) Important parts of the bronchial blocker include the occluding balloon (red star), loop to guide bronchoscopic positioning (red arrow), and the adapter (black star) with ventilation port (1), bronchial blocker port (2), and bronchoscopy port (3); (**b**) left-sided bronchial blocker (red arrow); (**c**) right-sided bronchial blocker (red arrow)

  - A common initial treatment is the instillation of ice-cold saline with dilute epinephrine into the affected airways.
  - Topical agents or local energy such as argon, laser, or electrocautery can be considered; however, it will not be useful if pathology is in the distal airways (which is often the case) and risks airway fire if patient is on high FI02.

- Embolization by interventional radiology.
  - Travel to interventional radiology for embolization should only be considered if the patient can maintain adequate ventilation and oxygenation with controlled bleeding.
  - Embolization has a high success rate of stopping the bleeding (64–100%, depending on institutional experience) in the short term.
  - Technique:

    Begin first with systemic circulation via arterial access, as the most likely source of bleeding is from the bronchial arteries (90%).

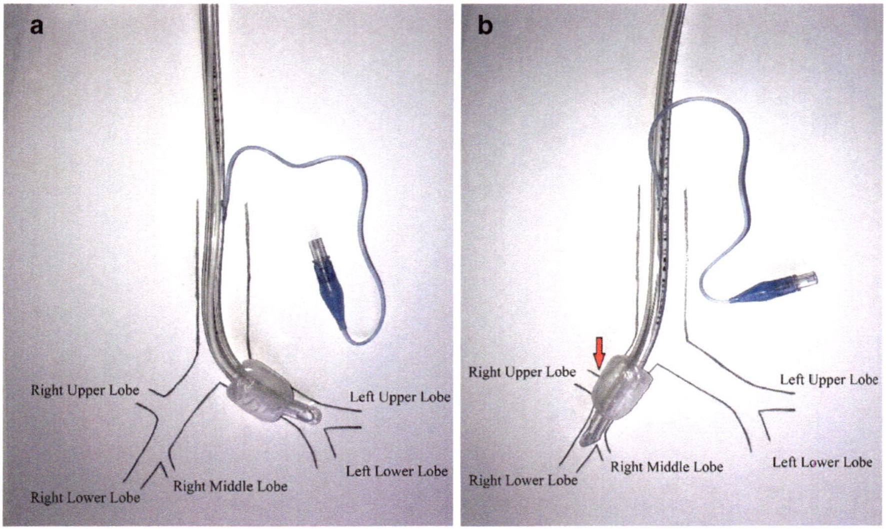

Fig. 16.5 Lung isolation by advancing standard single-lumen endotracheal tube. (**a**) Left mainstem bronchus intubation; (**b**) right mainstem bronchus intubation; note that due to the right main bronchus being short, the right upper lobe will likely not be ventilated as it will be blocked by the balloon (arrow)

Angiographic findings indicative of bleeding vessels (Fig. 16.6) include extravasation, aneurysm, hypertrophy and tortuosity, parenchymal hypervascularity, and bronchial artery to pulmonary vein or artery shunting.

All branches to the diseased side can be embolized without ischemic consequences as the lung has dual circulation, systemic and pulmonary.

Assess other systemic circulation arteries such as subclavian, internal mammary, and intercostal as these may provide collateral source to the disease process.

If bleeding persists despite interrogation/embolization of the systemic circulation, then assess the pulmonary artery circulation, which will require venous access.

The pulmonary artery can be interrogated first (before systemic circulation) in cases of obvious pulmonary artery bleeding such as Swan-Ganz catheter injury.

Beware of the rare complication of spinal ischemia due to proximal embolizing of a bronchial artery that has common origin with the anterior spinal artery.

– Despite the high immediate success rate of embolization, hemoptysis will recur if the pathology is not properly treated.

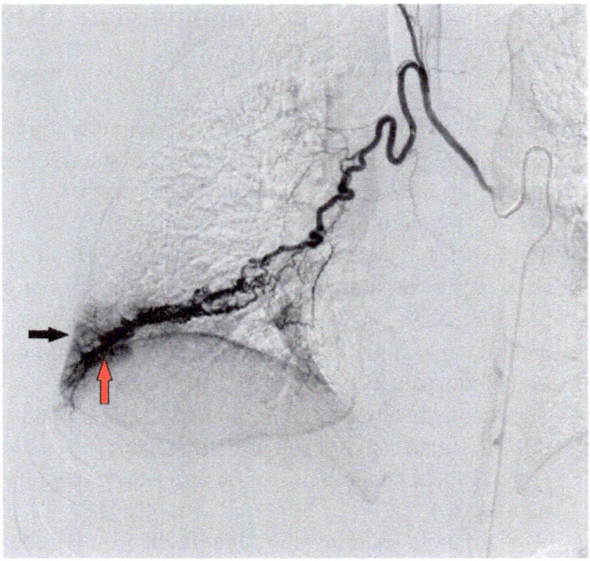

Fig. 16.6 Bronchial artery embolization. Patient with hemoptysis from bronchiectasis of the anterior/lateral basal segment right lower lobe. Note the dilated and tortuous bronchial artery (red arrow) that extends to the distal aspect of the segment, and the blush indicated active extravasation/bleed (black arrow)

- Surgical resection.
  - Emergent resection has a high risk for postoperative morbidity and mortality compared to elective resection; in addition, the patient's pulmonary function and stage of disease (if lung cancer) may not be known at the time.
  - Due to the high success rate of embolization, coupled with the high risk of emergent surgery, embolization is the preferred initial method to stop bleeding, which allows for patient recovery and the full workup to be completed.
  - Emergent resection is necessary in cases of hemodynamic instability and exsanguination, as in cases of parenchyma rupture and free bleeding into pleural space.

Definitive Management

Early recurrence following bronchial artery embolization may signal incomplete embolization, neovascularization, or disease progression. Late recurrence is reported in up to 40% of patients and is associated with pathologies not successfully treated with medical therapy alone, such as aspergilloma, tuberculosis, malignancy, and bronchiectasis. As such, bronchial artery embolization may serve as an effective temporizing measure to provide a bridge to surgery, thus allowing for patient recovery and the completion of preoperative workup. Surgical resection, if indicated and patient deemed a candidate, can then be performed in a more elective setting, minimizing postoperative morbidity and mortality.

Hemoptysis from Tracheoinnominate Fistula After Tracheostomy

- Tracheoinnominate fistula (TIF), communication between the innominate artery (also named brachiocephalic artery) and the trachea, is a rare complication after tracheostomy, reported in under 1% of cases.
- TIF has a high mortality of 75–100%.
- TIF usually manifests within 3 weeks of tracheostomy.
- Risk factors include low tracheostomy placement, below the third tracheal ring, pressure necrosis from overinflated tracheostomy cuff, prolonged intubation, anatomically high innominate artery, steroid and immunosuppressant use, radiation, and tracheitis.
- Sentinel hemorrhage may be an early sign that indicates the presence of TIF, just prior to the massive exsanguination event.
- High clinical suspicion is paramount for expedient simultaneous diagnosis and management.
- Workup includes removal of the tracheostomy tube to examining the entire anterior tracheal wall with bronchoscopy and contrast CT scan; however short of visualizing obvious hemorrhage and contrast extravasation, neither absolutely rule in or out TIF; thus there is frequently diagnostic dilemma prior to massive hemorrhage event.
- If massive bleeding occurs after tracheostomy:
  - Hyperinflation of the balloon cuff, in hopes that it will tamponade the bleeding.
  - If bleeding continues, then remove tracheostomy tube, and simultaneously intubate patient with oral endotracheal tube while placing a finger down the trachea through the stoma to pull against the posterior sternum in hopes that the compression will stop or slow the hemorrhage.
  - Definitive treatment is surgical, achieved by median sternotomy with artery ligation (for details see Chap. 37).

Key Reference

- Prey B, Francis A, Williams J, Krishnadasan B. Evaluation and treatment of massive hemoptysis. Surg Clin North Am. 2022;102(3):465–81.

Further Reading

Charya AV, Holden VK, Pickering EM. Management of life-threatening hemoptysis in the ICU. J Thorac Dis. 2021;13(8):5139–58.

Kathuria H, Hollingsworth HM, Vilvendhan R, Reardon C. Management of life-threatening hemoptysis. J Intensive Care. 2020;8:23.

Kaufman CS, Kwan SW. Bronchial artery embolization. Semin Intervent Radiol. 2022;39(3):210–7.

Reger B, Neu R, Hofmann HS, Ried M. High mortality in patients with Tracheoarterial fistulas: clinical experience and treatment recommendations. Interact Cardiovasc Thorac Surg. 2018;26(1):12–7.

Chapter 17
Infections of the Lung

Les James and Travis Geraci

Introduction

Familiarity with various infections of the lower respiratory tract is important in the practice of thoracic surgery because their complications may require procedural or surgical intervention. Additionally, the presence of intrathoracic infections in the preoperative or postoperative setting may complicate thoracic surgical procedures. While surgery has largely been replaced by medical therapy for various pulmonary infections, there is still a role for surgery in instances of worsening or uncontrolled disease, as well as in cases of diagnostic uncertainty. This chapter will cover lung abscesses, tuberculous and nontuberculous mycobacterial infections, and fungal infections prevalent in immunocompetent and immunocompromised patients.

Lung Abscess

- Lung abscesses are circumscribed, purulent infections contained within the lung parenchyma (Fig. 17.1).
- Lung abscesses can be classified as primary or secondary:

L. James
Division of Cardiac Surgery, Department of Cardiothoracic Surgery, New York University Langone Health, New York, NY, USA
e-mail: leslie.james@nyulangone.org

T. Geraci (✉)
Division of Thoracic Surgery, Department of Cardiothoracic Surgery, New York University Langone Health, New York, NY, USA
e-mail: travis.geraci@nyulangone.org

T. Ng, T. Geraci (eds.), *Thoracic Surgery Clerkship*, Contemporary Surgical Clerkships, https://doi.org/10.1007/978-3-031-44645-0_17

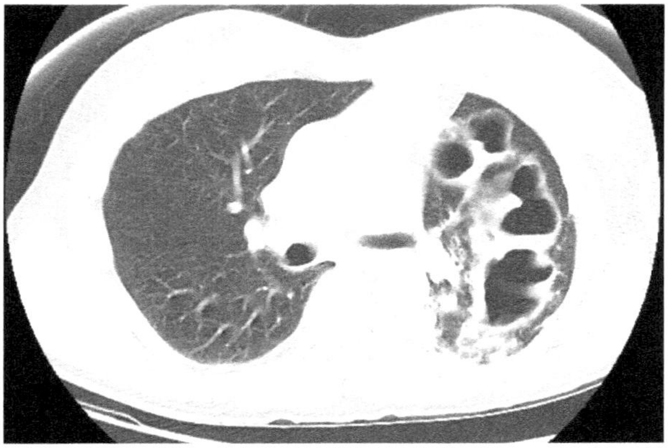

Fig. 17.1 Lung abscess of the left lower lobe after left upper lobectomy, from pulmonary infarction

- Primary lung abscesses: direct infection of the pulmonary parenchyma in an otherwise healthy person; most result from aspiration and, less commonly, from infection with pyogenic bacteria (*S. aureus*).
- Secondary lung abscesses: occur as a result of a predisposing condition such as bronchial obstruction (foreign body, neoplasm), hematogenous spread (empyema, right-sided endocarditis), or immunocompromised state.

Pathogenesis

- Aspiration: lung abscesses are most commonly caused by aspiration of oropharyngeal secretions in patients with risk factors for aspiration (e.g., advanced age, decreased level of consciousness, supine position, tracheal intubation and mechanical ventilation, presence of a nasogastric tube); typically polymicrobial.
- Hematogenous spread: lung abscesses can be a consequence of septic embolization during bacteremia such as right-sided infective endocarditis, intravenous drug use, or jugular vein suppurative thrombophlebitis (Lemierre syndrome).
- Direct extension: lung abscesses can develop as direct extension of an empyema, subphrenic or mediastinal abscess, or trachea- or broncho-esophageal fistula.
- Bronchial obstruction: endobronchial obstruction from a bronchogenic or mediastinal mass, bronchial stenosis, or an inhaled foreign body may all lead to post-obstructive pneumonia that progresses to abscess formation.
- Superinfection or spread of airway infection: lung abscesses can develop as a superinfection of pulmonary infarcts, congenital malformations, or lung contusion.

Microbiology

- Lung abscesses resulting from an aspiration event are typically polymicrobial; the most commonly isolated pathogens are anaerobes and streptococci.
  - Most common anaerobes include *Prevotella*, *Peptostreptococcus*, *Fusobacterium* spp., and *Bacteroides*.
  - Most common streptococci include *Streptococcus anginosus*, *Streptococcus milleri* group species, and *Streptococcus mitis*.
- Lung abscesses can also be a complication of acute monomicrobial infections with pyogenic bacteria (e.g., *Staphylococcus aureus*, *Klebsiella pneumoniae*, and *Pseudomonas aeruginosa*).
- Other bacteria can cause monomicrobial lung abscesses.
  - *Actinomyces* classically causes multiple abscesses throughout the body, including within the lungs; these infections are typically penicillin-sensitive.
  - *Klebsiella pneumoniae* typically presents with rapid onset tissue necrosis, a slow antibiotic response, and frequent bacteremia.
  - *Nocardia* is also a causative pathogen, especially in immunocompromised patients receiving steroids.
  - Fungal infections can also lead to formation of lung abscesses.

Clinical Presentation

- Patients with a lung abscess typically have nonspecific symptoms that mimic those of pneumonia, including fever and chills, productive cough with foul-smelling sputum (if the abscess drains into the tracheobronchial tree), dyspnea, chest pain, and hemoptysis.
  - Anaerobes are the most common culprit for foul-smelling sputum.
- Rupture into the pleural space may result in pyopneumothorax, with rapid onset of respiratory failure and septic shock.

Diagnosis

- Diagnosis of lung abscess relies on CT chest, which will demonstrate a cavity with an air fluid level and/or areas of parenchymal necrosis; malignancy should always be considered in the differential diagnosis.

Treatment

- First-line treatment for lung abscesses is broad-spectrum antibiotics, with therapy tailored to culture results.
  - Preferred antibiotic regimens include a beta-lactam plus a beta-lactamase inhibitor (ampicillin-sulbactam) or carbapenems (meropenem).
- Surgical drainage is not typically required for lung abscesses that drain into the bronchial tree; CT-guided or bronchoscopic-guided aspiration of the abscess can be performed to obtain accurate culture data.
- Surgery is reserved for suspected neoplasm, hemorrhage, or treatment failure.
  - Predictors of antibiotic failure include abscesses >6 cm in diameter, abscesses that result in an obstructed bronchus, and abscesses associated with highly resistant organisms (*Pseudomonas aeruginosa*).

Mycobacterial Infections

Tuberculous Mycobacterial Infections

- Tuberculosis (TB) is a leading cause of morbidity and mortality worldwide.
- Appropriate treatment requires prolonged antibiotic therapy with rifampin, isoniazid, and pyrazinamide; the optimal regimen depends on the susceptibility of a given patient's isolate.
  - Multidrug-resistant TB (MDR-TB) refers to TB isolates that are resistant to isoniazid and rifampin.
  - Extensively drug-resistant TB (XDR-TB) refers to TB isolates that are resistant to isoniazid, rifampin, and fluoroquinolones, as well as capreomycin and/or aminoglycosides.
- Surgical treatment for TB is reserved for patients with MDR-TB or XDR-TB who have:
  - Positive sputum cultures following 6 months of medical therapy.
  - Cases of XDR-TB that are not likely to be cured with medical management alone.
  - Complications, including persistent bronchopleural fistula or life-threatening hemoptysis.

- If surgical intervention is indicated, it is ideally performed following several months of antibiotic therapy and after cultures obtained from a patient no longer produce tuberculosis cell cultures.
  - Surgical intervention for TB is more likely to be successful when performed after culture conversion and with partial lung resections, but not with pneumonectomy.
  - A full course of antituberculosis therapy should be administered postoperatively.
- Several complications can arise from TB, including pericardial effusion, constrictive pericarditis, pleural lesions, hemoptysis, and endobronchial stenosis.
- High levels of adenosine deaminase activity in the pericardial fluid are indicative of TB.
- Standard treatment for TB-related pericardial effusion is drainage, in addition to antibiotic therapy.
- TB can result in constrictive pericarditis, diagnosed by pericardial biopsy; treatment includes pericardiectomy.
- Pleural lesions caused by TB can result in a lymphocyte-rich effusion; diagnosis is made by pleural biopsy, as fluid culture is often nondiagnostic.
  - Treatment includes antibiotic therapy, thoracostomy tube placement for large effusions, and decortication for trapped lung or empyema.
- TB can also result in hemoptysis, leading to cavitary lesions in the lung that can predispose patients to the formation of aspergillomas.
- Although rare, TB can cause endobronchial stenosis from scarring or from extrinsic compression of the airway by involved lymph nodes; treatment includes inhaled corticosteroids and incision and drainage of involved lymph nodes.

Nontuberculous Mycobacterial Infections

- Nontuberculous mycobacterial (NTM) infections include *Mycobacterium avium*, *Mycobacterium intracellulare*, and *Mycobacterium chimaera*; together, these represent the three main species that cause disease in *Mycobacterium avium* complex (MAC).
- NTM infections tend to occur in diseased lungs, women are more commonly affected than men, and they occur predominantly in Caucasian patients.
- Surgical resection of the diseased lung is effective in controlling infection; indications for surgery include:

  - Medically treated patients who fail to convert to negative sputum cultures after 6 months of therapy.
  - Patients with macrolide-resistant disease.
  - Patients with localized cavitary disease.

- Patients with MAC are often malnourished, and preoperative nutrition optimization (albumin >3 g/dL) should be considered prior to surgery.
- Surgery should be performed after sputum cultures are negative, as positive cultures at the time of resection are associated with postoperative complications.
- NTM infections can cause the formation of dense adhesions between parietal and visceral pleural, necessitating extrapleural dissection.
- Depending on the extent of disease, resection may involve lobectomy or pneumonectomy, with complete anatomic resection being the key to success.
- Tissue flaps are often used to attempt to reduce bronchial stump complications, as surgery for mycobacterial infections tend to have higher complication rates compared to resection for other disease processes; rates of persistent bronchopleural fistula are high.

Fungal Infections

- Fungal infections can be divided into those that cause infections in immunocompetent hosts and those that primarily occur in immunocompromised states (Table 17.1).
  - Fungal infections are a frequent complication in lung transplant recipients; fungal infection in a transplanted individual is associated with a mortality rate of greater than 50%.

Table 17.1 Fungal infections of the lung

Fungal infections that infect immuno*competent* hosts	Fungal infections that primarily occur in immuno*compromised* hosts
• Histoplasmosis • Coccidioidomycosis • Blastomycosis • Paracoccidioidomycosis	• Aspergillosis • *Cryptococcus neoformans* • Candidiasis • Mucormycosis • Pneumocystis

Histoplasmosis

- Causative agent is *Histoplasma capsulatum*, a dimorphic fungus: cold (20 °C) = mold, heat (37 °C) = yeast.
- Endemic to Midwestern states located in the Ohio and Mississippi River valleys; transmitted by the inhalation of spores from bat or bird feces.
  - Among endemic mycoses, it is the most common cause for hospitalization.
- Neutrophils and macrophages isolate histoplasmosis without destroying it.
- Acute pulmonary histoplasmosis is often asymptomatic, but may result in a self-limited, flu-like illness; no treatment is required.
- Disseminated histoplasmosis can occur in immunocompromised patients and should be treated with antifungals.
  - Chronic cavitary histoplasmosis occurs in patients with intrinsic lung disease and can mimic TB.
- Definitive diagnosis of histoplasmosis relies on isolation of the organism in culture; positive serology is nondiagnostic, as it can reflect a remote of exposure.
- Indications for surgery include a solitary nodule where cancer cannot be ruled out, pericarditis with effusion due to infection, cavitary disease that is resistant to antifungals, and mediastinal granuloma with obstruction of the mediastinal vessels, esophagus, and bronchi (Fig. 17.2).

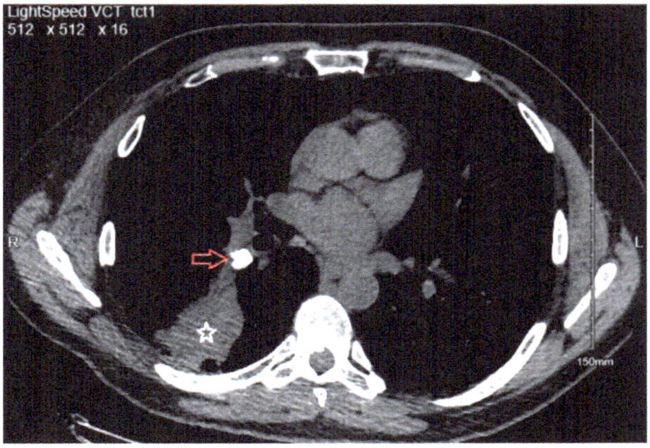

Fig. 17.2 Calcified granulomatous hilar adenopathy (broncholith), obstruction superior segment right lower lobe bronchus (arrow), leading to atelectasis and post-obstructive pneumonia (star)

Coccidioidomycosis

- *Coccidioidomycosis* is the infection caused by the fungi *Coccidioides immitis* and *Coccidioides posadasii*; dimorphic fungi: cold (20 °C) = mold, heat (37 °C) = yeast.
- *Coccidioides* is found in the southwestern United States, including south-central Arizona, the San Joaquin Valley and adjacent areas of California, regions of southern Nevada and Utah, southwestern New Mexico, and western Texas; *Coccidioides* is also endemic to northern Mexico and parts of Central and South America.
- Spores are found in the soil, inhaled, and can result in self-limited acute pneumonia (primary pulmonary coccidioidomycosis, "valley fever") or extrathoracic disseminated infection.
- Majority of patients who develop primary pulmonary infection are either asymptomatic or mildly symptomatic.
  - Symptomatic infection has a similar presentation to pneumonia, with the most common presenting symptoms being fever, cough, and chest pain.
  - Some patients develop systemic symptoms that last for weeks to months, including fevers, drenching night sweats, weight loss, and extreme fatigue.
  - Rheumatologic complaints are common, including symmetric arthralgias ("desert rheumatism") and erythema nodosum, characterized by tender, red bumps that form on the shins, which is a positive prognostic sign of cell-mediated immunity.
- Diagnosis should be made by serology and culture.
- In immunocompetent patients, the disease is self-limited; however, if symptoms persist, treatment with antifungal therapy should be initiated.
- Chronic infection can lead to cavitation or formation of granulomatous nodules; these cavities are often located peripherally and can rupture into the pleural space, resulting in effusion, pneumothorax, empyema, or bronchopleural fistula.
- Surgical intervention may be required for chronic coccidioidomycosis or to differentiate *Coccidioides* nodules from malignancy.

Blastomycosis

- Blastomycosis is the infection caused by the fungi *Blastomyces dermatitidis* or *Blastomyces gilchristii*; dimorphic fungi: cold (20 °C) = mold, heat (37 °C) = yeast.
- Endemic areas include the southeastern and south-central states bordering the Mississippi and Ohio River basins and the Midwestern states and Canadian provinces bordering the Great Lakes.
- Spores in the soil are inhaled, resulting in disease.

- Half of cases are symptomatic, presenting with flu-like illness.
- Like *Histoplasma* and *Coccidioides*, *Blastomyces* also induces a granulomatous reaction.
- *Blastomycosis* can lead to pulmonary blastomycosis, cutaneous blastomycosis (multiple ulcerated skin nodules in disseminated cases), and disseminated blastomycosis (involving the bone and meninges).
- Diagnosis is made by microscopy and DNA-based diagnosis (cultures are time-consuming and serology is often nondiagnostic).
- Mainstay of treatment is antifungals; limited role for surgical intervention, except to rule out malignancy.

Paracoccidioidomycosis

- Dimorphic fungi: cold (20 °C) = mold, heat (37 °C) = yeast
- Endemic to Latin America
- Rarely requires surgical intervention other than for diagnosis

Aspergillosis

- *Aspergillus fumigates* is a fungus found in soil; it is the most common fungal infection in lung transplant recipients.
- Invasive pulmonary aspergillosis is the most severe form and carries a significant mortality rate; it can cause pulmonary infarcts and cavitation with hemoptysis.
- Patients with asthma and cystic fibrosis can have a hypersensitivity reaction to the fungus that results in allergic bronchopulmonary aspergillosis (associated with eosinophilia and elevated IgE elevation).
- Aspergillomas typically form in preexisting cavities, and cross-sectional imaging shows a fungus ball within a thick-walled cavity, sometimes surrounded by a crescent of air (Monod sign) (Fig. 17.3).

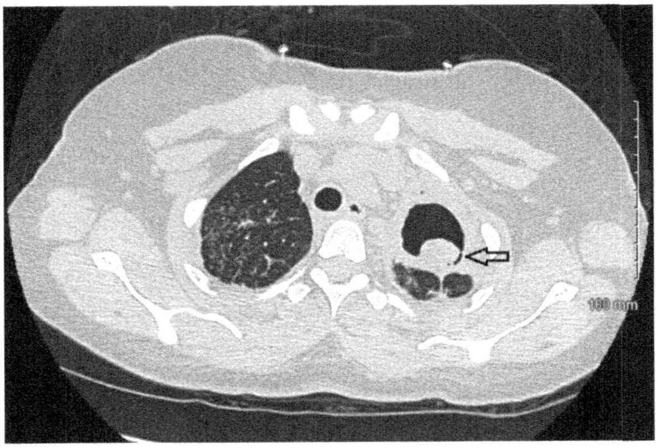

Fig. 17.3 Monod sign: gas that surrounds a mycetoma (most commonly an aspergilloma) in a preexisting pulmonary cavity; implies a freely mobile mass (arrow), which moves on mobilizing the patient and is best demonstrated by acquiring images in a prone position

- Diagnosis is made with a combination of clinical presentation and imaging, as well as positive serology or cultures.
- Asymptomatic aspergillomas should not be treated, as most resolve spontaneously.
- If the patient is symptomatic and a surgical candidate, aspergillomas should be surgically removed.
  - Hemoptysis is the most common symptom of aspergillomas and often responds well to bronchial artery embolization; however, recurrence of bleeding and hemothorax can occur and resection of the mass should be attempted.
- For invasive pulmonary aspergillosis, indications for surgery include failure of medical management, an enlarging fungal mass, hemoptysis, proximity to major vascular structures, and evidence of fungal disease distant from a localized cavity.

Cryptococcus neoformans

- Encapsulated yeast found in pigeon and chicken droppings; transmitted via inhalation.
- *Cryptococcus* induces a granulomatous reaction that forms a nodule or mass that can mimic lung cancer (Fig. 17.4).
- It tends to invade the meninges, especially in patients with impaired immunity (e.g., AIDS).
- Diagnosis relies on microscopy, which shows capsule and narrow budding, as well as cultures.
- If pathology of a lung mass demonstrates *Cryptococcus neoformans*, spinal tap and analysis of CSF should be performed; amphotericin is the treatment of choice if there is evidence of meningitis.

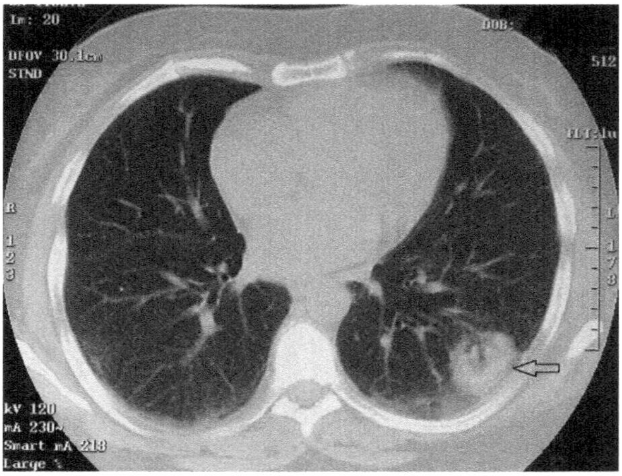

Fig. 17.4 *Cryptococcus neoformans*, left lower lobe (arrow)

Candidiasis

- *Candida* endocarditis is the most common cause of fungal endocarditis and is usually the result of candidemia.
  - Targets patients with prosthetic heart valves, IV drug users, and patients with prolonged candidemia and indwelling venous catheters.
  - Septic emboli are common.
- *Candida* mediastinitis can occur as a complication of thoracic surgery and presents as fever, chest wall erythema and drainage, and sternal instability.
- *Candida* empyema is most often found in patients with malignancies and commonly occurs as a healthcare-associated infection.

Mucormycosis

- Mucormycosis is caused by yeast found in soil that thrive in acidic, hyperglycemic environments.
  - Patients with uncontrolled diabetes (i.e., diabetic ketoacidosis) are particularly susceptible.
  - Other risk factors: corticosteroid use, neutropenia.
- Pulmonary form of disease presents as pneumonia that is refractory to antibiotic treatment.
- Pulmonary mucormycosis causes infarction of lung tissue (Fig. 17.5) and can cause pulmonary artery rupture and hemoptysis, as well as invasion of the chest wall and mediastinum.

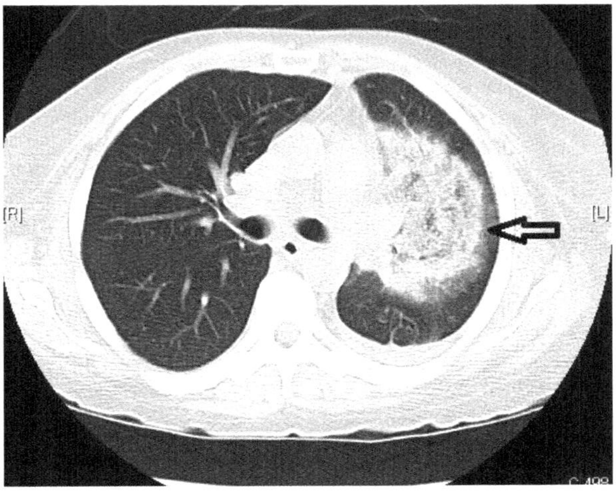

Fig. 17.5 Necrotizing infection from mucormycosis, rapidly destroying the left upper lobe (arrow)

- Diagnosis is made by microscopy; *Mucor* is characterized by broad aseptate hyphae with right-angled projections.
- Treatment includes correction of hyperglycemia, reversal of immunosuppression if possible, granulocyte-macrophage colony-stimulating factor (GM-CSF) if the patient is neutropenic, amphotericin, and immediate, aggressive surgical resection.

Pneumocystis

- *Pneumocystis jirovecii* pneumonia (formerly called *Pneumocystis carinii* pneumonia, PCP) is a yeast-like fungus (originally classified as protozoan).
- In healthy individuals, it is generally asymptomatic.
- *Pneumocystis jirovecii* is the most common opportunistic respiratory infection in patients with AIDS and typically occurs in patients with a CD4 count <200 cells/microL who are not on antiretroviral therapy or appropriate prophylaxis.
- Treatment for *Pneumocystis* is trimethoprim-sulfamethoxazole (TMP/SMX).

Key Reference

- Yu JA, Weyant MJ, Mitchell JD. Surgical treatment of atypical mycobacterial infections. Thorac Surg Clin. 2012;22(3):277–85.

Further Reading

Bradsher. Mycology, pathogenesis, and epidemiology of blastomycosis. In: Kauffman CA, Bogorodskaya M, editors. UpToDate. Waltham, MA: UpToDate; Accessed 26 May 2022.

Cox GM. Mucormycosis (zygomycosis). In: Kauffman CA, Hall KK, editors. UpToDate. Waltham, MA: UpToDate; Accessed 26 May 2022.

Egyud M, Suzuki K. Post-resection complications: abscesses, empyemas, bronchopleural fistulas. J Thorac Dis. 2018;10(Suppl 28):S3408–s3418.

Fox GJ, et al. Surgery as an adjunctive treatment for multidrug-resistant tuberculosis: an individual patient data metaanalysis. Clin Infect Dis. 2016;62(7):887–95.

Kauffman CA. Pathogenesis and clinical features of pulmonary histoplasmosis. In: Baddley JW, Bogorodskaya M, editors. UpToDate. Waltham, MA: UpToDate; Accessed 26 May 2022.

Klompas M. Lung abscess in adults. In: UpToDate, Calderwood SB, Dieffenbach P, Bond S (eds), UpToDate, Waltham, MA; Accessed 26 May 2022.

Limper AH, et al. An official American Thoracic Society statement: treatment of fungal infections in adult pulmonary and critical care patients. Am J Respir Crit Care Med. 2011;183(1):96–128.

Mitchell JD, et al. Anatomic lung resection for nontuberculous mycobacterial disease. Ann Thorac Surg. 2008;85(6):1887–92; discussion 1892–3.

Skiada A, et al. Challenges in the diagnosis and treatment of mucormycosis. Med Mycol. 2018;56(suppl_1):93–101.

Yusen RD, et al. The registry of the International Society for Heart and Lung Transplantation: thirty-third adult lung and heart-lung transplant report-2016; focus theme: primary diagnostic indications for transplant. J Heart Lung Transplant. 2016;35(10):1170–84.

Chapter 18
Congenital Malformations of the Lung

Travis Geraci and T. K. Susheel Kumar

Lung Embryology

The development of the airways and lungs is divided into five stages: embryonic, pseudoglandular, canalicular, saccular, and alveolar. The process occurs from approximately 3 weeks through birth with full maturation occurring around 8 years of age.

- Embryonic stage (3–6 weeks): the primitive foregut produces a respiratory diverticulum, which progresses to form the trachea anteriorly and esophagus posteriorly. The bronchial buds form from the primitive trachea.
- Pseudoglandular stage (5–17 weeks): generation and branching of the bronchial tree.
- Canalicular stage (16–25 weeks): division of the conducting airways and the respiratory units. Extensive angiogenesis creates a dense capillary bed.
- Saccular stage (24 weeks to birth): expansion of the gas-exchange surface area with creation of the saccular terminal units of the lungs. Pulmonary surfactant production begins.
- Alveolar stage (36 weeks–8 years): the final division of saccular units to alveoli.

T. Geraci (✉)
Division of Thoracic Surgery, Department of Cardiothoracic Surgery, New York University Langone Health, New York, NY, USA
e-mail: travis.geraci@nyulangone.org

T. K. S. Kumar
Division of Pediatric and Adult Congenital Cardiothoracic Surgery, Department of Cardiothoracic Surgery, New York University Langone Health, New York, NY, USA
e-mail: tksusheel.kumar@nyulangone.org

T. Ng, T. Geraci (eds.), *Thoracic Surgery Clerkship*, Contemporary Surgical Clerkships, https://doi.org/10.1007/978-3-031-44645-0_18

Congenital Pulmonary Airway Malformation (CPAM)

Congenital pulmonary airway malformations are developmental defects of the lower respiratory tract with cystic and/or adenomatous pulmonary lesions (hamartomatous lesions) of variable size and distribution.

- Result from abnormal branching morphogenesis of the lung.
- Incidence: 1 per 10–35,000 births (most common congenital lung lesion).
- Lesions occur sporadically without a known genetic predisposition or maternal factors.

Anatomy

- Arise from the tracheal, bronchial, or alveolar tissues.
- Equal distribution between the right and left lungs.
- Typically limited to a single lobe, but may infrequently involve multiple lobes.
- Lesions have a pulmonary arterial supply; connections to systemic vessels are rare.
- Cysts can be small (< 0.5 cm) to massive (> 10 cm) involving the entire lung lobe.
- Typically, they do not communicate with the tracheobronchial tree.

Stocker's Classification

- Type 0 (1–3%).
  - Arise from the trachea or bronchial tissues.
  - Small (< 0.5 cm), diffuse cystic lesions that replace the entire lung.
  - Lung function is severely affected typically resulting in death at birth.
- Type 1 (60–70%).
  - Arise from the distal bronchi and/or proximal bronchioles.
  - Cysts are typically single, but may be multiple.
  - Limited malignant potential.
- Type 2 (15–20%).
  - Multiple small cysts (2 cm), often with solid tissue elements.
  - Associated with other congenital anomalies.
- Type 3 (5–10%).

- Large cysts (> 5 cm) with solid tissue elements (may be entirely solid).
- Lung function is severely affected typically resulting in death in the neonatal period.

- Type 4 (5–10%).
  - Large cysts (> 5 cm) arising from acinar tissue.
  - May occupy the entire lung lobe.
  - Significant risk of malignant degeneration, most commonly associated with pleuropulmonary blastoma.

Presentation

- Variable presentation dependent on type, size, and number of cystic lesions.
- Prenatal period.
  - Commonly identified on prenatal ultrasound.
  - Fetal hydrops may develop from compression of the adjacent heart or vena cava.
- Neonatal period.
  - Twenty-five percent are symptomatic at birth: abnormal breathing, hypoxia, tachypnea, and respiratory distress.
- Childhood period.
  - Approximately one-third of CPAMs are diagnosed in childhood.
  - May present with symptoms (cough, dyspnea), recurrent pneumonia, or pneumothorax (cystic rupture).

Imaging

- Most commonly visualized as single or multiple air-filled cysts, but may have solid tissue components (Type 3 may be completely solid).
- Prenatal ultrasound.
  - CPAM volume ratio (CVR) evaluates cyst size to fetal head size and provides a prognostic index.
  - A limited number of lesions resolve during gestation.
- Chest radiograph (CXR).
  - Obtained in all neonates with a prenatal diagnosis of CPAM.

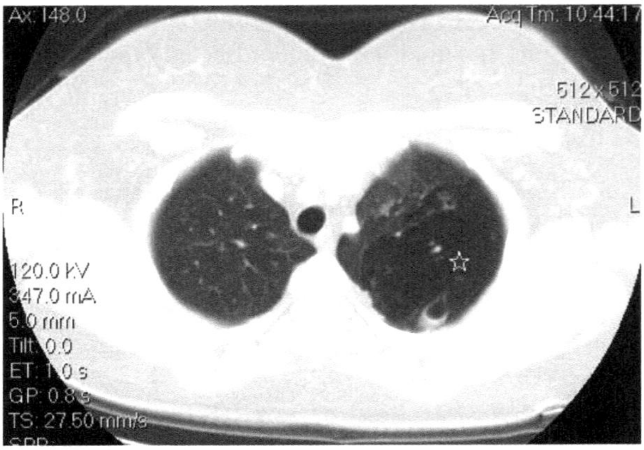

Fig. 18.1 CT scan images of a left upper lobe congenital pulmonary airway malformation, showing a cystic lesion replacing the left upper lobe (star)

- Magnetic resonance imaging (MRI) or computed tomography (CT) scan (Fig. 18.1).
  - Obtained in symptomatic neonates.
  - Used to distinguish between other anomalies (such as bronchopulmonary sequestration or congenital lobar emphysema).

Management

- Prenatal:
  - Assess for other congenital abnormalities.
  - Serial ultrasound studies to monitor for progression of disease and/or development of fetal hydrops.
  - Pleuroamniotic shunts can be performed to drain the cysts.
- Postnatal:
  - Symptomatic lesions are treated by surgical resection; typically patients undergo a pulmonary lobectomy.
  - Although there is some controversy, prophylactic surgical resection (to reduce risk of complication, infection, or malignant degeneration) may be preferred over observation for asymptomatic lesions.
- Long-term outcomes following successful resection are excellent.

Bronchopulmonary Sequestration

A bronchopulmonary sequestration is abnormal parenchymal lung tissue that lacks communication with the tracheobronchial tree and has irregular pulmonary arterial vasculature (typically, from the systemic circulation). Pulmonary sequestrations are classified as intralobar or extralobar.

Intralobar Sequestration (Fig. 18.2a–c)

- Abnormal lung tissue located within a normal lung lobe; does not have a visceral pleura.
- Most common form (75–90%) of sequestration.
- Most common in lower lobes; left more common than right.

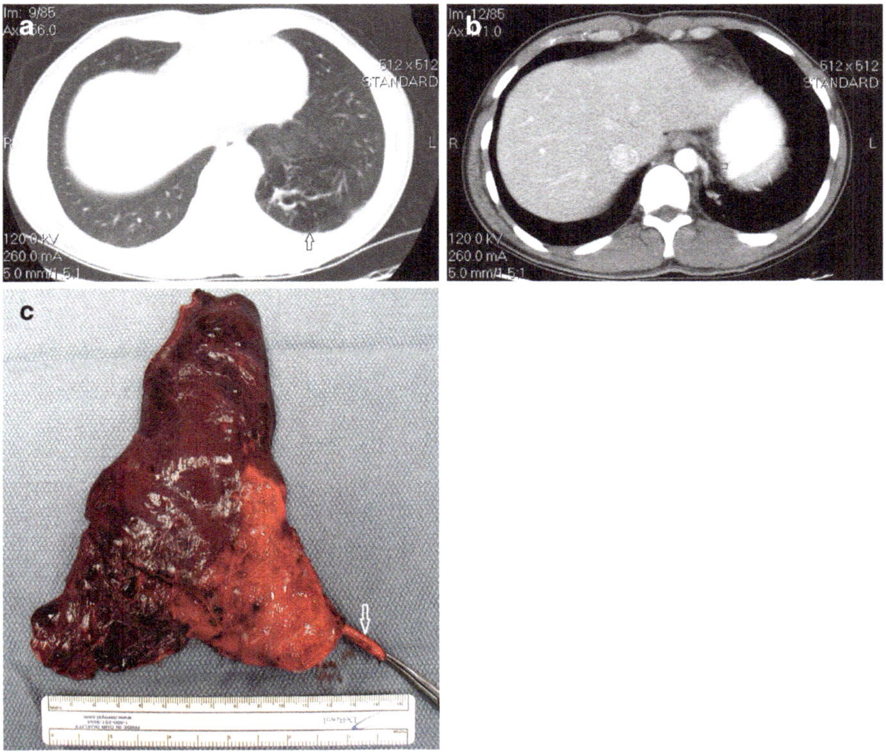

Fig. 18.2 Intralobar sequestration. (**a**) CT scan shows partially cystic lesion in the posterior-inferior aspect of the left lower lobe (arrow); (**b**) CT angiogram showing systemic artery supply from the aorta (arrow); (**c**) resected specimen showing ligated systemic artery off the aorta (arrow)

- Typically (90%) do not have a bronchial connection to the airway. Only rarely present as pores of Kohn.
- Arterial supply from branches of the descending thoracic aorta.
- Venous drainage is usually normal, to the pulmonary veins or left atrium.
- Rarely, have an anomalous connection to the gastrointestinal tract (also known as a bronchopulmonary foregut malformation).

Extralobar Sequestration (Fig. 18.3a, b)

- Abnormal lung tissue that is separated from the remaining lung by its own visceral pleural investment.
- Most commonly occur inferior to the left lower lobe, above the hemidiaphragm; they rarely can arise below the diaphragm.
- Arterial supply from branches of the descending thoracic or abdominal aorta.
- Venous drainage is typically abnormal, to the azygous or hemiazygous vein, right atrium, vena cava, or portal vein.
- Rarely, there are fistulous connections to the esophagus.
- Associated with other congenital anomalies: diaphragmatic hernia, pericardial defects, anomalous pulmonary venous drainage.

Presentation

- Variable presentation dependent on type, size, and anatomy.
- Prenatal period.
  - Homogeneous echogenic thoracic mass of variable size.
  - Lesions may remain stable or regress over gestation.

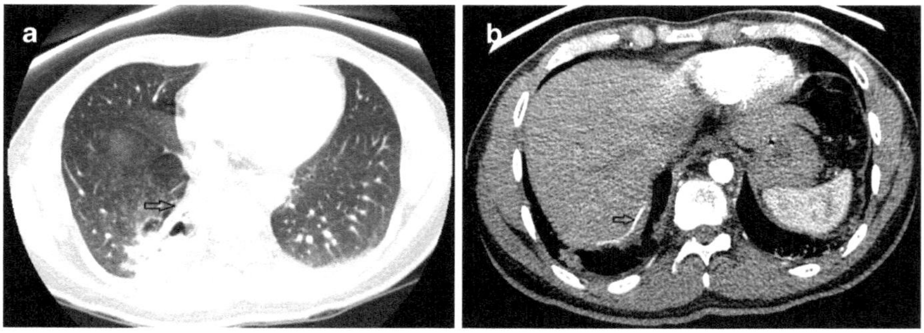

Fig. 18.3 Extralobar sequestration. (**a**) CT scan shows cystic/solid lesion in the posterior inferior thorax with its own pleura (arrow); (**b**) CT angiogram showing systemic arterial supply (arrow) which eventually leads to the abdominal aorta

- Neonatal period.
  - Large lesions (> 20% of the hemithorax) may be symptomatic.
- Childhood and older period.
  - Most common presentation is recurrent pneumonia (more common in intralobar sequestration) and hemoptysis.

Imaging

- CXR: triangular dense mass, typically in or adjacent to the lower lobes.
- CT scan: soft tissue density; may have cystic changes (Figs. 18.2a and 18.3a).
- CT angiography: can demonstrate the aberrant vascular arterial supply and venous drainage if present (not typically visualized on non-contrast CT) (Figs. 18.2b and 18.3b).

Management

- Symptomatic:
  - Lobectomy or segmentectomy with inclusion of the sequestration.
  - All vessels must be identified and ligated (Fig. 18.2c); preoperative embolization of large arterial vessels may reduce the risk of perioperative bleeding.
- Asymptomatic:
  - There is no definitive guideline for observation versus surgical intervention, but surgical resection may be preferred to prevent future complications.

Foregut Cysts: Bronchogenic and Esophageal

Abnormal development of the tracheobronchial tissue from the foregut may result in closed cystic spaces lined by bronchial or esophageal mucosa. Bronchogenic cysts are foregut malformations that can arise at any location throughout the tracheobronchial anatomy. When these cysts form adjacent or within the esophageal wall, they are lined with esophageal epithelium and are termed esophageal duplication cysts.

Anatomy

- There are two major forms, mediastinal and parenchymal, although they may manifest in other locations such as the inferior pulmonary ligament, retroperitoneum, and neck.
- Cystic structure (typically single) lined with respiratory or esophageal epithelium. Often filled with fluid or mucous.
- No communication with the tracheobronchial tree or esophagus.
- Rare case reports of malignant tissue in the cyst wall.

Presentation

- Mostly asymptomatic and discovered as incidental findings.
- May become symptomatic in infancy throughout adulthood and result from compression of adjacent structures or secondary infection.
- Symptoms: cough, chest discomfort, dyspnea, wheezing (misdiagnosis of asthma), dysphagia, fever.

Imaging

- CXR (Fig. 18.4a and b) or CT (Fig. 18.5a and b): round, low-density, homogeneous, well-circumscribed lesions, may have air-fluid levels.

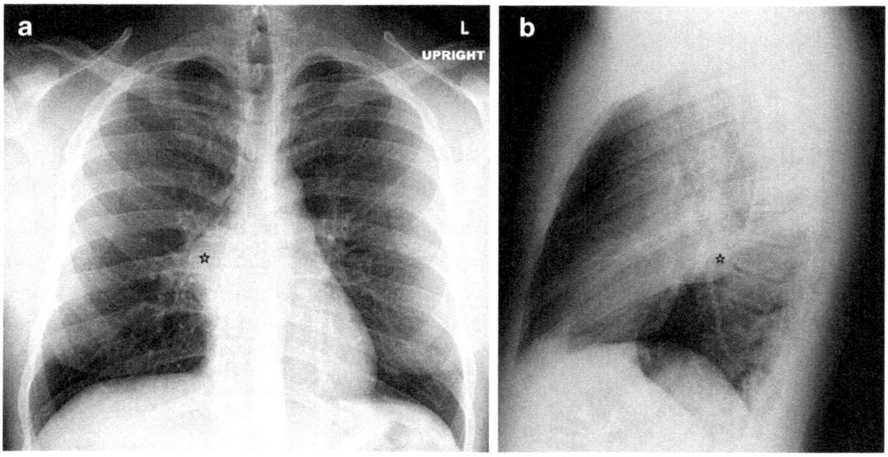

Fig. 18.4 Chest radiograph of bronchogenic cyst, showing a well-circumscribed mediastinal lesion (star). (**a**) Posterior-anterior view; (**b**) lateral view

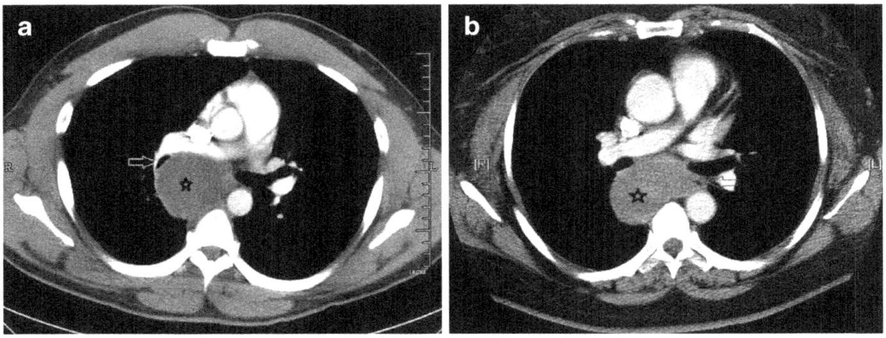

Fig. 18.5 CT scan of foregut cysts showing low-density, homogenous, and well-circumscribed lesions (star). (**a**) Bronchogenic cyst in the subcarinal position, compressing the bronchus intermedius (arrow); (**b**) esophageal duplication cyst compressing the esophagus (arrow)

Fig. 18.6 Barium esophagram showing smooth lesion compressing the esophagus (arrow)

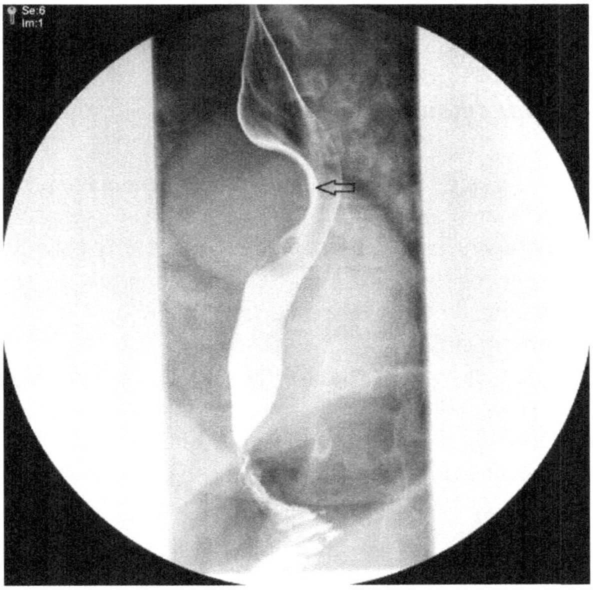

- Esophagram (Fig. 18.6): may show esophageal compression from an extrinsic or intramural cyst.
- MRI (Fig. 18.7): bright lesion on T2-weighted images confirms the fluid-filled cystic nature.
- Endoscopic ultrasound or endobronchial ultrasound: can confirm cystic nature; if this is the case, then avoid needle biopsy or aspiration as this can introduce infection.

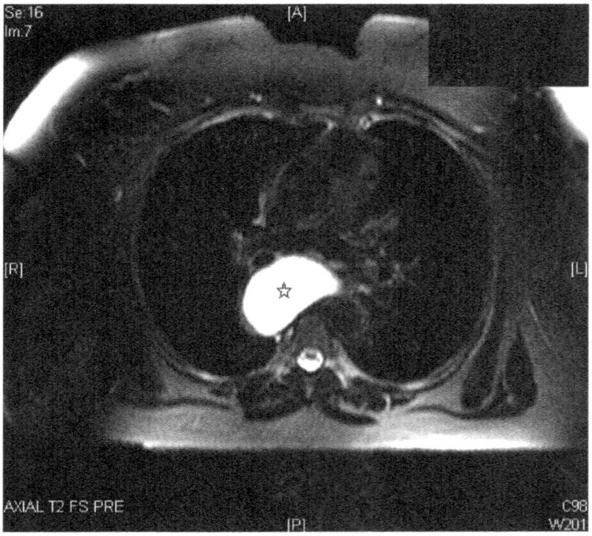

Fig. 18.7 MRI of esophageal duplication cyst shows the lesion to be completely bright on T2-weighted image (star), confirming its fluid-filled cystic nature

Management

- Surgical resection is indicated in symptomatic patients.
- Although there may be some controversy, asymptomatic patients may be observed, especially in high-risk or elderly patients; for young healthy patients, resection to prevent future complications can be considered.
- Minimally invasive approach (thoracoscopic or robotic) for resection is preferred over open.
- Bronchogenic cysts: attempt complete resection; however if part of the cyst is densely adherent to vital structures, then resect all, but leaving the adherent portion behind, ablating the residual lining mechanically, chemically, or with energy.
- Esophageal duplication cysts: resect by enucleation, leaving underlying mucosa intact, closing the muscle layer over. There is no indication for esophageal resection.

Congenital Lobar Emphysema

Congenital lobar emphysema is an anomalous hyperinflation of the pulmonary parenchyma, most commonly attributed to compression of a developing airway.

- Rare pulmonary malformation (10% of thoracic congenital malformations).
- Male predominance (3:1).

- The lung tissue is normal, although it may have an increased number of alveoli, but the airspaces are enlarged/overinflated.
- The pulmonary vasculature to the affected lobe is preserved.

Anatomy

- Extrinsic compression (most common): thoracic mass or cyst, pulmonary vascular malformation, congenital heart diseases such as tetralogy of Fallot or pulmonary stenosis associated with pulmonary artery dilation.
- Intrinsic compression ("ball-valve" obstruction phenomenon): abnormal bronchial cartilage, bronchomalacia, mucous or meconium plugging, redundant tissue/mucosa.
- In approximately 50% of cases, a definitive obstruction cannot be identified.
- Large regions of emphysema may cause mediastinal shift.
- Typically affects a single lobe. Upper lobes more affected than the lower lobes. The left upper lobe is the most common location (40–50%).

Presentation

- May become symptomatic infancy through adulthood.
- Symptoms: cough, chest discomfort, dyspnea, wheezing (misdiagnosis of asthma).
- Mistaken for pneumothorax.

Investigation

- Prenatal US or MRI may establish the diagnosis.
- CXR (Fig. 18.8a) or CT scan (Fig. 18.8b and c): hyperinflated lobe with compression of the remaining lung and mediastinal shift to the contralateral side due to the hyperinflation.
- CT scan can rule out extrinsic causes.
- Bronchoscopy in the stable patient, to rule out endobronchial lesion and to assess bronchial wall quality.

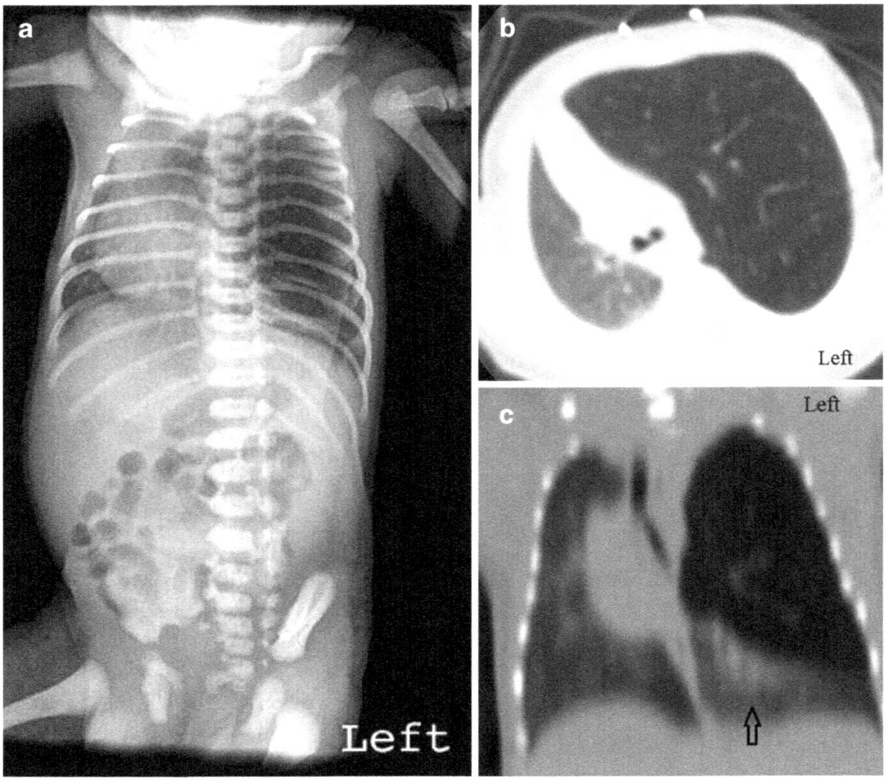

Fig. 18.8 Congenital lobar emphysema. (**a**) Plain radiograph showing hyperinflation of the lung in the left lung with mediastinal shift to the right and compression of the right lung; (**b**) CT scan axial view showing hyperinflation of the left upper lobe with mediastinal shift and compression of the right lung; (**c**) CT scan coronal view showing hyperinflation of the left upper lobe with compression of the left lower lobe (arrow), mediastinal shift, and compression of the right lung

Management

- Close observation is an option for mildly symptomatic patients; otherwise surgical is indicated.
- Resection is often by thoracotomy as minimally invasive approaches are difficult in this disease.
- Extent of resection is by lobectomy, less commonly segmentectomy, to entirely resect the diseased lung.
- Surgeon must be aware that emergent thoracotomy may be needed during induction of anesthesia as hyperinflation and mediastinal shift can worsen to cause hemodynamic compromise.
- Good long-term prognosis.

Pulmonary Arteriovenous Malformation

A pulmonary arteriovenous malformation (PAVM) is an abnormal direct communication between the pulmonary artery and pulmonary vein without traversing an intervening capillary system. The vascular connection allows blood to return directly to the heart creating a right-to-left shunt. In bypassing the pulmonary circulation, a varying degree of cyanosis may occur.

- Developmental abnormality of the pulmonary vascular terminal capillary loops.
- Strongly associated with hereditary hemorrhagic telangiectasia (HHT, also known as Osler-Weber-Rendu syndrome) with multiple sites of involvement.
- The majority are congenital; however, PAVM may also be acquired (hepatic cirrhosis, chest trauma, postsurgical such as Fontan patients).

Anatomy

- Typically only one (PAVM) is present (90%), most commonly located in the lower lobes.
- The majority of PAVM have a single feeding artery (90%). Lesions with multiple feeding arteries are considered "complex."
- Lesions progress in size over time; rare regression.

Presentation

- Prenatal US or MRI: Large/growing lesions may cause esophageal compression leading to polyhydramnios. Compression of the heart or great vessels may lead to cardiac failure. Compression of the surrounding lung tissue may lead to pulmonary hypoplasia.
- Asymptomatic (60%), found incidentally on postnatal chest imaging.
- Symptomatic:
  - Respiratory: dyspnea, hemoptysis, hypoxemia, hemothorax.
  - Symptoms related to HHT: cutaneous telangiectasias, epistaxis, gastrointestinal bleeding, central nervous system symptoms.
  - Secondary to anomalous vascular connection: paradoxical embolization, stroke, or brain abscess.

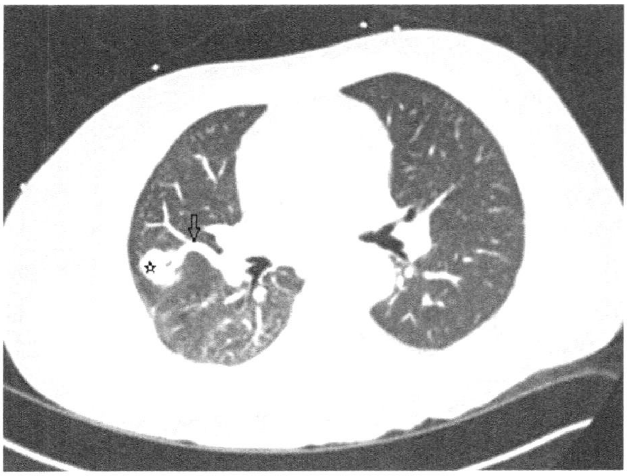

Fig. 18.9 CT scan of pulmonary arteriovenous malformation, showing a smooth well-demarcated lesion (star) with a clear feeding arterial vessel (arrow)

Imaging

- Prenatal US or MRI: May establish the diagnosis.
- CXR or CT scan (Fig. 18.9): Smooth, demarcated, round or oval mass with a clear feeding artery, draining vein often not visualized. May be difficult to differentiate from a cancerous nodule.
- CT angiography: Used to confirm diagnosis and further define vascular communication.
- Transthoracic contrast echocardiography ("bubble echocardiography").
- Tests for presence of (PAVM)-associated right-to-left shunt.

Management

- Asymptomatic: observation is an option if feeding artery less than 2 mm; however intervention can be considered to prevent future complications for all asymptomatic patients who are good candidates.
- Symptomatic:
  - Embolization.

    Often preferred as it is less invasive than surgery, especially if there are multiple PAVMs.

    Low risk of complication: pulmonary infarction, pleural reaction, systemic embolization.

    Risk of (PAVM) recurrence (persistent perfusion, missed feeding artery, recanalization, migration of embolic material) with possible development of complications due to the recurrent PAVM.

    Procedure may be repeated for failure/recurrence.

– Surgical resection.

Most definitive treatment, but results in pulmonary parenchymal loss of varying degrees.
May be considered for single PAVM.
Indicated if embolization not successful or unavailable.
Can be performed by minimally invasive approaches (thoracoscopy or robotic) for excision, wedge resection, segmentectomy, or lobectomy as indicated.

Tracheoesophageal Fistula

A tracheoesophageal fistula (TEF) is a congenital malformation connecting the trachea and esophagus, with various anatomic configurations.

- Incidence: 1 in 2500–4000 births.
- Associated with esophageal atresia.
- Associated with VACTERL (vertebral defects, imperforate anus, cardiac anomalies, TEF, renal anomalies, and limb defects) and CHARGE syndrome (coloboma, heart defects, atresia choanae, growth retardation, genital abnormalities, and ear abnormalities).

Anatomy (Fig. 18.10)

- Type A: Esophageal atresia without TEF.
- Types B, C (most common 85%), D: Esophageal atresia with proximal (B), distal (C), or proximal and distal (D) TEF.
- Type E: TEF without esophageal atresia; fistula is typically in the neck.

Presentation

- Prenatal: Polyhydramnios commonly occurs in patients with esophageal atresia as the fetus is unable to swallow amniotic fluid.
- Neonatal: Respiratory symptoms, difficulty feeding, gastric air distention, aspiration pneumonia.
- Small defects may present months to years after birth.
- Symptoms and signs unrelated to TEF, associated with other congenital defects and syndromes.

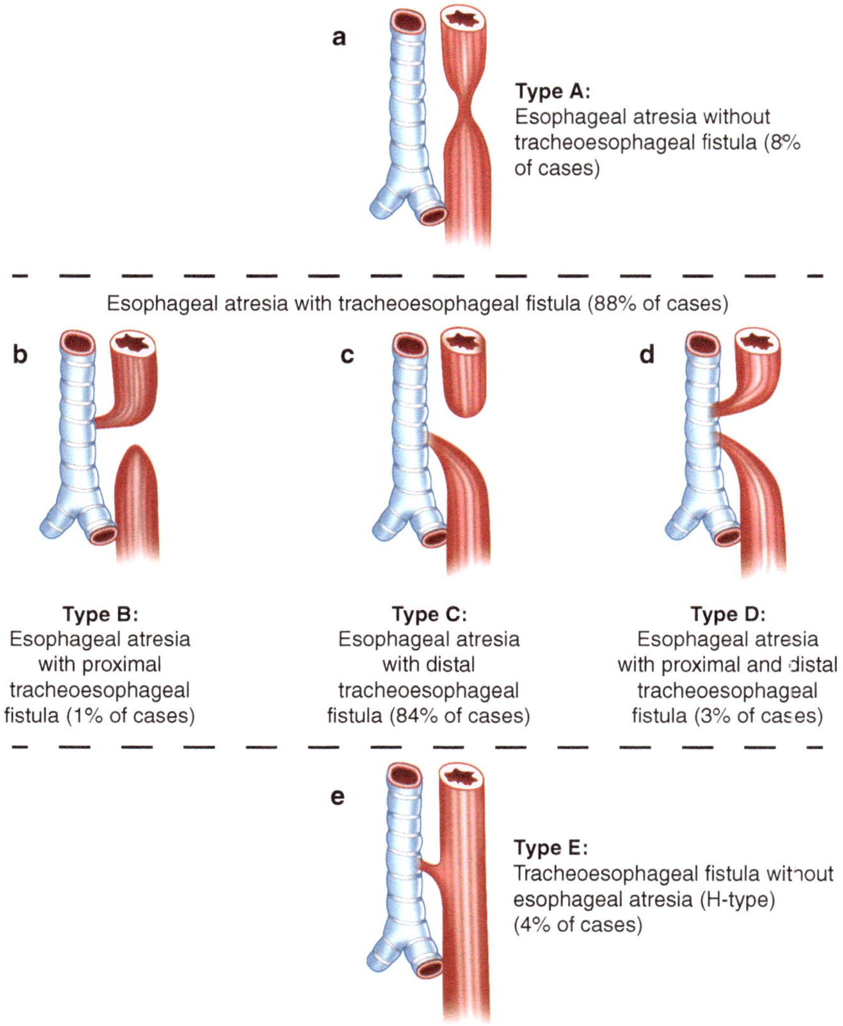

Fig. 18.10 Types of tracheoesophageal fistula

Diagnosis

- Esophageal atresia can be investigated by attempting to place a nasogastric tube, which, if present, may not be able to be passed and may be seen coiled in the proximal esophagus on imaging.
- Contrast can be injected into the nasoesophageal tube and assessed under fluoroscopic imaging to detail the anatomy of the esophageal pouch.
- Bronchoscopy is often used to diagnose proximal fistulae.

Management

- Surgical ligation of the fistula with or without repair of the trachea (as needed) and primary anastomosis of the separated esophageal segments.
- Access is typically via a muscle-sparing posterior right thoracotomy. A minimally invasive approach may be appropriate for patients with a short-gap esophageal atresia.
- If the esophageal segments are too distant to repair ("long-gap esophageal atresia," typically greater than 2 cm between esophageal segments), surgery is delayed to allow for growth. If excessive gap between esophageal segments persists despite growth, lengthening procedures by traction or myotomy or alternative conduits such as the stomach or jejunum may be utilized.
- Proton pump inhibitors are given in the postoperative period to reduce reflux attributed to impaired esophageal peristalsis.

Surgical Complications

- Anastomotic stricture (35–60%): Risk factors for stricture include long-gap esophageal atresia, tension and ischemia at the anastomosis, and postoperative anastomotic leak. Initial management is with serial esophageal dilations. Recalcitrant strictures may require steroid injections or, rarely, surgical resection with reconstruction.
- Anastomotic leak (10–20%): Initial management is with chest tube drainage and cessation of oral feeding. Surgical exploration and washout is indicated for patients with large fluid collections or sepsis.
- Recurrent TEF (5–10%): Requires reoperative surgical repair.

Key Reference

- Baird R, Puligandla PS, Laberge JM. Congenital lung malformations: informing best practice. Semin Pediatr Surg. 2014; 23:270.

Further Reading

Abbey P, Das CJ, Pangtey GS, et al. Imaging in bronchopulmonary sequestration. J Med Imaging Radiat Oncol. 2009;53:22.

Baird R, Lal DR, Ricca RL, et al. Management of long gap esophageal atresia: a systematic review and evidence-based guidelines from the APSA outcomes and evidence based practice committee. J Pediatr Surg. 2019;54:675.

Cassina M, Ruol M, Pertile R, et al. Prevalence, characteristics, and survival of children with esophageal atresia: a 32-year population-based study including 1,417,724 consecutive newborns. Birth Defects Res A Clin Mol Teratol. 2016;106:542.

Cottin V, Chinet T, Lavolé A, et al. Pulmonary arteriovenous malformations in hereditary hemorrhagic telangiectasia: a series of 126 patients. Medicine (Baltimore). 2007;86:1.

Gezer S, Taştepe I, Sirmali M, et al. Pulmonary sequestration: a single-institutional series composed of 27 cases. J Thorac Cardiovasc Surg. 2007;133:955.

Kapralik J, Wayne C, Chan E, Nasr A. Surgical versus conservative management of congenital pulmonary airway malformation in children: a systematic review and meta-analysis. J Pediatr Surg. 2016;51:508.

Nagano M, Ichinose J, Sasabuchi Y, Nakajima J, Yasunaga H. Surgery versus percutaneous transcatheter embolization for pulmonary arteriovenous malformation: analysis of a national inpatient database in Japan. J Thorac Cardiovasc Surg. 2017;154(3):1137–43.

Orford J, Cass DT, Glasson MJ. Advances in the treatment of oesophageal atresia over three decades: the 1970s and the 1990s. Pediatr Surg Int. 2004;20:402.

Pollak JS, Saluja S, Thabet A, et al. Clinical and anatomic outcomes after embolotherapy of pulmonary arteriovenous malformations. J Vasc Interv Radiol. 2006;17:35.

Swendiman RA, Nance ML. Pediatric mediastinal tumors. In: Darling GE, Baumgartner WA, Jacobs JP, editors. Pearson's general thoracic surgery. STS cardiothoracic surgery e-book. Chicago, IL: Society of Thoracic Surgeons; 2022; ebook.sts.org. Accessed 13 Dec 2022.

Taghavi K, Tan Tanny SP, Hawley A, et al. H-type congenital tracheoesophageal fistula: insights from 70 years of the Royal Children's Hospital experience. J Pediatr Surg. 2021;56:686.

Tander B, Yalçin M, Yilmaz B, et al. Congenital lobar emphysema: a clinicopathologic evaluation of 14 cases. Eur J Pediatr Surg. 2003;13:108.

Thakral CL, Maji DC, Sajwani MJ. Congenital lobar emphysema: experience with 21 cases. Pediatr Surg Int. 2001;17:88.

Van Raemdonck D, De Boeck K, Devlieger H, et al. Pulmonary sequestration: a comparison between pediatric and adult patients. Eur J Cardiothorac Surg. 2001;19:388.

Wong HH, Chan RP, Klatt R, Faughnan ME. Idiopathic pulmonary arteriovenous malformations: clinical and imaging characteristics. Eur Respir J. 2011;38:368.

Chapter 19
Chronic Obstructive Pulmonary Disease

Travis Geraci and Andrew J. DeMaio

Chronic Obstructive Pulmonary Disease

Chronic obstructive pulmonary disease (COPD) encompasses a number of pulmonary disorders, which are unified by chronic respiratory symptoms and airflow limitation. Persistent airway inflammation is central to its pathogenesis, which results in a progressive decline in pulmonary function and exacerbations of respiratory symptoms:

- COPD is the third leading cause of death in the United States and its prevalence is increasing worldwide.
- Approximately 10% of people over age 40 have COPD.
- COPD is a chronic, progressive lung disease accentuated by exacerbations in which treatment is both acute and lifelong.
- Although COPD has been classically described as a relentlessly progressive lung disease, a subgroup of patients may have pulmonary function which stabilizes (or rarely improves) over time.

T. Geraci (✉)
Division of Thoracic Surgery, Department of Cardiothoracic Surgery, New York University Langone Health, New York, NY, USA
e-mail: travis.geraci@nyulangone.org

A. J. DeMaio
Division of Pulmonary, Critical Care and Sleep Medicine, New York University Langone Health, New York, NY, USA
e-mail: andrew.demaio@nyulangone.org

T. Ng, T. Geraci (eds.), *Thoracic Surgery Clerkship*, Contemporary Surgical Clerkships, https://doi.org/10.1007/978-3-031-44645-0_19

Pathogenesis of COPD

- The airways and lung parenchyma mount an inflammatory response to an inhaled irritant, most commonly cigarette smoke, resulting in damage and remodeling of affected tissues.
  - Worldwide, only about 50% of COPD is due to cigarette smoking.
  - Other potential causes include air pollution, environmental tobacco smoke, and occupational exposures.
- Chronic inflammation leads to destruction of terminal airways and loss of elastic recoil of the lungs and increased airway resistance, both of which contribute to airflow limitation.
- Long-standing airway obstruction and remodeling leads to hyperinflation and abnormal respiratory mechanics including depression of the diaphragms, which further increase work of breathing and dyspnea.
- Further destruction of terminal airways and lung parenchyma reduces capacity for gas exchange, which can lead to chronic hypoxic and hypercapneic respiratory failure in advanced disease.
- Only about 20% of cigarette smokers develop COPD, suggesting that there are genetic components which are associated with its development.
- Alpha-1-antitrypsin deficiency is the best characterized genetic risk factor for COPD.
  - Alpha-1-antitrypsin inhibits neutrophil elastase which can degrade structural proteins of the lung if unopposed.

COPD is a heterogeneous disease with disease manifestations in both small airways (bronchitis/bronchiolitis) and lung parenchyma (emphysema):

- *Chronic bronchitis* is characterized by chronic mucus hypersecretion from gland hyperplasia and/or hypertrophy, resulting in a chronic productive cough:
  - The classic "blue bloater" phenotype describes an overweight patient with severe hypoxemia and hypercarbia, secondary polycythemia, and right heart failure (cor pulmonale).
- *Emphysema* is defined as non-fibrotic parenchymal destruction of the lungs from enlargement of the airspaces distal to the terminal bronchioles:
  - The classic "pink puffer" phenotype describes a thin patient with breathlessness, hyperinflation, and mild hypoxemia.
- Emphysema may also be classified radiographically based on the location in which it occurs, as this has diagnostic and prognostic implications:
  - Centrilobular emphysema is defined by abnormal destruction of the respiratory bronchiole and is most commonly associated with COPD from inhaled irritants.

- Panlobular emphysema refers to destruction of all parts of the secondary respiratory lobule. This is most commonly described in cases of alpha-1-antitrypsin deficiency.
- Paraseptal emphysema describes dilation and/or destruction of the alveolar ducts.

Clinical Presentation and Diagnosis

- Symptoms: Dyspnea, cough (often productive), wheezing, exercise intolerance.
- Coexistent disease states: Cardiovascular disease, pulmonary hypertension, coronary artery disease, lung cancer, anxiety, depression.
- Risk factors: Cigarette smoking, occupational inhalational exposures, asthma, genetics (alpha-1-antitrypsin deficiency), reduced developmental lung maturity.
- Radiography.
  - Chest radiograph may demonstrate hyperinflated lungs with a depressed diaphragm, emphysema, or regions of atelectasis from mucous impaction, especially in severe disease (Fig. 19.1). Mild disease may demonstrate normal chest radiography.
  - Chest computed tomography (CT) may demonstrate airway disease, define regions of emphysema, or identify concomitant pulmonary nodules.

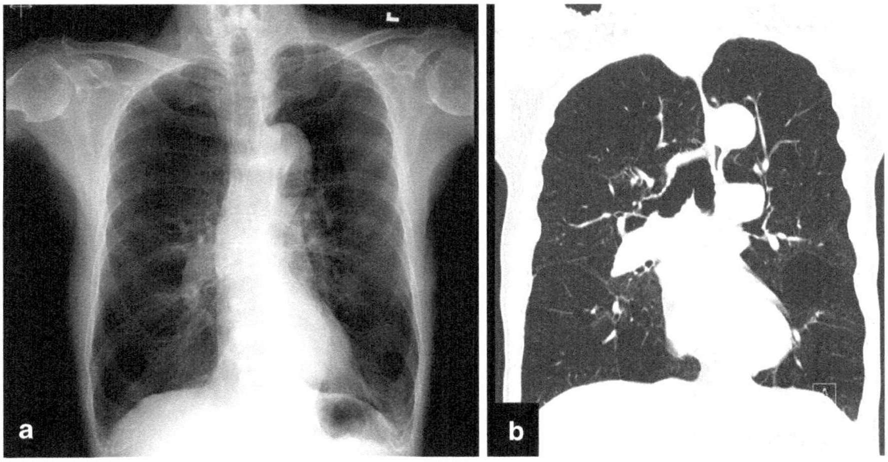

Fig. 19.1 A patient with advanced emphysematous COPD revealing diffuse hyperinflation of the lungs, increased lucency of lung fields, and depression/flattening of the diaphragms. (**a**) Anteroposterior chest radiography; (**b**) coronal CT image

Spirometry

- Required for the diagnosis of COPD based on Global Initiative for Chronic Obstructive Lung Disease (GOLD) guidelines:
  - GOLD classification requires FEV1/FVC < 0.7 *after administration of inhaled bronchodilator* to establish the diagnosis of COPD.
  - The FEV1 is then used to determine severity of airflow obstruction.

GOLD 1	Mild	FEV1 ≥ 80% predicted
GOLD 2	Moderate	FEV1 50–79% predicted
GOLD 3	Severe	FEV1 30–49% predicted
GOLD 4	Very severe	FEV1 < 30% predicted

- Forced expiratory volume in 1 s (FEV1) is associated with disease severity, symptoms, and clinical outcomes including overall survival:
  - FEV1 declines approximately 30 mL per year but is variable.
  - Risk factors for accelerated decline include ongoing tobacco use, emphysema, and bronchodilator reversibility.
- BODE index is used as a prognostic indicator:
  - Combines body mass index (BMI), FEV1, Medical Research Council Dyspnea Score, and 6-min walk test.
  - Points are assigned to each component assessment, and the aggregate score is correlated to a 52-month survival rate.

Medical Management

- All patients should have the following interventions as they have been shown to reduce mortality in COPD:
  - Smoking cessation.
  - Vaccination (influenza and pneumococcal).
  - Supplemental oxygen if SpO_2 < 88% on ambient air.
- Inhalers may improve symptoms and reduce exacerbation frequency but do not affect mortality.
- Any ongoing triggers or inhaled irritants should be identified and minimized.
- GOLD guidelines for pharmacologic therapy:
  - Group A: mild symptoms short-acting and/or long-acting bronchodilator.

- Group B: moderate/severe symptoms dual long-acting bronchodilators (long-acting beta-agonists (LABA) + long-acting muscarinic antagonists (LAMA)), ideally as a combination inhaler.
- Group E (formerly group C + D): characterized by frequent exacerbations dual inhaled bronchodilator (LAMA + LABA); consider LAMA+LABA+inhaled corticosteroids if eosinophils >300.

Smoking Cessation

- Greatest impact on clinical outcomes in patients who continue to smoke.
- Associated with a reduced mortality and rate of decline of lung function.
- The success of behavioral modifications and/or medications for nicotine addiction are limited with long-term cessation rates generally less than 25%.

Pulmonary Rehabilitation

- Pulmonary rehabilitation includes breathing and physical exercise testing and training, nutritional optimization, and disease education.
- Improves symptoms, exercise capacity, and quality of life across all grades of COPD.
- Longer courses of treatment (greater than 6 weeks) generally confer a superior clinical benefit.

Inhaled Bronchodilators

- Bronchodilators provide symptom relief by increasing expiratory airflow, reducing hyperinflation, and increasing exercise capacity.
- Inhaled bronchodilators, including LABA and LAMA, are the primary inhaled therapy for COPD.
- All patients should have a short-acting bronchodilator (e.g., albuterol) for use as a rescue inhaler in case of dyspnea or wheezing.
- Adverse effects are often minor (tachycardia, urinary retention).
- Inhaler therapy should be supervised by caregivers as incorrect use of inhalers is common and often associated with poor treatment response.

Inhaled Corticosteroids

- Not first line for treatment of COPD as chronic use has been associated with increased risk of pneumonia.
- Use of inhaled corticosteroids is considered in patients with frequent exacerbations, features of asthma, or elevated eosinophil counts.
- Oral steroids are only given in case of exacerbation.

Prophylactic Antibiotics

- Not indicated for the majority of patients with stable COPD.
- Azithromycin prophylaxis has been evaluated in select patients with frequent exacerbations, as limited data have shown slight decrease in the risk of exacerbations, albeit with potential increased risk of hearing loss and bacterial resistance.

Supplemental Oxygen

- In patients with severe hypoxia defined as arterial partial pressure of carbon dioxide (PaO_2) 55 mmHg or less or an oxygen saturation (SpO_2) of 88% or less, continuous supplemental oxygen reduces 5-year mortality.
- Supplemental oxygen does not improve mortality in patients with mild hypoxemia (88–94% on ambient air) or mild exertional hypoxemia ($SpO_2 > 80\%$).
- Excessive oxygen supplementation may precipitate hypercapnia by ventilation-perfusion mismatch and decreased respiratory drive.
  - Goal of SpO_2 88–92% at rest.
  - Consider a slightly higher goal of SpO_2 92–96% only if associated with significant pulmonary hypertension.

COPD Exacerbation

- Defined as an acute increase in pulmonary symptoms that cannot be attributed to another diagnosis and leads to a change in medical management and/or hospitalization.

- Classically defined if two of three of the following criteria are met:
  - Increased dyspnea.
  - Increased sputum volume.
  - Increased sputum purulence.
- Typically caused by bacterial or viral infections, inhaled exposures or treatment interruption.
- "Frequent" exacerbations are defined as two or greater episodes per year.
- In patients hospitalized with a COPD exacerbation, oral corticosteroids improve symptoms, reduce hospital length of stay, and accelerate recovery of FEV1:
  - Prednisone 40 mg by mouth daily for 5 days often provided, as a randomized controlled trial suggested non-inferiority to a 14-day course with reduced steroid exposure.
- Antibiotics also recommended if bacterial is suspected (particularly in patients with increased sputum production and respiratory failure):
  - Choose antibiotic based on prior susceptibility (if available).
  - Examples include amoxicillin/clavulanate, TMP-SMX, azithromycin, doxycycline, and fluoroquinolones.
- In patients with severe disease complicated by respiratory failure, supplemental oxygen or noninvasive positive pressure ventilation may be needed.
  - Goal SpO_2 88–92% desired to avoid hypoventilation.

Blebs, Bullae, and Pneumothorax

Patients with emphysematous COPD may develop blebs (small cystic subpleural collections of air) and/or bulla (blebs greater than 1 cm in diameter). These cystic collections form from deformation or destruction of the terminal alveoli in the setting of increased intrathoracic pressure in the lung parenchyma, loss of elastic recoil, and decreased strength of interstitial connective tissues.

- Blebs and bullae may be found incidentally on imaging (Fig. 19.2) or may rupture, presenting with spontaneous pneumothorax.
- Most commonly form in the upper lobe apices and the superior segments of the lower lobes.
- Surgical resection of blebs and bullae is most often performed after pneumothorax and involves stapled resection of the target bleb.
  - In patients with severe emphysema, utilizing a buttressed surgical stapler may prevent postoperative air leak.
  - Concomitant mechanical pleurodesis or pleurectomy to help reduce the likelihood of subsequent episodes.

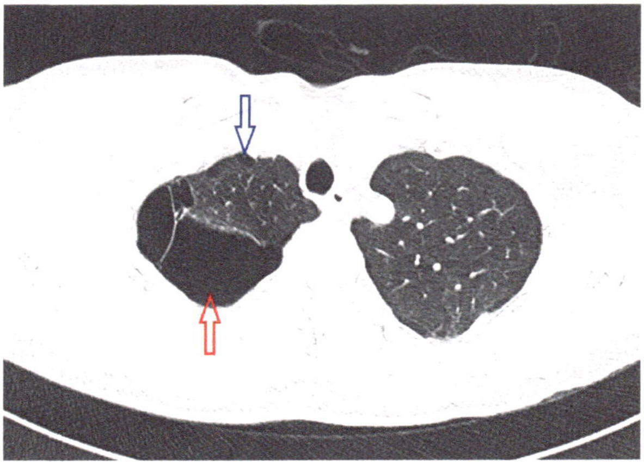

Fig. 19.2 Axial chest CT image demonstrating pulmonary blebs (blue arrow) and bulla (red arrow) of the right upper lobe

Lung Volume Reduction Surgery

Lung volume reduction surgery (LVRS) is an option for select patients with severe emphysematous COPD refractory to maximal medical therapy. The goal of the operation is to reduce symptoms and improve pulmonary function, thereby improving overall quality of life. It is theorized that removal of severely diseased emphysematous lung parenchyma may decrease hyperinflation, reduce ventilation-perfusion mismatch, and improve respiratory mechanics.

The National Emphysema Treatment Trial (NETT)

- Prospective, randomized study that established the risks and benefits for LVRS for end-stage emphysema.
- LVRS was associated with a greater chance of improved exercise capacity, lung function, and quality of life and reduced dyspnea, but changes after surgery were variable and returned to perioperative values at around 2 years after surgery.
- Patients with heterogenous, predominantly upper lobe emphysema with low maximal workload capacity after rehabilitation had lower mortality and greater improvement in symptoms and exercise capacity after LVRS than medical therapy.
- Patients with homogenous, non-upper lobe emphysema had a higher mortality rate with LVRS than medical therapy.

Candidates for LVRS

- Age less than 75 years.
- Body mass index (BMI) less than 32 kg/m^2.
- Forced expiratory volume in 1 s (FEV1) less than 45%, but greater than 20%.
- $PaCO_2$ of less than 60 mmHg.
- PaO_2 greater than 45 mmHg.
- Six-minute walk distance greater than 140 m, but low maximal exercise capacity (measured in watts; less than 40 watts for men, 25 watts for women).
- Smoking cessation for at least 6 months.

There are numerous contraindications to LVRS, including significant cardiac disease, prior thoracic surgery, and severe pulmonary insufficiency and/or pulmonary hypertension. Patients that are not candidates for LVRS may be recommended for lung transplantation.

- Oxygen supplementation to greater than 6 L/min.
- Pulmonary function testing with an FEV1 and DLCO <20% of predicted.
- Hypercapnia to a $PaCO_2$ > 60 mmHg.
- Pulmonary hypertension.

Surgical Technique for LVRS

- Unilateral or bilateral (more common) procedure via a minimally invasive approach.
- Adhesions are dissected with cautery mobilizing the upper lobe. A clamp is used across the apex to demarcate the anticipated wedge resection. A generous wedge resection is performed above the hilum.
- Utilizing a buttressed surgical stapler (with polytetrafluoroethylene or bovine pericardium strips) may help prevent postoperative air leak. Since the lung rarely will fill the superior aspect of the chest, a pleural tent may further decrease the risk of air leak.
- Complications (major morbidity rate of 59% in the NETT): 90-day mortality (5.5%), air leak, respiratory insufficiency/failure, pneumonia, cardiopulmonary complications.
- LVRS is substantially more expensive than medical therapy.

Bronchoscopic Lung Volume Reduction

Patients who are not medically fit for LVRS or have homogenous emphysema may be candidates for bronchoscopic lung volume reduction with the use of endobronchial valves (Fig. 19.3). Randomized trials have demonstrated improvements in dyspnea, lung function, exercise tolerance, and quality of life following bronchoscopic lung volume reduction in appropriately selected patients. Other techniques for bronchoscopic lung volume reduction (including endobronchial coils and bronchoscopic thermal vapor ablation) are experimental and not currently approved by the United States Food and Drug Administration.

- Endobronchial valves prevent airflow distal to the valve, thereby promoting atelectasis of the emphysematous lung, improving ventilation-perfusion mismatch and respiratory mechanics.
- Atelectasis may not occur following endobronchial valve placement if collateral ventilation between lobes is present.
- Careful patient selection is essential for procedural success. Some commonly applied criteria include:
  - Respiratory symptoms due to COPD rather than other medical condition.
  - FEV1 between 15% and 45% predicted.
  - Hyperinflation (total lung capacity >100% predicted and residual volume > 175% predicted).
  - Completion of pulmonary rehabilitation program.

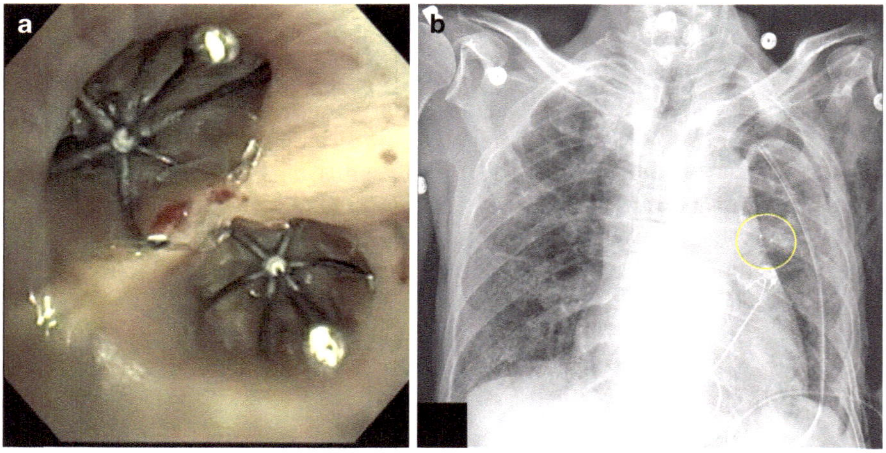

Fig. 19.3 Endobronchial valves in the anterior and apicoposterior segments of the left upper lobe. (**a**) Bronchoscopic view; (**b**) anteroposterior chest x-ray (valves shown in yellow circle), which additionally demonstrates a left pneumothorax (which occurs in around 25% of patients following bronchoscopic lung volume reduction) with subcutaneous emphysema and a Blake drain in place

  - Smoking cessation for at least 6 months.
  - Absence of collateral ventilation determined by fissure completeness (based on CT) or during bronchoscopy (Chartis System) prior to valve placement.

- The target lobe(s) are selected based on character/degree of emphysema and hyperinflation, fissure completeness, and occasionally results of ventilation/perfusion scanning.
- The risk of pneumothorax is around 25% following endobronchial valve placement:
  - Inpatient observation is often performed for 72 h following valve placement so pneumothorax can be managed acutely if it occurs.
- There must be no concerning lung nodules in the lung distal to the endobronchial valve, as subsequent atelectasis will prevent radiologic surveillance.

Lung Transplantation

Lung transplantation is occasionally considered for end-stage COPD without other treatment options. Due to complexity and potential morbidity, lung transplantation in this context is a complex decision that involves multiple factors including disease severity, comorbid conditions, and socioeconomic variables.

- Over one-third of lung transplants are performed for patients with end-stage COPD (31%) or COPD with alpha-1-antitrypsin deficiency (5%).
- Patients may undergo single or bilateral (double) lung transplantation, although bilateral transplant may result in superior clinical outcomes and long-term survival.
- Transplantation results in marked improvement in pulmonary function, symptoms, and quality of life.
- While patients with COPD have the best 1-year survival postsurgery, a long-term survival benefit has not been definitively established with a median survival of 7.1 years. Given this, lung allocation scoring prioritizes patients with the most advanced disease with a high risk of mortality without transplantation.

Key Reference

- Global Initiative for Chronic Obstructive Lung Disease (GOLD). Global strategy for the diagnosis, management and prevention of chronic obstructive pulmonary disease: 2023 report. http://www.goldcopd.org.

Further Reading

Agustí A, Hogg JC. Update on the pathogenesis of chronic obstructive pulmonary disease. N Engl J Med. 2019;381(13):1248–56.

Celli BR, Cote CG, Marin JM, et al. The body-mass index, airflow obstruction, dyspnea, and exercise capacity index in chronic obstructive pulmonary disease. N Engl J Med. 2004;350:1005–12.

Celli B, Locantore N, Yates JC, Evaluation of COPD Longitudinally to Identify Predictive Surrogate Endpoints (ECLIPSE) Investigators, et al. Markers of disease activity in COPD: an 8-year mortality study in the ECLIPSE cohort. Eur Respir J. 2021;57(3):2001339.

Celli BR, Wedzicha JA. Update on clinical aspects of chronic obstructive pulmonary disease. N Engl J Med. 2019;381(13):1257–66.

Criner GJ, Sue R, Wright S, Dransfield M, Rivas-Perez H, et al. A Multicenter randomized controlled trial of zephyr endobronchial valve treatment in heterogeneous emphysema (LIBERATE). Am J Respir Crit Care Med. 2018;198(9):1151–64.

Fishman A, Martinez F, Naunheim K, National Emphysema Treatment Trial Research Group, et al. A randomized trial comparing lung-volume-reduction surgery with medical therapy for severe emphysema. N Engl J Med. 2003;348(21):2059–73.

Hurst JR, Vestbo J, Anzueto A, et al. Susceptibility to exacerbation in chronic obstructive pulmonary disease. N Engl J Med. 2010;363:1128–38.

Jacobs SS, Krishnan JA, Lederer DJ, et al. Home oxygen therapy for adults with chronic lung disease. An official American Thoracic Society clinical practice guideline. Am J Respir Crit Care Med. 2020;202(10):e121–41.

Leard LE, Holm AM, Valapour M, et al. Consensus document for the selection of lung transplant candidates: an update from the International Society for Heart and Lung Transplantation. J Heart Lung Transplant. 2021;40(11):1349–79.

Leuppi JD, Schuetz P, Bingisser R, Bodmer M, Briel M, et al. Short-term vs conventional glucocorticoid therapy in acute exacerbations of chronic obstructive pulmonary disease: the REDUCE randomized clinical trial. JAMA. 2013;309(21):2223–31.

Lipson DA, Barnhart F, Brealey N, IMPACT Investigators, et al. Once-daily single-inhaler triple versus dual therapy in patients with COPD. N Engl J Med. 2018;378(18):1671–80.

Masmoudi H, Etienne H, Sylvestre R, et al. Three hundred fifty-one patients with pneumothorax undergoing Uniportal (single port) video-assisted thoracic surgery. Ann Thorac Surg. 2017;104(1):254–60.

QuickStats: percentage of adults aged ≥18 years with diagnosed chronic obstructive pulmonary disease, †by urbanization level§ and age group—National Health Interview Survey, United States, 2019. MMWR Morb Mortal Wkly Rep. 2021;70(26):959.

Nici L, Mammen MJ, Charbek E, Alexander PE, Au DH, Boyd CM, et al. Pharmacologic management of chronic obstructive pulmonary disease: an official American Thoracic Society clinical practice guideline. Am J Respir Crit Care Med. 2020;201:e56–69.

Sciurba FC, Ernst A, Herth FJ, Strange C, Criner GJ, Marquette CH, Kovitz KL, Chiacchierini RP, Goldin J, McLennan G, VENT Study Research Group. A randomized study of endobronchial valves for advanced emphysema. N Engl J Med. 2010;363(13):1233–44.

van Agteren JE, Carson KV, Tiong LU, Smith BJ. Lung volume reduction surgery for diffuse emphysema. Cochrane Database Syst Rev. 2016;10(10):CD001001.

Chapter 20
Spontaneous Pneumothorax

Darren S. Bryan and John S. Young

Introduction

A pneumothorax, colloquially known as a "collapsed lung," occurs with the introduction of air into the intrapleural space and subsequent loss of visceral and parietal pleural apposition. This chapter focuses on "spontaneous" pneumothorax, those without a known etiology, such as traumatic, purposeful, and iatrogenic pneumothorax. Generally, treatment is aimed at the evacuation of air to allow for the re-establishment of pleural apposition. Surgical intervention is warranted in patients with persistent or recurrent pneumothorax refractory to less invasive interventions.

Anatomy

- Visceral and parietal pleura line the surface of the lung and thoracic cavity, respectively.
- The visceral and parietal pleura are composed of mesothelial cells, elastin, and collagen.
- The potential space between the pleural surfaces is termed the pleural space.
- The pleural space is normally under negative pressure with respect to the atmospheric and alveolar pressure, generated by the elastic recoil of the lungs and rigidity of the chest wall.
- The transpulmonary pressure is the difference between the alveolar pressure and the intrapleural pressure (Palv-Ppl).

D. S. Bryan (✉) · J. S. Young
Division of Thoracic and Cardiac Surgery, Brigham and Women's Hospital, Boston, MA, USA
e-mail: Dbryan@bsd.uchicago.edu; jyoung0@bwh.harvard.edu

T. Ng, T. Geraci (eds.), *Thoracic Surgery Clerkship*, Contemporary Surgical Clerkships, https://doi.org/10.1007/978-3-031-44645-0_20

Pathogenesis

- With introduction of air into the pleural space, the intrapleural pressure and alveolar pressure equilibrate, and the lung collapses under its own recoil.
- The source of intrapleural air can be atmospheric (traumatic pneumothorax, or purposeful when the chest is opened during surgical procedures) or from the lung and/or airways themselves.
- The degree of pneumothorax is poorly quantified based on standard chest radiograph.
- In the absence of drainage and with ongoing introduction of air, the pressure of the pleural space will progressively increase.
- Increased intrapleural pressure leads to further lung collapse and compression of other structures in the hemithorax, including the mediastinum which shifts to the contralateral side impairing venous return to the heart, leading to hypotension and ultimately pulseless electrical activity (PEA) arrest—a condition termed "tension" pneumothorax.

Primary Spontaneous Pneumothorax

- Occur in patients with no identified cause or underlying lung disease
- Most frequently in thin, young men of tall stature as well as patients with Marfan's syndrome
- Frequently found to be secondary to rupture of an air containing sac on the surface of the lung, termed a subpleural "bleb" (Fig. 20.1), with a resultant parenchymal-pleural fistula (air leak)

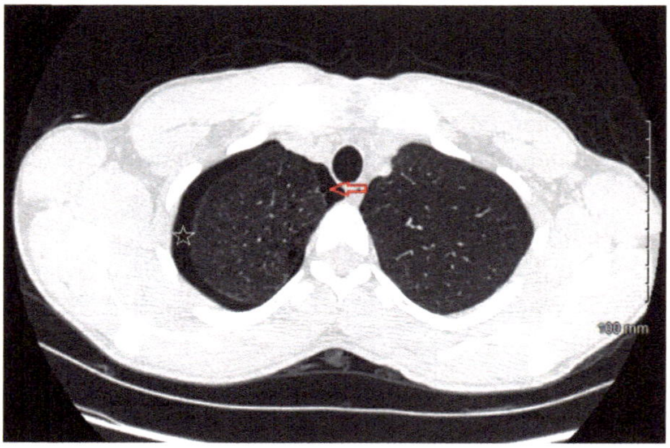

Fig. 20.1 CT scan of a patient with primary spontaneous pneumothorax, demonstrating pneumothorax (star) and normal lung parenchyma with the exception of a small subpleural bleb (arrow)

Secondary Spontaneous Pneumothorax

- Pneumothoraces that occur in patients with underlying lung disease or condition suspected to be causative of a parenchymal-pleural fistula (Fig. 20.2), most common etiology being chronic obstructive pulmonary disease (COPD); other causes include:
  - Airway disease

    COPD
    Cystic fibrosis
    Status asthmaticus
    COVID-19
  - Infectious

    Necrotizing pneumonia
    Pneumocystis carinii pneumonia
- Interstitial lung disease
  - Interstitial lung disease

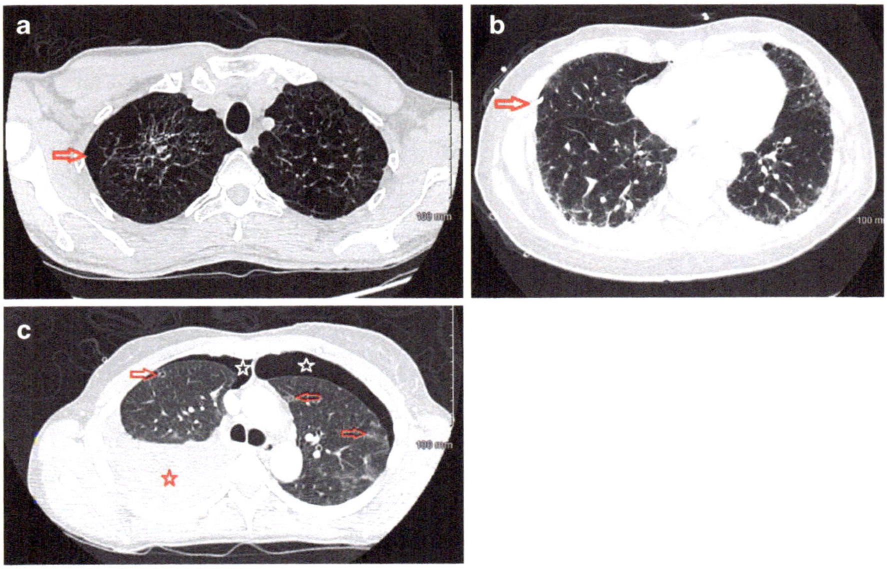

Fig. 20.2 CT scan of patients with secondary spontaneous pneumothorax. (**a**) Patient with severe bilateral emphysema and a small pneumothorax (arrow); (**b**) patient with idiopathic pulmonary fibrosis (or usual interstitial pneumonia) with pneumothorax that has been treated with pigtail chest catheter (arrow); (**c**) patient with multiple small cystic parenchymal lesions (arrows), bilateral pneumothoraces (white stars), and right chylous effusion (red star), common presentation of lymphangiomyomatosis

    - Sarcoidosis
    - Idiopathic pulmonary fibrosis
    - Langerhans cell histiocytosis
    - Lymphangioleiomyomatosis
    - Tuberous sclerosis

- Connective tissue disease

    - Rheumatoid arthritis
    - Ankylosing spondylitis
    - Polymyositis and dermatomyositis
    - Scleroderma
    - Marfan's syndrome
    - Ehlers-Danlos syndrome

- Malignancy

    - Metastatic sarcoma
    - Lung cancer

- Thoracic endometriosis/catamenial pneumothorax

History

- Typically symptom onset is sudden without an eliciting activity or event.
- Symptoms range in severity (and may be mild) depending on degree of pneumothorax, baseline pulmonary function, and presence/absence of tension physiology.
- Most common symptoms are shortness of breath, dyspnea with exertion, and pleuritic chest pain.
- Risk factors for pneumothorax: cigarette or marijuana smoking.

Physical Examination

- Key finding: diminished/absent breath sounds on affected side
- Other findings: hyper-resonant to percussion on affected side, tracheal shift away from affected side (with tension physiology)

Imaging

- Clinically significant pneumothorax is primarily a clinical diagnosis that can be supported or confirmed radiographically.

- Treatment of suspected tension pneumothorax or of patients in extremis, suspected to be due to pneumothorax, should not be delayed by obtaining confirmatory imaging (tension pneumothorax should never be diagnosed radiographically; it is a clinical diagnosis that when made, treatment should be immediately instituted).
- Chest radiograph (Fig. 20.3):
  - Best first study for evaluation of the chest
  - Difficult to determine the degree of lung collapse
  - Difficult to discern anterior or posterior components of pneumothorax
- CT scan (without contrast):
  - Excellent test to evaluate anatomy and better define the thoracic pathology
  - Useful to identify parenchymal lung cysts
- Ultrasound:
  - Useful and fast bedside test when pneumothorax is suspected
  - Should be followed by a chest radiograph or CT scan for treatment planning, provided the patient is stable
  - High degree of practitioner variability

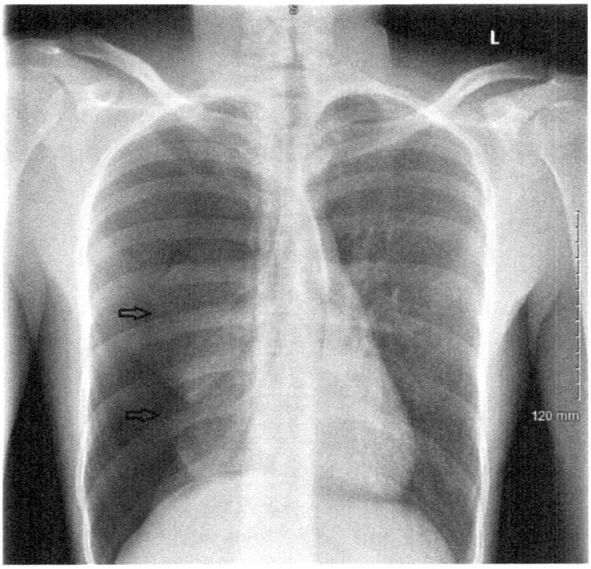

Fig. 20.3 Chest radiograph of a patient with primary spontaneous pneumothorax, showing the visceral pleural line of the collapse lung (arrows)

Immediate Treatment

- Immediate treatment aimed at evacuating intrapleural space of air, which serves two purposes:
  - Allows for lung expansion and re-establishment of visceral-parietal apposition, as parenchymal defects close faster with pleural apposition
  - Relieves any compressive or tension effect of positive pressure within pleural space
- Pleural drainage via large-bore chest tube or pigtail chest catheter (see Chap. 2) is considered for all situations:
  - A large-bore chest tube can be placed in all circumstances.
  - A small-bore pigtail chest catheter (14 Fr) is more comfortable for the patient; however, if a very small-bore tube is used (less than 14 Fr) or if the tube is placed inferiorly, the pneumothorax may not evacuate completely, confounding further management decisions.
  - In selected patients who are healthy, asymptomatic, and with small pneumothorax (confined only to the apex), observation or aspiration of air with a syringe with repeat chest radiograph in 4–6 h may be appropriate.
  - In patients with suspected tension physiology, chest radiograph should not be performed to confirm the diagnosis. Rather, upon clinical suspicion, the pleural space should be quickly drained through needle decompression or immediate chest tube placement.

Subsequent Intervention Versus Observation

- First-episode spontaneous pneumothorax
  - There is a 15–30% chance of recurrence, and an informed decision is made regarding proceeding with intervention to lower the risk of recurrence versus observation.
  - Factors that lean toward intervention after first episode include persistent air leak more than 3 or 4 days, resides or works in a remote/isolated setting, occupation that involved change in air pressure (pilot, submarine operator), simultaneous bilateral pneumothorax, and comorbidities that may make a small pneumothorax life threatening.
  - Counseling regarding smoke cessation (of any substance) is required, not only to decrease the risk of recurrence, but to reinforce the negative cardiac, pulmonary, and cancer effects of smoke.

- Second-episode spontaneous pneumothorax
  - Due to high risk (> 50%) of third recurrence, intervention is recommended.
  - Counseling regarding smoke cessation is recommended, not only to decrease the risk of recurrence, but to reinforce the negative cardiac, pulmonary, and cancer effects of smoking.

Intervention to Decrease Pneumothorax Recurrence

- Bedside Pleurodesis
  - Obliteration of the pleural space through induced adhesions between visceral and parietal pleura.
  - Agents instilled into the chest tube bedside include talc slurry, doxycycline, or bleomycin.
  - Although less effective than surgery, this option has less risk; thus it may be appropriate for patients with significant comorbidities, which is often the case with secondary spontaneous pneumothorax.
  - Bedside pleurodesis can be quite painful, especially with doxycycline.
- Surgery
  - More effective than bedside pleurodesis, with recurrence rates of 5% or less.
  - Requires general anesthesia with single-lung ventilation, and together with the possibility of complications, surgical option represents the higher-risk option as compared with bedside pleurodesis; thus it may not be appropriate for patients with significant comorbidities.
  - The lung parenchyma is evaluated for the source of the air leak (bleb, bullae), and this is sealed or removed by wedge resection using the endoscopic stapler, with or without buttress material depending on the quality/fragility of the lung parenchyma.
  - In primary spontaneous pneumothorax, the source of air leak (subpleural bleb) is usually located in the apex of the upper lobe or superior segment of the lower lobe; in the event this is not clearly identified, then the apex of the upper lobe is empirically resected by wedge using the endoscopic stapler, presuming the offending apical subpleural bleb has ruptured and thus not identified.
  - A pleurodesis procedure should then follow, which may be by delivering 5 g sterile talc with an atomizer, mechanical abrasion of the parietal pleura, partial parietal pleurectomy (resection of the apical parietal pleura), or a combination of these.
  - A large-bore chest tube is placed intraoperatively (for management of chest tubes, see Chap. 2).

Key Reference

- Brown SGA, Ball EL, Perrin K, Asha SE, Braithwaite I, Egerton-Warburton D, Jones PG, Keijzers G, Kinnear FB, Kwan BCH, Lam KV, Lee YCG, Nowitz M, Read CA, Simpson G, Smith JA, Summers QA, Weatherall M, Beasley R, PSP Investigators. Conservative versus interventional treatment for spontaneous pneumothorax. N Engl J Med. 2020;382(5):405–415.

Further Reading

Baumann MH, Strange C, Heffner JE, Light R, Kirby TJ, Klein J, Luketich JD, Panacek EA, Sahn SA, AACP Pneumothorax Consensus Group. Management of spontaneous pneumothorax: an American College of Chest Physicians Delphi consensus statement. Chest. 2001;119(2):590–602.

Cerfolio RJ. Pneumothorax and pneumomediastinum. In: Sugarbaker DJ, Bueno R, Burt BM, Groth SS, Loor G, Wolf AS, et al., editors. Sugarbaker's adult chest surgery. New York, NY: McGraw-Hill Education; 2020.

Sahn SA, Heffner JE. Spontaneous pneumothorax. N Engl J Med. 2000;342(12):868–74.

Schnell J, Beer M, Eggeling S, Gesierich W, Gottlieb J, Herth FJF, Hofmann HS, Jany B, Kreuter M, Ley-Zaporozhan J, Scheubel R, Walles T, Wiesemann S, Worth H, Stoelben E. Management of spontaneous pneumothorax and post-interventional pneumothorax: German S3 guideline. Respiration. 2019;97(4):370–402.

Walker SP, Bibby AC, Halford P, Stadon L, White P, Maskell NA. Recurrence rates in primary spontaneous pneumothorax: a systematic review and meta-analysis. Eur Respir J. 2018;52(3):1800864.

Chapter 21
Pleural Empyema and Effusions

Michael A. Wright and Thomas Ng

Introduction

The pleural fluid that collects can be characterized as transudative or exudative based on the cause and composition of the fluid. Transudative effusions contain little protein and are often related to problems with hydrostatic pressure, oncotic pressure, and fluid balance. Exudative effusions are protein-rich and may be related to disruption of lymphatic reabsorption or to capillary permeability from inflammation or infection. Most effusions present with dyspnea due to compression and collapse of the adjacent lung. Physical exam may demonstrate decreased tactile fremitus, dullness to percussion, or diminished breath sounds on auscultation. Additional symptoms and signs will be dependent on the specific etiology.

Anatomy

- The pleural cavity is a potential space separating the visceral and parietal pleura within the chest. It contains a small amount of pleural fluid that provides lubrication and aids in lung expansion and contraction during respiration.

M. A. Wright
Department of Surgery, University of Tennessee Health Science Center, College of Medicine, Memphis, TN, USA
e-mail: mwrigh86@uthsc.edu

T. Ng (✉)
Division of Thoracic Surgery, University of Tennessee Health Science Center, College of Medicine, Memphis, TN, USA
e-mail: tng4@uthsc.edu

T. Ng, T. Geraci (eds.), *Thoracic Surgery Clerkship*, Contemporary Surgical Clerkships, https://doi.org/10.1007/978-3-031-44645-0_21

- Although several liters of fluid are produced and cross this space daily, almost all the fluid is reabsorbed through the lymphatics of the parietal pleura.
- A small imbalance in the production or reabsorption processes can lead to an accumulation of fluid or pleural effusion.

Workup

- Workup focuses on history, clinical exam, imaging, and diagnosis by pleural fluid analysis or by pleural biopsy.
- Chest radiograph (Fig. 21.1a) and computed tomography (CT) (Fig. 21.1b) of the chest will show opacity of the effusion with mediastinal shift to the contralateral side, lung atelectasis, and consolidation.
- Pleural fluid obtained by thoracentesis, often with image guidance (ultrasound or CT scan), is characterized by its gross appearance and odor, and analysis is sent for cell count, cell differential, pH, total protein, lactate dehydrogenase (LDH), glucose, amylase, triglycerides, gram stain, culture, and cytology.
- Light's criteria can be used to differentiate an exudative from transudative effusions. Based on Light's criteria, an exudative effusion is defined by:
  - Pleural fluid-to-serum total protein ratio greater than 0.5.
  - Pleural fluid-to-serum LDH ratio greater than 0.6.
  - Pleural fluid LDH greater than two-thirds of the normal serum level.
- If diagnosis is still in question, then consider pleural biopsy, by needle with image guidance (CT scan or ultrasound) or by surgery with thoracoscopy.

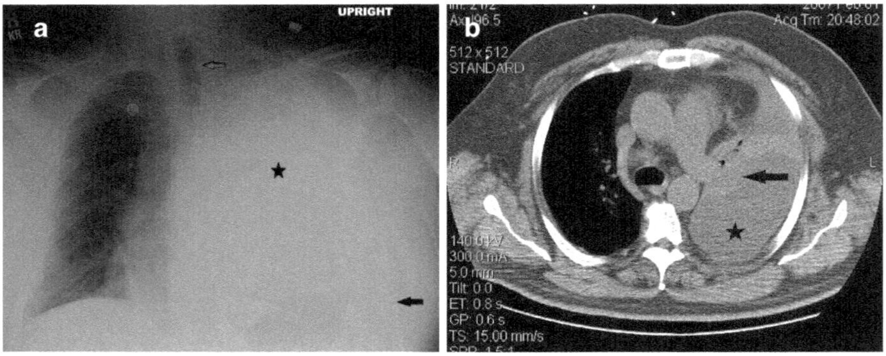

Fig. 21.1 Imaging of a patient with parapneumonic effusion. (**a**) Chest X-ray showing opacity from the effusion (star), mediastinal shift to the contralateral side (red arrow), and placement of pigtail catheter for drainage (black arrow); (**b**) CT scan showing loculated effusion (star) and collapse/compressed lung (arrow)

Table 21.1 Differential diagnosis of pleural effusions

Causes of transudative effusion	Causes of exudative effusion
Congestive heart failure	Infection (bacterial, tuberculosis, fungal, parasitic, viral)
Cirrhosis	Malignancy (metastatic, mesothelioma)
Nephrotic syndrome	Collagen-vascular disease (rheumatoid arthritis, systemic lupus erythematosus, Wegener's granulomatosis)
Peritoneal dialysis	Esophageal perforation
Glomerulonephritis	Pancreatitis
Hypoalbuminemia	Intra-abdominal infection
Myxedema	Radiation
Pulmonary embolism	Drug-induced
	Pulmonary embolism
	Asbestosis
	Post-pericardiotomy/cardiac surgery
	Post-myocardial infarction
	Hemothorax
	Chylothorax

Transudative Effusions

- Transudative effusions have a narrow differential diagnosis (Table 21.1) and are often the result of underlying medical conditions such as congestive heart failure, cirrhosis, or nephrotic syndrome. The fluid that collects is often bilateral and free-flowing and lacks the loculations that are commonly found in exudative effusions.
- Treatment is aimed at treating the underlying condition with medical therapy, but occasionally drainage may be required to relieve symptomatic large effusions.

Exudative Effusions

- A wide differential diagnosis is seen with exudative effusions (Table 21.1).
- Compared to transudative effusion, invasive investigative procedures (including pleural biopsy) should be considered if diagnosis is not clearly obvious, and a more aggressive approach for complete effusion drainage should be taken due to risk of developing trapped lungs with exudative effusions.
- A detailed discussion of two exudative effusions commonly managed by thoracic surgeons, parapneumonic effusion/empyema and malignant effusion, is provided below.

Parapneumonic Effusion/Empyema

- Empyemas are an infection of the pleural space.
  - They most often occur in association with pneumonia.
  - They can occur following trauma, thoracic procedures, esophageal perforations, or extension of infection from adjacent compartments (neck, mediastinum, chest wall, spine, and abdomen).
- Exudative effusion associated with pneumonia can be classified as parapneumonic (noninfected fluid) or empyema (infection of pleural fluid – purulence, gram stain positive, culture positive, low pH). Approach to treatment for both is often similar.
- Symptoms include shortness of breath, productive cough, chest pain, fever, malaise, anorexia, and weight loss. In addition to signs of effusion discussed above, patients will have signs of sepsis including fever, tachypnea, and tachycardia.
- Further diagnostic tests include bloodwork, imaging with chest X-ray (Fig. 21.1a) and CT scan (Fig. 21.1b), and thoracentesis for pleural fluid analysis as discussed above.
- Common pathogens.
  - Community-acquired: *Streptococcus pneumoniae*, *Haemophilus influenzae*, *Staphylococcus aureus*, *Mycoplasma pneumoniae*, *Streptococcus pyogenes*.
  - Hospital-acquired: *Klebsiella pneumoniae*, *Escherichia coli*, *Pseudomonas aeruginosa*, *Staphylococcus aureus*.
- Treatment includes fluid resuscitation, intravenous antibiotics, and an intervention for source control/effusion evacuation. Choice of intervention depends on the stage of disease.
  - Stage I: Exudative phase (weeks 1–2).

    The pleural fluid in this early stage is free-floating without loculations. Treatment goal is to evacuate all pleural fluid. This can be achieved with thoracentesis or by chest tube (commonly small-bore pigtail chest catheter placed with image guidance; see Chap. 2).
  - Stage II: Fibrinopurulent phase (weeks 2–3).

    Loculations begin to form as the fluid contains heavy fibrin deposits. Treatment may be by chest tube drainage or with surgery by thoracoscopy. There is debate regarding the optimal approach; certain circumstances that may favor one approach over the other are discussed below.

    For chest tube drainage, although counterintuitive due to the thick loculated nature, pigtail catheters are ideal as they can be placed in the precise location of the loculated effusion using image guidance (ultrasound or CT scan), which allows for delivery of lytic therapy into the center of the effusion for effective lyses and drainage (Fig. 21.2). The advantage of this is

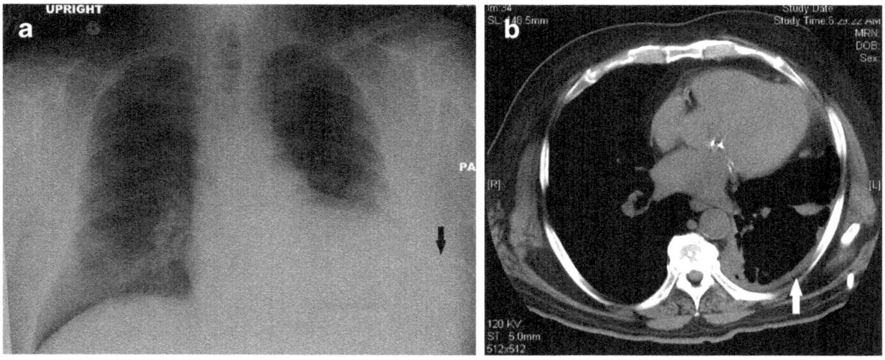

Fig. 21.2 Imaging after lytic therapy of the same patient as in Fig. 21.1. (**a**) Chest X-ray, as compared to Fig. 21.1a, shows near-complete resolution of the parapneumonic effusion after lytic therapy via pigtail catheter (arrow); (**b**) CT scan, as compared to Fig. 21.1b, shows near-complete resolution of effusion after lytic therapy via pigtail catheter with small residual fluid and/or pleural thickening (arrow)

that if successful, surgery can be avoided, especially in patients who are poor surgical candidates due to comorbidities. The disadvantage is that it may require placement of more than one catheter to evacuate the pleural space, or if it fails, it would then require surgery, both of which will prolong hospitalization.

For surgery, minimally invasive technique by thoracoscopy is preferred over open thoracotomy to completely clear all fluid and material in the pleural space, along with any visceral pleural peel that may be beginning to form on the surface of the lung. The advantage is that the pleural space can be cleared with a single procedure, which can provide rapid source control in severely septic patients and may shorten hospitalization. Since this is a major procedure, with potential for blood loss and major fluid shifts, even if completed by thoracoscopy, the disadvantage is the risk of the procedure, especially in patients with significant comorbidities.

– Stage III: Organizing phase (>3–4 weeks).

Ingrowth of fibroblast with collagen deposition creates a thick rind that encases and traps the lung, which not only results in loss of lung function but also sets up the presence of a space for infected fluid/empyema to persist (Fig. 21.3).

Treatment options include long-term drainage of the empyema space with large-bore chest tube, surgical decortication, or rib resection for open thoracic window drainage. Treatment selection is based on patient comorbidities and risk-benefit discussion between surgeon and patient regarding each option.

Drainage with a large-bore chest tube is the least invasive and lowest-risk option, with the goal of controlling sepsis by maintaining drainage of the

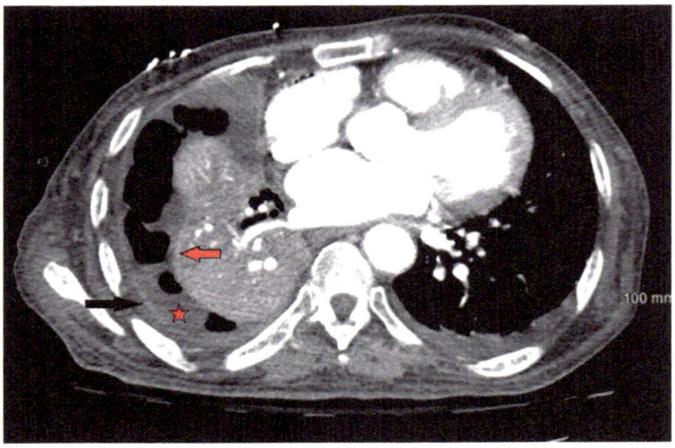

Fig. 21.3 CT scan image of stage III empyema. Despite partial evacuation of the empyema, as noted by air and fluid in the pleural space (star), the lung fails to expand as it is trapped by a pleural peel which enhances with intravenous contrast (red arrow). The parietal pleural also enhances with intravenous contrast (black arrow)

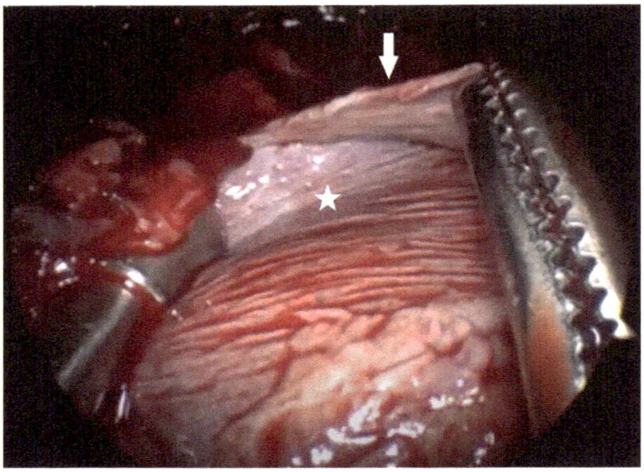

Fig. 21.4 Surgical decortication by thoracoscopy, with removal of the thick pleural peel (arrow) that has entrapped the lung (star)

infected pleural space. The lung, however, will likely remain trapped and thus not regain function. In addition, maintaining a functioning chest tube free from dislodging and clogging long term is difficult.

Surgical decortication may be performed by thoracoscopy (Fig. 21.4) or open thoracotomy. The goal of surgery is to remove the rind that traps the lung. Allowing the lung to expand both restores lung function and obliterates the empyema space, thus minimizing the risk of recurrent empyema (the dictum "no space, no infection"). This option imparts the most stress and risk onto the patient as there is potential for blood loss and injury to adjacent structures, therefore it may not be an ideal option for patients with significant comorbidities.

Rib resection for thoracic window drainage (Fig. 21.5) is a more definitive method to maintain drainage of the empyema space as compared to long-

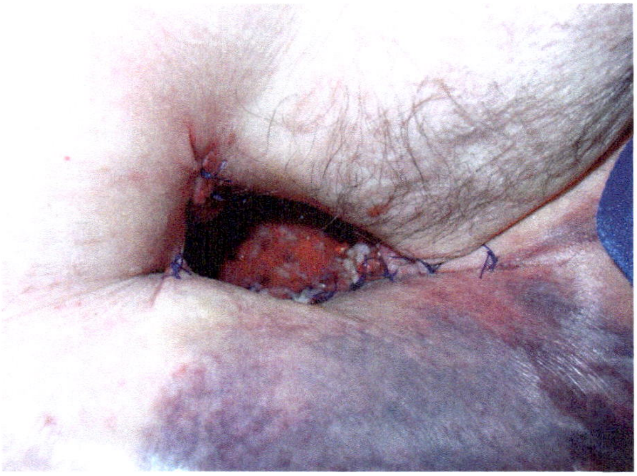

Fig. 21.5 Rib resection for open thoracic window drainage of stage III empyema

term large-bore chest tube. After resection of two or three ribs over the empyema space, skin flaps are turned in and sutured to the pleura, thus preventing its closure as an epithelialized opening is created. Daily dressing changes to pack the empyema space are required. The thoracic window can be a permanent situation or can be closed if the space is well cleaned after long-term debridement with the dressings and the patient is deemed a candidate for a second major procedure. Closure may be by muscle flap, omental flap, thoracoplasty, or a combination of these or by reversal skin flap to close the window followed by filling of the space with antibiotic solution (Clagett procedure, which has modest success rate).

Malignant Pleural Effusion

- Malignant pleural effusion may be due to primary pleural malignancy or secondary due to pleural metastasis originating from elsewhere. Effusion develops due to blockage of pleural lymphatic drainage and pleural permeability. These effusions are typically exudative and frequently bloody.
- The most common cause of malignant effusion is lung cancer. Breast cancer, ovarian cancer, gastric cancer, and lymphoma are other possible primary sites.
- Malignant effusion presents most commonly with dyspnea. Chest pain, cough, fatigue, anorexia, and weight loss are other possible symptoms. Signs of effusion are as discussed above. Other symptoms and signs will be specific to the origin of the primary.

Diagnosis

- Clinical evaluation with complete history and physical examination.
- Imaging modalities such as chest X-ray, ultrasound, CT scan (Fig. 21.6), and PET as indicated.
- Cytologic analysis of pleural fluid obtained by thoracentesis can confirm malignancy; however, in 25% of patients with malignant pleural effusion, thoracentesis will not identify malignant cells, in which case biopsy for tissue diagnosis will be necessary.
- Biopsy may be by needle with CT scan guidance of the pleural nodules/mass or by thoracoscopy (Fig. 21.7) which also allows for the option of performing pleurodesis at the same time.

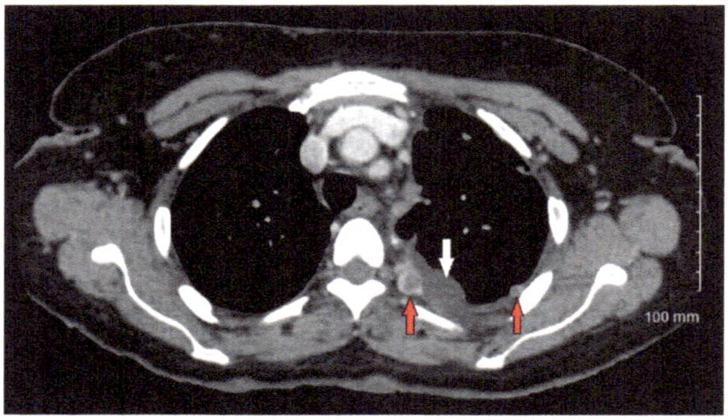

Fig. 21.6 CT scan of a patient with malignant effusion (white arrow) with intravenous contrast enhancing the malignant pleural nodules (red arrow)

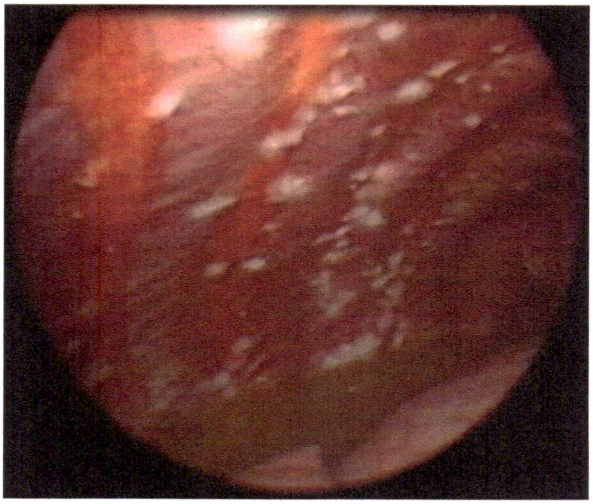

Fig. 21.7 Intraoperative picture during thoracoscopy, of a patient with malignant effusion, showing diffuse pleural nodules

Treatment

- Treatment of malignant effusion focuses on treating the underlying cancer, removal of pleural fluid for symptomatic relief, and preventing recurrence of the effusion. Small asymptomatic effusions do not require drainage and can be managed with observation.
- For symptomatic or recurrent malignant effusions, options include intermittent thoracentesis, pleurodesis, or indwelling tunneled chest catheter for home drainage. Choice of therapy is dependent on patient preference and cancer factors as discussed below.
- A note of caution regarding the development of re-expansion pulmonary edema when draining a large malignant effusion; this occurs when a chronic large effusion is drained too rapidly, especially if active suction is applied. To prevent this complication, clamp thoracentesis catheter or chest tube immediately after insertion, release 1 L at a time (i.e., every 6 hours) then re-clamp, and avoid the use of suction.
- Intermittent thoracentesis may be appropriate if there is an expectation that the malignancy will respond well with therapy (such as lymphoma). Otherwise, if frequent thoracentesis is required due to rapid reaccumulation of effusion, the patient's quality of life will be adversely affected by the frequent trips for drainage.
- Pleurodesis can be completed surgically by thoracoscopy or performed at bedside. Surgical pleurodesis is preferred if the patient can tolerate brief anesthesia as it is more comfortable and more effective than bedside pleurodesis.
  - Bedside pleurodesis involves placing a chest tube, either large-bore or pigtail catheter, followed by delivery of talc slurry or doxycycline into the pleural space via the chest tube. Awake chest tube placement is uncomfortable, but the greatest source of discomfort is from the sclerosing agent, notably doxycycline. As complete effusion drainage and distribution of the sclerosing agent are less effective than surgery, the success of pleurodesis is likely inferior to surgery.
  - Surgical pleurodesis via thoracoscopy is performed under general anesthesia; thus, it is more comfortable for the patient. Under direct vision, complete drainage of the effusion and a wide distribution of the sclerosing agent can be achieved; thus, pleurodesis is likely more successful than bedside procedure. Sterile talc powder is commonly used and can be effectively delivered to all areas of the pleural space using an atomizer (Fig. 21.8). Other techniques of pleurodesis during thoracoscopy, such as mechanical abrasion or pleurectomy, are rarely performed as these can result in blood loss for the malignant pleura, thus increasing the risk of the procedure for these fragile patients.
- Indwelling tunneled chest catheter (Fig. 21.9) can be placed under general or local anesthesia and is used for long-term home drainage of malignant effusion. This is ideal for patients who are comfortable with having an indwelling device

Fig. 21.8 Intraoperative picture of thoracoscopic pleurodesis using sterile talc powder

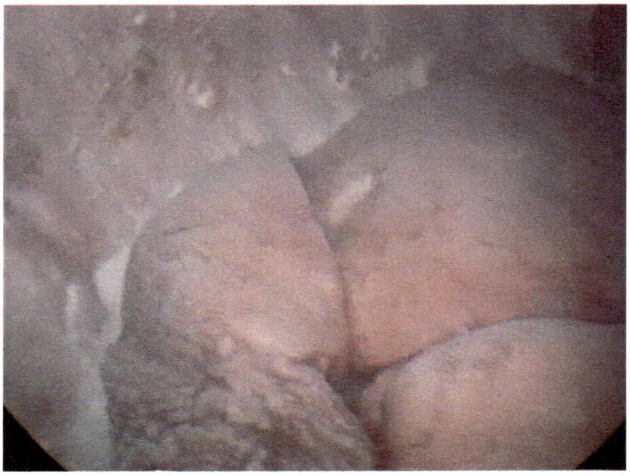

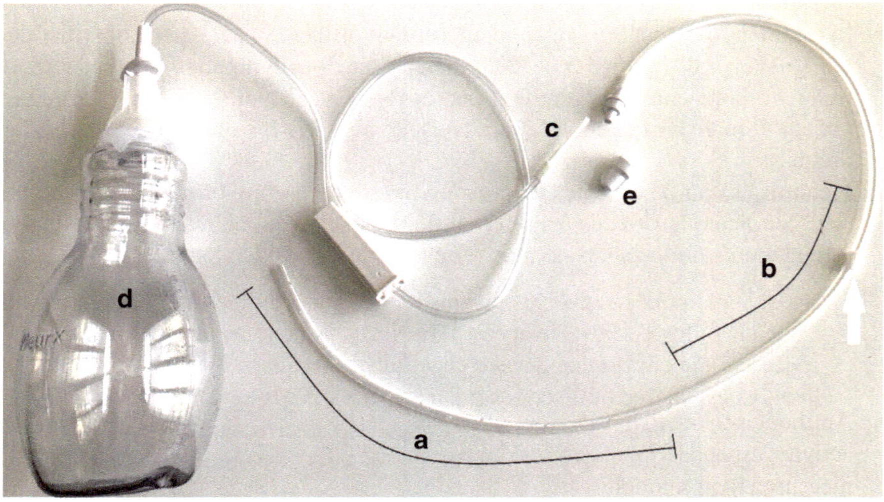

Fig. 21.9 Tunneled chest catheter for long-term home drainage; portion in pleural space (**a**); subcutaneous portion (**b**), with cuff (arrow) that holds this in place; connector from vacuum bottle to tunneled catheter (**c**); vacuum bottle (**d**); catheter cap when tube not in use (**e**)

at home for intermittent drainage when symptomatic and for patients with trapped lung due to malignant pleural disease (in which case pleurodesis will not be successful due to lack of visceral-to-parietal pleural apposition). The catheter can be removed if the effusion resolves. As this is a foreign body in the pleural cavity, catheter infection and empyema are risks.

Key Reference

- Rahman NM, Maskell NA, West A, Teoh R, Arnold A, Mackinlay C, Peckham D, Davies CW, Ali N, Kinnear W, Bentley A, Kahan BC, Wrightson JM, Davies HE, Hooper CE, Lee YC, Hedley EL, Crosthwaite N, Choo L, Helm EJ, Gleeson FV, Nunn AJ, Davies RJ. Intrapleural use of tissue plasminogen activator and DNase in pleural infection. N Engl J Med. 2011;365(6):518–26.

Further Reading

Davies HE, Lee YC. Management of malignant pleural effusions: questions that need answers. Curr Opin Pulm Med. 2013;19(4):374–9.

Feller-Kopman DJ, Reddy CB, DeCamp MM, Diekemper RL, Gould MK, Henry T, Iyer NP, Lee YCG, Lewis SZ, Maskell NA, Rahman NM, Sterman DH, Wahidi MM, Balekian AA, Management of Malignant Pleural Effusions. An official ATS/STS/STR clinical practice guideline. Am J Respir Crit Care Med. 2018;198(7):839–49.

Light RW, Macgregor MI, Luchsinger PC, Ball WC Jr. Pleural effusions: the diagnostic separation of transudates and exudates. Ann Intern Med. 1972;77(4):507–13.

Shen KR, Bribriesco A, Crabtree T, Denlinger C, Eby J, Eiken P, Jones DR, Keshavjee S, Maldonado F, Paul S, Kozower B. The American Association for Thoracic Surgery consensus guidelines for the management of empyema. J Thorac Cardiovasc Surg. 2017;153(6):e129–46.

Chapter 22
Chylothorax

Haley Leesley and Steven Milman

Overview

- Chylothorax is the accumulation of chyle within the pleural space.
- Iatrogenic disruption of the thoracic duct or its tributaries during surgery (esophageal, pulmonary, or cardiac) is the most common etiology.
- A persistent chyle leak results in immunosuppression, malnutrition, and eventual death from sepsis.
- Low-output leaks can be managed nonoperatively, whereas large disruptions most often require embolization and/or surgical ligation.

Pathogenesis

- Fatty acids (except medium-chain triglycerides) enter the lacteals in the small bowel and travel as chylomicrons along the lymphatic channels to the cisterna chyli.
- The thoracic duct originates at the cisterna chyli and travels superiorly in the right side of the mediastinum against the vertebral body, between the esophagus, aorta, and azygos vein. The thoracic duct crosses the chest to the left side at approximately the level of the T6 vertebral body and eventually empties into the left subclavian at the confluence with the internal jugular vein confluence (Fig. 22.1).

H. Leesley
Department of Surgery, University of Texas Medical Branch Galveston, Galveston, TX, USA
e-mail: haleesle@utmb.edu

S. Milman (✉)
Department of Surgery, Signature Healthcare, Brockton, MA, USA

T. Ng, T. Geraci (eds.), *Thoracic Surgery Clerkship*, Contemporary Surgical Clerkships, https://doi.org/10.1007/978-3-031-44645-0_22

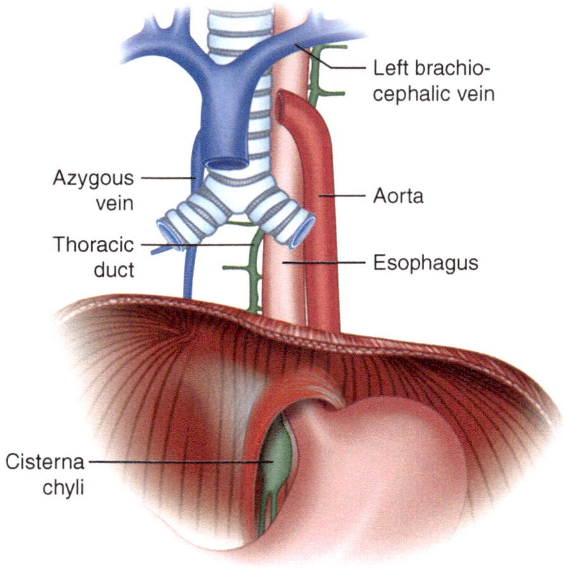

Fig. 22.1 Anatomy of the thoracic duct

- Thoracic duct anatomy is highly variable, both in number of branches and their exact location, with the most consistent anatomy being entry into the chest close to the diaphragmatic hiatus.
- Disruption of the duct leads to spillage of chyle into the pleural space, with resultant depletion of immunoglobulins and leukocytes which eventually results in immunosuppression and susceptibility to infection and sepsis.
- Nontraumatic causes include diseases of the lymphatic system, such as lymphangioleiomyomatosis. However, by far the most common nontraumatic etiology is malignancy, particularly lymphoma.
- Traumatic etiologies are typically iatrogenic injuries, with correction of congenital heart defects and esophagectomy being the most likely. Mediastinal node dissection during pulmonary resection is also a known risk for chylothorax.
- Pseudochylothorax (also referred to as cholesterol pleurisy or chyliform effusion) is a cholesterol-rich pleural effusion (PE) that is commonly associated with chronic inflammatory disorders.

Evaluation

History

- Obtain a detailed history with a particular focus on any recent intrathoracic procedures, B-symptoms of possible lymphoma, and history of conditions such as tuberculosis or rheumatoid arthritis that may cause a "pseudochylothorax."
- High-output pleural fluid volume from a chest tube in a patient without oral intake (NPO) in the postoperative phase should raise a suspicion of chylothorax.

Physical Examination

- Physical exam will likely reveal diminished breath sounds and dullness to percussion in the affected hemithorax.
  - Evidence of nutritional depletion should be noted.
- If a chest drain is present, the fluid turning "milky" in consistency after initiation of a diet (Fig. 22.2) and becoming serous again when the patient is made NPO is nearly pathognomonic for chylothorax.

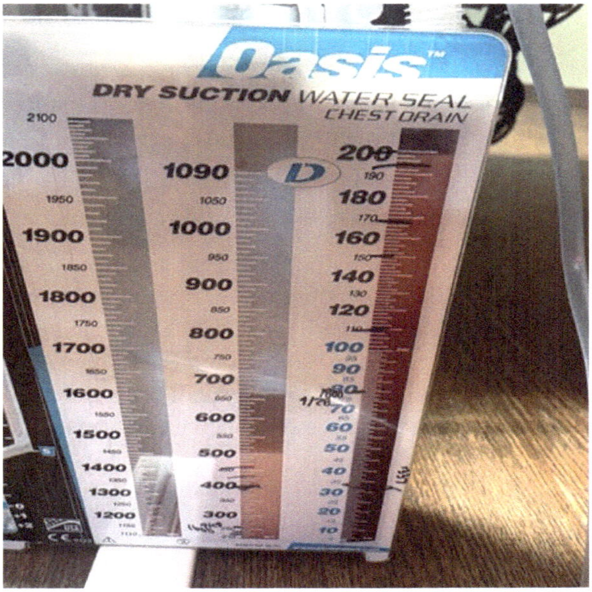

Fig. 22.2 Typical appearance of a chylous effusion

Laboratory Studies

- Serum laboratory values will likely be normal, but a baseline CBC, LDH, and triglyceride levels may be useful for comparison purposes.
- Cell count in the pleural fluid should show a lymphocyte predominance.
- Pleural fluid triglyceride level > 110 mg/dL and/or the presence of chylomicrons on microscopy confirm the diagnosis.

Imaging

- Plain radiography will show a pleural effusion if a chest drain is not present.
- For non-iatrogenic chylothoraces on initial presentation, a chest CT with IV contrast is used to look for lymphadenopathy and masses that would suggest malignancy as the cause.
- Traditional as well as magnetic resonance lymphangiography is used for better anatomic delineation of the duct and site of disruption for planning of embolization.

Treatment

- Placement of a drain to relieve dyspnea and quantify chyle output should be done if not already performed.
  - The chest tube should be kept on water seal (avoid suction settings, as this theoretically precipitates fluid egress from the lymphatics).
- Initial trial of NPO for 48–72 h will help stratify the patients into those who are more likely to resolve without further intervention and those that may not:
  - Patients whose output becomes serous and decreases in volume (typically to under 500 mL/day) in that time period likely have only a small tributary disruption and are more likely to heal with nonoperative intervention.
  - If drainage improves to <500 mL/day, then consider starting total parenteral nutrition (TPN) or low-fat enteral feeds with medium-chain triglycerides, and reassess in a week, after which resume po and remove chest tube if no recurrent chylothorax.
  - Octreotide may be added to reduce the volume of drainage although its data regarding efficacy is limited.
- If the drainage does not subside with NPO status, > 500 mL/day over 2–3 days, then the main duct is likely disrupted (as after an esophagectomy), and intervention to close the duct should not be delayed. Once again, excessive loss of immune cells will lead to infection, sepsis, and eventual death.

- Interventions to close the thoracic duct include surgical ligation or embolization.
  - Surgical duct ligation (Fig. 22.3) is typically performed via a right chest approach, with mass ligation of all the tissues between the vertebral body, aorta, azygos vein, and esophagus just above the diaphragm so that any duplicate ducts and tributaries are encompassed in the ligation.
  - Embolization by interventional radiology involves cannulating the cisterna chyli followed by placement of coils or glue into the duct (Fig. 22.4).
  - Choice of surgery or embolization depends on the clinical context and availability of local expertise.

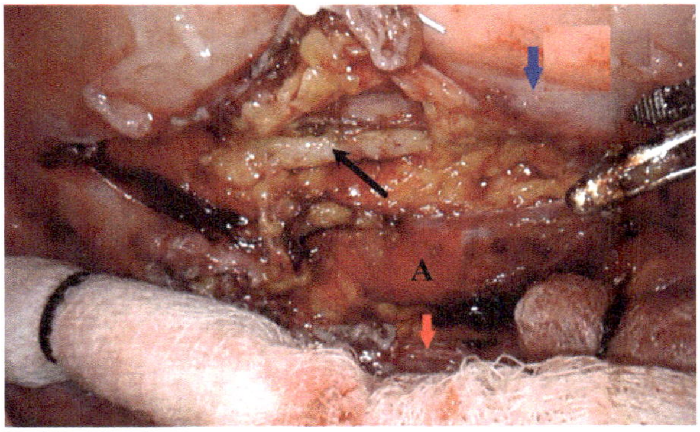

Fig. 22.3 Intraoperative picture via the right chest. Mass ligation of the thoracic duct (black arrow) would involve ligation of all the mediastinal tissues between the esophagus (red arrow), aorta (**A**), azygos vein (blue arrow), and vertebral body (behind the thoracic duct and mediastinal fat)

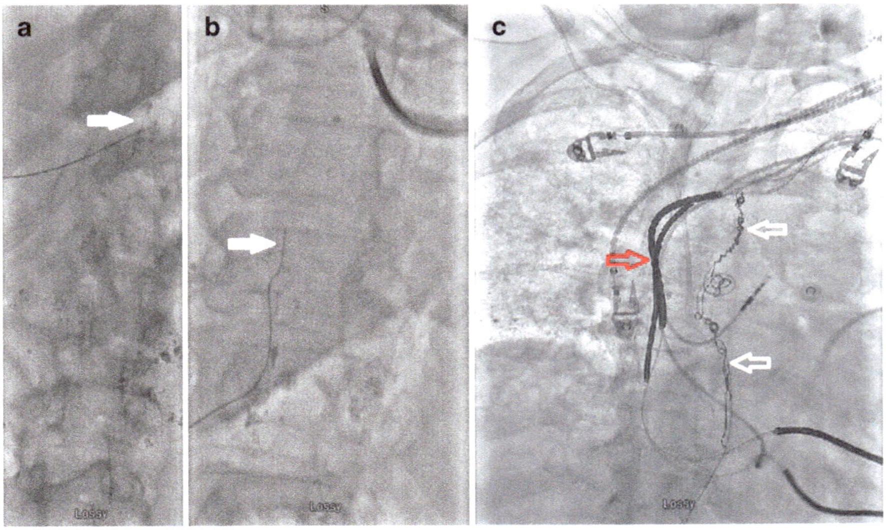

Fig. 22.4 Thoracic duct embolization. (**a**) Access of the cisterna chyli which has been opacified by lymphangiogram (arrow); (**b**) after access, guidewire and catheter are advanced up the thoracic duct (arrow); (**c**) coil and glue embolization of the thoracic duct (white arrow); other radiopaque structures represent patient's defibrillator leads (red arrow)

Key Reference

- Agrawal A, Chaddha U, Kaul V, Desai A, Gillaspie E, Maldonado F. Multidisciplinary management of chylothorax. Chest. 2022;162(6):1402–12.

Further Reading

Chen C, Wang Z, Hao J, Hao X, Zhou J, Chen N, Liu L, Pu Q. Chylothorax after lung cancer surgery: a key factor influencing prognosis and quality of life. Ann Thorac Cardiovasc Surg. 2020;26(6):303–10.

Darling GE, Allen MS, Decker PA, et al. Randomized trial of mediastinal lymph node sampling versus complete lymphadenectomy during pulmonary resection in the patient with N0 or N1 non-small cell carcinoma: results of the ACOSOG Z0030 trial. J Thorac Cardiovasc Surg. 2011;141:662–70.

Gilyard SN, Khaja MS, Goswami AK, Kokabi N, Saad WE, Majdalany BS. Traumatic chylothorax: approach and outcomes. Semin Intervent Radiol. 2020;37(3):263–8.

Low DE, Kuppusamy MK, Alderson D, et al. Benchmarking complications associated with esophagectomy. Ann Surg. 2019;269(2):291–8.

Riley LE, Ataya A. Clinical approach and review of causes of a chylothorax. Respir Med. 2019;157:7–13.

Yasuura Y, Konno H, Hayakawa T, et al. Chylothorax after pulmonary resection and lymph node dissection for primary lung cancer; retrospective observational study. J Cardiothorac Surg. 2022;17:11–6.

Chapter 23
Thoracic Trauma

Aaron Zuckerman and Leslie S. Tyrie

Anatomy of the Chest

Chest Wall

- All patients with significant blunt traumatic mechanism or penetrating trauma to the thorax should be considered for thoracic injury.
- "The box" is the anatomic region bounded by (Fig. 23.1):
  - Superior: the clavicles and sternal notch.
  - Lateral: the midclavicular lines.
  - Inferior: a line connecting the intersection between the midclavicular lines and the costal margin of the ribs.
- Penetrating injury to the box should prompt concern for cardiac injury, and workup in the stable patient should include transthoracic echocardiography (TTE).
- The thoracoabdominal region is bounded by:
  - Superior: the level of the nipples (anterior) or tip of the scapula (posterior).
  - Inferior: the level of the umbilicus (anterior) or T10 (posterior).
- Penetrating wounds involving this area should prompt concern for the chest, diaphragm, or abdominal organs.

A. Zuckerman · L. S. Tyrie (✉)
Department of Surgery, New York University Langone Health, New York, NY, USA
e-mail: aaron.zuckerman@nyulangone.org

T. Ng, T. Geraci (eds.), *Thoracic Surgery Clerkship*, Contemporary Surgical Clerkships, https://doi.org/10.1007/978-3-031-44645-0_23

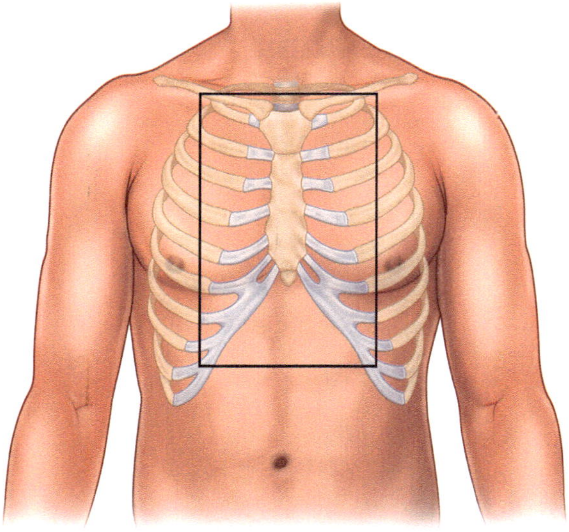

Fig. 23.1 The borders of the cardiac box

Heart and Great Vessels

- The right ventricle is the most anterior part of the heart and is the most prone to penetrating stab injuries.
- Acceleration/deceleration injuries can cause blunt aortic injury, usually around the fixed point of the ligamentum arteriosum.
- A normal cardiac silhouette on CXR should be no more than half of the chest diameter.
- The mediastinum on CXR should be 8 cm or less and occupy less than 1/3 of the chest diameter.

Lungs and Pleura

- The left main bronchus is normally higher and shallower than the right main bronchus.
- The right diaphragm is normally the same height as the left or slightly higher.
- Normal costophrenic angles are sharp on CXR.
- Mediastinal shift on CXR implies increased pressure in the thoracic cavity.

Trachea

- The trachea bifurcates at the angle of Louis (second sternocostal joint).
- The cricothyroid membrane can be palpated between the thyroid cartilage (superior) and the cricoid cartilage (inferior). Emergent airways are performed through the cricothyroid membrane.

Esophagus

- The proximal esophagus courses posteriorly in the neck towards the left.
- The mid-thoracic esophagus is most easily approached through the right chest.
- The distal thoracic esophagus is most easily approached through the left chest.

Thoracic Outlet

- The subclavian vein and phrenic nerve are found anterior to the anterior scalene muscle.
- The subclavian artery and brachial plexus are found between the anterior and middle scalene muscles.

Approach to the Trauma Patient

The initial approach to all trauma patients is the same: the primary survey followed by the secondary survey and adjuncts. These surveys are repeated any time the patient has a change in clinical status.

Airway

- Ask the patient to speak. Clear speech usually indicates an intact airway and may indicate adequate breathing mechanics.
- Inspect the trachea for any obvious deformities or deviation.
- Concern for airway compromise should prompt immediate endotracheal intubation.

Breathing

- Observe respiratory effort and rate, look for chest symmetry, listen to breath sounds bilaterally, check oxygen saturation, and palpate the chest wall to assess for fractures or deformity.
- Diminished breath sounds may indicate pneumothorax or hemothorax.
- Penetrating wounds to the chest can be covered with a three-sided occlusive dressing, since a completely occlusive dressing may cause development of tension physiology.
- Simple pneumothorax may become a tension pneumothorax with intubation and positive pressure ventilation.

Circulation

- Check central and peripheral pulses, assess heart rate and blood pressure, and control any obvious external hemorrhage.
- Jugular venous distention (JVD) may indicate increased intrathoracic pressure from either developing tension pneumothorax or pericardial tamponade.
- Patients may be in shock secondary to hemorrhage and/or tension pneumothorax or pericardial tamponade.
- Penetrating injury to the box should warrant prompt TTE or operative exploration depending on the patient's hemodynamic status.
- Immediate return of 1000 mL from a chest tube should prompt operative thoracic exploration.

Disability

- Consider traumatic brain injury or spinal cord injury when a patient presents with an abnormal neurologic exam.

Exposure

- All clothes should be removed, and the patient should be rolled to check for any injuries to the back and axillae.
- Penetrating objects should be left in place for exploration and removal in the operating room.

Secondary Survey

- After completing the primary survey, a head-to-toe assessment must be performed to assess for any further lacerations, hematomas, tenderness, skeletal deformities, or neurological deficits. Inspect all orifices, and document all injuries.

Adjuncts to the Primary and Secondary Survey

- A screening CXR should be routinely performed early in the assessment of chest injury.
- CXR can rapidly help identify significant rib fractures, pulmonary contusion, hemo- and/or pneumothorax, blunt aortic injury, and diaphragmatic hernia.
- If safe, CXR is ideally performed upright. Markers may be used to help identify the location of wounds.
- Focused abdominal sonography for trauma (FAST) should be performed to assess for the presence of pericardial fluid after any penetrating injury to the box. It may also be indicated for thoracoabdominal trauma. Blunt cardiac rupture is rare, but the cardiac window should be included in all patients with significant traumatic mechanism and unexplained hypotension.
- Extended FAST (E-FAST) additionally assesses the chest for pneumothorax or hemothorax.
- Electrocardiography (EKG) is useful in the workup of blunt cardiac injury.

Rib Fractures/Pulmonary Contusion

Presentation

- Usually result from blunt trauma.
- Often find localized chest pain with focal chest wall tenderness.
- Flail chest (3 or more ribs broken in 2 places) may have paradoxical motion of that segment of chest wall.
- Pulmonary contusion can be mild (incidentally seen on CT scan) or severe causing both hypoxic and hypercapnic respiratory failure.

Workup

- CXR is a good screening test. This must be followed by a delayed CXR or a CT scan.
- Contusion to the lung appears as a white consolidation on CXR that does not layer at the costophrenic angles.
- CT is more sensitive for rib fractures than CXR and can demonstrate occult pulmonary contusion, hemothorax, or pneumothorax.

Management

- The greatest risk to respiratory status is the underlying pulmonary contusion.
- Mortality is higher in elderly patients, and even a small number of rib fractures may require monitoring in an intensive care setting.
- Multimodal pain control is essential. Minimize opioids (respiratory depression), and consider a rib block or an epidural if needed.
- Encourage incentive spirometry and trend performance.
- Rib plating is appropriate for the management of some fracture patterns. Indications are varied but include flail segment, significant chest wall deformity, or inability to control pain.

Pneumothorax

Presentation

- Can be secondary to penetrating or blunt trauma.
- May be asymptomatic or associated with varying degrees of dyspnea or chest pain.
- Tension pneumothorax is characterized by hypotension; it can be rapidly fatal if unrecognized.

Workup

- Tension pneumothorax is a clinical diagnosis, and a chest tube or needle decompression should be performed when suspected before obtaining a CXR.

- Stable patients should undergo screening CXR (upright if possible) and follow-up with a delayed CXR or a CT scan.
- Deep sulcus sign (the inferior lateral border of the diaphragm is pushed down below the level of the CXR) may indicate pneumothorax.

Management

- A small, asymptomatic pneumothorax can be observed in carefully selected patients.
- A large or symptomatic pneumothorax should be evacuated with a chest tube (tube thoracostomy).
- Tension pneumothorax requires immediate decompression with a large-bore angiocatheter (needle decompression) or a chest tube. Needle decompression should be followed by a chest tube.

Hemothorax

Presentation

- Usually occurs secondary to bleeding from the chest wall, lungs, intercostal vessels, or internal mammary vessels.
- Patients may complain of dyspnea, and breath sounds may be diminished or absent on the affected side.
- Massive hemothorax leads to hemorrhagic shock.

Workup

- Start with a screening CXR, upright if possible.
- In the setting of trauma, blunting of the costophrenic angle usually indicates blood in the pleural space.
- Follow up with a delayed CXR or a CT scan. CT is more sensitive for smaller amounts of fluid and may identify intravenous (IV) contrast extravasation at the site of injury.

Management

- Most hemothorax will be treated with a chest tube, but small amounts of fluid can be observed. Chest tubes are usually inserted in the fourth or fifth intercostal space in the anterior or midaxillary line.
- Chest tube drainage >1000 mL initially or > 200 mL/hour for 4 h should prompt surgical exploration.
- If hemothorax is still present >48 h after chest tube insertion, surgical evacuation should be considered.
- Options for surgical evacuation and control of hemorrhage include video-assisted thoracoscopic surgery (VATS) or thoracotomy. Unstable patients should undergo thoracotomy.

Penetrating Cardiac Injury

Presentation

- Patients may be asymptomatic or complain of chest pain/pressure.
- They may be hemodynamically stable or unstable.
- JVD may represent increased intrathoracic pressure.
- Pericardial tamponade is characterized by hypotension. Beck's triad is the finding of JVD, muffled heart sounds, and hypotension. Even a small amount of pericardial blood can cause tamponade physiology, and these patients can decompensate into cardiac arrest quickly.

Workup

- Diagnosis should be made by pericardial view of the FAST exam or a formal echocardiography. This may be falsely negative for cardiac injury if blood is decompressing into another space (i.e., hemothorax) or if there is a small amount of blood posterior to the heart.
- CXR should be performed and may identify a widened cardiac silhouette or important pulmonary pathology.
- CT can identify associated injuries if they are suspected but should only be obtained in stable patients.

Management

- The presence of pericardial fluid suggests cardiac injury, and patients should be taken for operative repair most often through a median sternotomy.
- Stable patients with pericardial fluid may be considered for subxiphoid pericardial window with a low threshold to convert to sternotomy.
- A patient in extremis or who lost vital signs within 15 min of arrival to the hospital should be considered for a left anterolateral thoracotomy (*resuscitative thoracotomy*) in the emergency department. The pericardium is opened (parallel to and avoiding the phrenic nerve) to release any hemopericardium. Injuries to the heart are controlled via digital pressure, sutures, or other means until definitive therapy in the operating room.
- Echocardiogram should be obtained prior to discharge, to rule out intracardiac injury such as septal defects or valve injuries.

Blunt Cardiac Injury

Presentation

- Uncommon; includes varied presentations ranging from asymptomatic, chest pain, dyspnea, arrhythmia, cardiogenic shock, to sudden death.

Workup

- Often includes EKG and troponin, but abnormal values are not always specific.
- A normal EKG and troponin are highly suggestive that a patient does not have a significant blunt cardiac injury.
- Obtain TTE if structural or functional abnormalities are suspected.

Management

- Patients should be observed on telemetry if blunt cardiac injury is suspected.
- Indications for operative management include structural injury such as rupture (rare in a living patient) or injuries that involve valvular function or the coronary vessels.

Diaphragm Injury

Presentation

- From direct penetrating trauma to the thoracoabdominal region or rupture from high-energy blunt trauma due to increased intrathoracic pressure.
- More prevalent on the left side as the right is protected by the liver.
- Patients may have varying degrees of chest pain or dyspnea.

Workup

- CXR may show an elevated hemidiaphragm or abdominal organs in the chest. Noting the course of a nasogastric tube (NGT) may help identify abnormalities.
- CT is more sensitive than CXR, but neither can completely rule out diaphragm injury.
- The gold standard for diagnosing diaphragm injury is direct visualization through thoracoscopy (VATS) or laparoscopy, which should be considered for all patients with penetrating thoracoabdominal wounds – especially on the left.

Management

- Left-sided diaphragm injuries should be repaired to prevent the risk of developing a diaphragmatic hernia in the future.
- Traditional surgical closure is performed with nonabsorbable horizontal mattress sutures with pledgets.
- Depending on the size, diaphragm injuries on the right can be observed since the liver prevents most diaphragmatic hernias.

Esophageal Injury

Presentation

- Variable and includes odynophagia or hematemesis.
- Cervical esophagus injuries may cause localized tenderness or crepitus.

- Intrathoracic injuries can cause fever, tachycardia, pneumomediastinum, or pleural effusion. Mediastinitis is a feared complication of missed injury in the chest.
- Intraabdominal injuries may lead to free intraperitoneal air or peritonitis.
- Delayed presentation generally results in more severe symptoms as well as increased morbidity and mortality.

Workup

- Screening CXR may identify pneumomediastinum, pleural effusion, or free air.
- Stable patients usually undergo a CT with IV contrast.
- If esophageal injury is suspected but not confirmed, additional testing includes contrast esophagogram and/or esophagoscopy.

Management

- Cervical esophageal injuries are usually approached through a longitudinal neck incision along the anterior border of the sternocleidomastoid muscle, on the side of injury. The main goal is a wide drainage. Primary repair with buttress (strap muscle) if possible, but not mandatory.
- Mid-thoracic esophageal injuries are approached through a right posterolateral thoracotomy and distal thoracic esophageal injuries through a left posterolateral thoracotomy. The main goal is primary repair in two layers (with the mucosa/submucosa layer the most important) and buttress with local tissue (intercostal muscle flap (preferred), pericardial fat flap, pleural flap). If the esophagus is not repairable, then perform diversion.

Injury to the Great Vessels/Blunt Aortic Injury

Presentation

- Major injuries to the great vessels usually lead to death at the scene, so the vast majority of these patients will have low or moderate grade injuries.
- Signs of great vessel injury in the chest include evidence of bleeding (found on imaging, hemodynamic compromise), absent pulses, or neurologic deficit.

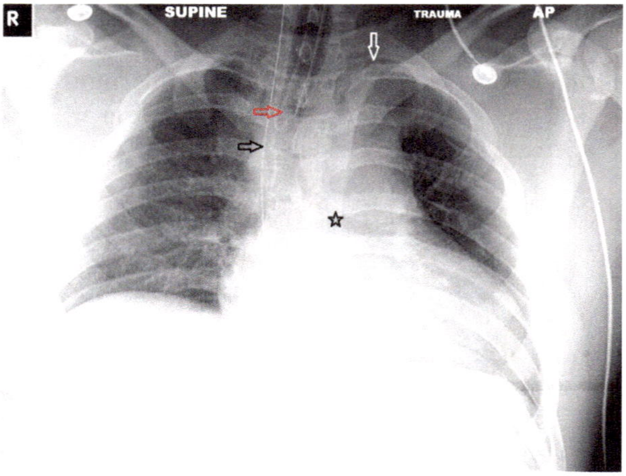

Fig. 23.2 Chest X-ray demonstrating widened mediastinum, apical cap (white arrow), left mainstem bronchus depression (star), rightward deviation of tracheal (red arrow), and deviated esophagus with nasogastric tube (black arrow). Blunt aortic injury was confirmed by CT scan

Workup

- There are many signs of aortic injury on screening CXR, including (Fig. 23.2):
  - Widened mediastinum.
  - Presence of an apical cap.
  - Depression of the left mainstem bronchus.
  - Deviation of the esophagus (as seen by NGT) or trachea to the right.
  - Loss of the aortopulmonary window.
  - Abnormal contour of the aorta or aortic knob.
  - Hemothorax.
- Unstable patients should proceed directly to the operating room.
- Stable patients should undergo CT angiogram of the chest.

Management

- The most common identified injury that requires treatment will be a blunt aortic injury, which can usually be repaired endovascularly after any other immediately life-threatening injury is dealt with.
- During delayed management, the risk of rupture is minimized with blood pressure control and heart rate management. An esmolol infusion may be useful for this purpose.
- For hemodynamically unstable patients with great vessel injury, operative management will be required. Different incisions may be necessary to access necessary structures.

- A median sternotomy is used to access the proximal aortic arch, innominate artery, origin of the right subclavian artery, and superior and inferior vena cavae as they insert into the heart, left and right brachiocephalic veins, and the main pulmonary artery and its branches.
- The right subclavian vessels can be further exposed via a supra- or infraclavicular incision or right anterolateral thoracotomy.
- Access to the proximal left subclavian artery can be very challenging, and approaches include a high left anterolateral thoracotomy, supra- or infraclavicular incision, or a combination of these (trap door).
- A clamshell thoracotomy provides the best exposure to all structures in the chest and can be done in the emergency department for patients in extremis when injury to the great vessels is suspected.

Airway Injury

Presentation

- Patients with major airway injury in the chest will usually be symptomatic. Signs include hemoptysis, crepitus, pneumothorax, pneumomediastinum, and/or respiratory failure.
- Beware that intubation may exacerbate injury or cause tension physiology.
- Blunt airway injuries commonly occur within 1–2 cm of the carina.

Workup

- Air decompresses into the chest or tissues, so initial management usually includes chest tube insertion. Suspect major airway injury in the chest when there is a large air leak from the chest tube or persistent pneumothorax after chest tube placement.
- Stable patients often get a CT scan initially to rule out associated injuries.
- Bronchoscopy is the best method to identify airway injury when suspected.

Management

- If possible, the endotracheal tube may be pushed past the site of injury. Other devices such as dual lumen tubes or bronchial blockers may help stabilize the patient until definitive repair can be performed.

- Operative exploration is performed via cervical incision, median sternotomy (partial or complete), or thoracotomy depending on the location of the airway injury. Initial goal is primary repair and buttress using local tissue, but if not repairable then resection with primary anastomosis.
- Small tracheobronchial tears resulting from blunt trauma may be observed or stented.

Key Reference

- Dennis BM, Bellister SA, Guillamondegui OD. Thoracic trauma. Surg Clin North Am. 2017;97(5):1047–64.

Further Reading

Bruner DI, Pritchard A, Hubert A. Pulmonary contusions Relias Media. 2011 [cited 2022 Jul 9]. https://www.reliasmedia.com/articles/131881-pulmonary-contusions.

Desalegn M, Chew C, Chew A. Traumatic diaphragmatic injury: a retrospective review of 14 cases managed at a regional hospital in Wolaita, Ethiopia. East Cent Afr J Surg. 2020;25(3):1.

Dixon A. Traumatic aortic rupture [Internet]. Radiopaedia. 2022. [cited 2022 Jul 9]. https://radiopaedia.org/cases/traumatic-aortic-rupture-1.

Dogrul BN, Kiliccalan I, Asci ES, Peker SC. Blunt trauma related chest wall and pulmonary injuries: an overview. Chin J Traumatol. 2020;23(3):125–38.

Gillman L, Ball C, Panebianco N, Al-Kadi A, Kirkpatrick A. Clinician performed resuscitative ultrasonography for the initial evaluation and resuscitation of trauma. Scand J Trauma Resusc Emerg Med. 2009;17(1):1.

Grewal HS, Dangayach NS, Ahmad U, Ghosh S, Gildea T, Mehta AC. Treatment of tracheobronchial injuries: a contemporary review. Chest. 2019;155(3):595–604.

Tesoriero R. Cardiac injury: techniques. In: Scalea TM, editor. The shock trauma manual of operative techniques. Cham: Springer; 2020.

Chapter 24
Thoracic Outlet Syndrome

Jason C. Zhang and Michael E. Barfield

Introduction

Thoracic outlet syndrome (TOS) encompasses a broad group of disorders resulting in symptoms of the shoulder and upper extremity. These symptoms of pain, weakness, and paresthesia are caused by compression of the neurovascular bundle as it exits the thoracic girdle. The diagnosis of the various forms of TOS (arterial, venous, neurogenic) can be complex and necessitates a good physical examination and clinical judgment to optimize treatment, which can be both surgical and nonsurgical. This chapter will discuss TOS anatomy, pathogenesis, presentation, diagnosis, and management.

Anatomy

- The thoracic outlet is defined as the space from the supraclavicular fossa to the axilla (Fig. 24.1). Important structures that course through this space include the brachial plexus, subclavian artery and vein, and axillary artery and vein. Compression of these structures leads to the classic symptoms of TOS described in a later section. Compression can occur in any of the three compartments within the thoracic outlet:

J. C. Zhang · M. E. Barfield (✉)
Division of Vascular and Endovascular Surgery, Department of Surgery, New York University Langone Health, New York, NY, USA
e-mail: jason.zhang@nyulangone.org

T. Ng, T. Geraci (eds.), *Thoracic Surgery Clerkship*, Contemporary Surgical Clerkships, https://doi.org/10.1007/978-3-031-44645-0_24

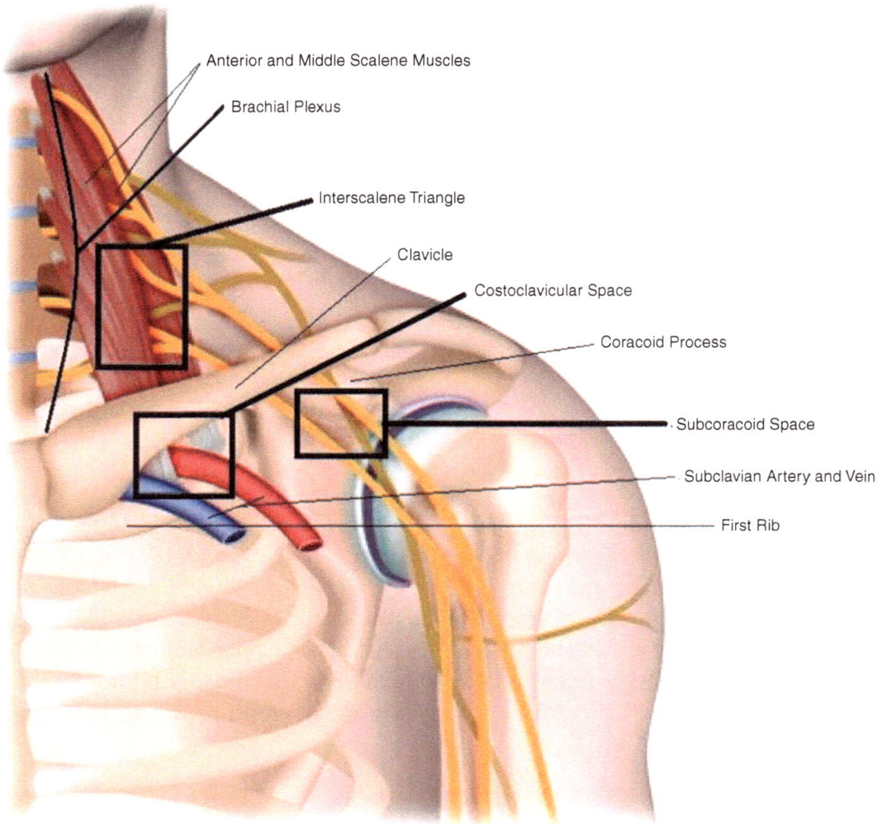

Fig. 24.1 Diagram of the thoracic outlet compartments and relative anatomy. Image reproduced as permitted by Creative Commons License (http://creativecommons.org/licenses/by-nc/4.0/). (Original image from Jones et al. (2019))

- Interscalene triangle: Bordered by the anterior scalene muscle anteriorly, first rib inferiorly, and middle scalene muscle posteriorly. The subclavian artery and brachial plexus course through this compartment.
- Costoclavicular space: Bordered by the middle third of the clavicle superiorly, first rib and anterior scalene muscle inferiorly and posteriorly, and subclavius muscle anteriorly. The brachial plexus, subclavian artery, and subclavian vein all pass through this space.
- Subcoracoid or pectoralis minor space: Bordered by the pectoralis minor anteriorly, ribs 2–4 posteriorly, and coracoid process superiorly. This is the most lateral compartment and contains the brachial plexus, axillary artery, and axillary vein.

Pathogenesis

- Several etiologies are thought to cause compression of the thoracic outlet. Though most factors predispose to all forms of TOS, some may be more classically associated with arterial TOS (aTOS), venous TOS (vTOS), or neurogenic TOS (nTOS).
- Trauma may cause TOS, as active hemorrhage, hematoma, whiplash, or displaced fractures may cause compression of arteries, veins, and/or nerves. Chronically, these injuries can lead to scarring and fibrosis, which may cause compression even after the initial injury is healed.
- Repetitive overhead motions (baseball, swimming, hair stylists, auto mechanics) may cause TOS through muscle hypertrophy and fibrosis leading to compression. This is typically seen in nTOS and vTOS.
- Anatomic variations may cause compression of the thoracic outlet. A cervical rib is an extra rib that grows from the cervical spine above the first rib (1–3% of population) and increases the chance of nerve or blood vessel compression. Cervical ribs increase the risk of aTOS. Other variations include anomalous first ribs and supernumerary scalene muscles.
- Malignancies may also compress the thoracic outlet. Most commonly, Pancoast tumors may compress the brachial plexus.

Epidemiology

- The true prevalence of TOS is unclear given difficulty in diagnosis and nonspecific symptoms; however, estimated incidence of nTOS and vTOS is 25 and 8 cases per 1,000,000 people per year, respectively.
- Historically, age at onset of symptoms is 20–50 years and is more prevalent in women.
- nTOS is the most common type, comprising 90–95% of all TOS patients. It is more common in women and tends to be unilateral.
- vTOS is the second most common, comprising 3–5% of all TOS patients. Patients typically present in 20s through 30s; it has a higher preponderance in men and typically presents unilaterally.
- aTOS is the least common, comprising 1–2% of all TOS patients. It typically presents unilaterally and affects both genders equally.

Evaluation (History)

Neurogenic TOS

- Neurogenic TOS is caused by compression of the C5-T1 brachial plexus nerve roots.

- Patients often present with upper extremity paresthesias, arm heaviness, neck pain, trapezius pain, shoulder/arm pain, occipital headaches, and paresthesias of the fingers on the affected side. Muscle wasting may be present in more advanced presentations.
- Frequently seen in patients with a history of trauma, commonly whiplash, that causes scarring of the thoracic outlet. Also frequently seen in young, active individuals who participate in repetitive overhead activity, such as swimming or baseball.
- Classically, patients report reproducible symptoms when performing aggravating activities, and symptoms correspond to the location of nerve impingement.

Venous TOS

- Venous TOS is caused by compression of the subclavian vein. Repeated compression and injury of the vein can cause thrombosis, known as "effort thrombosis" or "Paget-von Schroetter syndrome."
- Like nTOS, vTOS is frequently associated with repetitive overhead motion or trauma.
- Thrombosis can be acute or chronic and either occlusive or nonocclusive.
- Acute thrombosis can present as acute upper extremity swelling, cyanosis, heaviness, and pain. Patients with chronic disease will note swelling, dull aching pain of the extremity, heaviness, and visibly dilated superficial veins across the shoulder, chest, back, and neck.
- Symptoms tend to be stable for vTOS, whereas symptoms for nTOS can be exacerbated by overhead positioning.
- Pulmonary embolism can be seen in 10–20% of patients with effort thrombosis.

Arterial TOS

- Arterial TOS is caused by subclavian artery compression, commonly by an anomalous first rib or cervical rib.
- Chronic, repetitive compression of artery can cause stenosis, leading to formation of post-stenotic aneurysm (Fig. 24.2). Thrombosis may occur in the setting of stenosis or aneurysmal disease.
- Patients with chronic disease may have claudication with arm usage.
- Patients may present with acute distal embolization or complete thrombosis of the subclavian artery, leaving patients with a threatened limb. Symptoms include the "6 P's": pain, pallor, poikilothermia (cool skin), pulselessness, paresthesia, and paralysis.

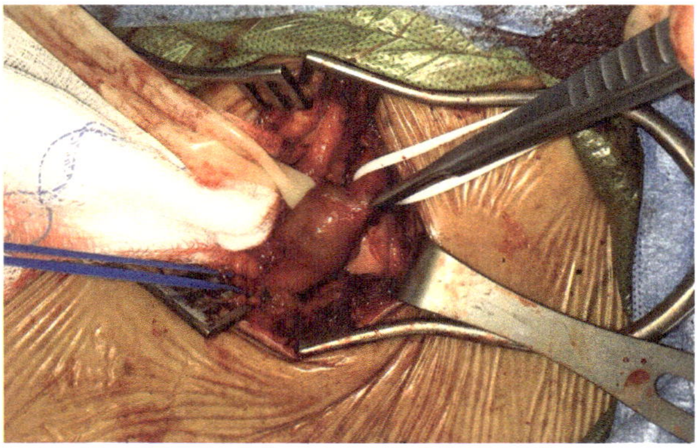

Fig. 24.2 Example of post-stenotic aneurysm of subclavian artery. (Courtesy of author Michael E Barfield MD)

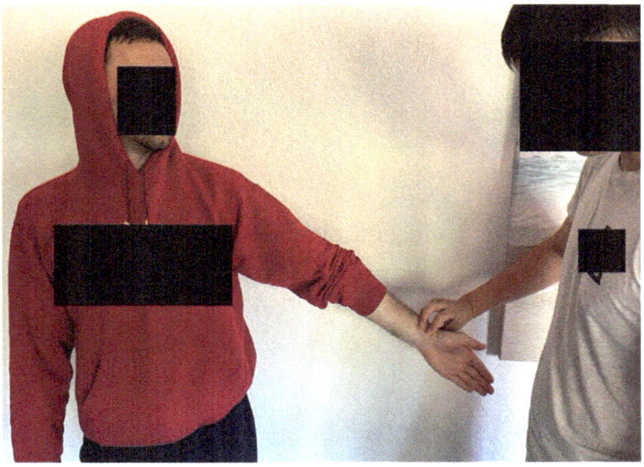

Fig. 24.3 Demonstration of Adson maneuver. A positive test notes a decrease or extinguishment of radial pulse with deep inspiration and head turn towards the affected arm

Physical Exam

- A complete physical exam of the upper extremity on both sides is crucial to diagnosis.
- Patients with nTOS may have weakness, pain, and wasting on the affected side.
- Patients with aTOS may have cool or cyanotic extremities and may have differences in blood pressure readings of both arms (>20 mmHg). Patients with vTOS may have swelling of the arm and significant varicosities over the neck, shoulder, and chest.
- Several common provocative maneuvers exist to help diagnose TOS, though the sensitivity and specificity of these exams are unclear.
  - Adson maneuver (Fig. 24.3): Used to diagnose aTOS. The affected arm is abducted 30° with the elbow flexed, and the practitioner should have fingers on the radial pulse. The patient is asked to take a deep breath and to extend the neck and turn his/her head towards the ipsilateral shoulder. A positive test notes a decrease or absence of the ipsilateral radial pulse.

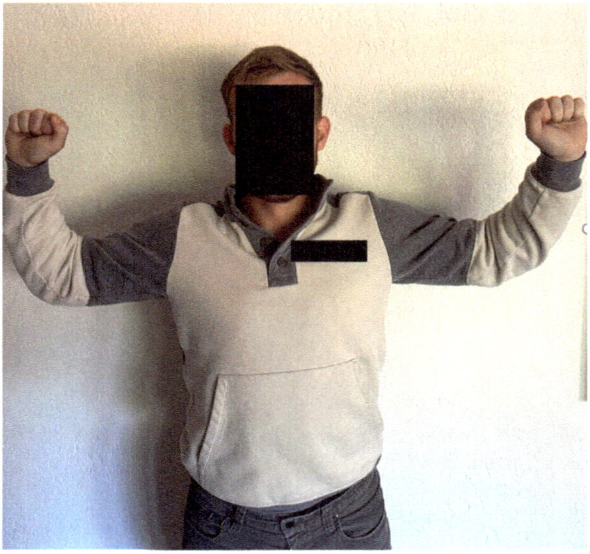

Fig. 24.4 Demonstration of elevated arm stress test

- Elevated arm stress test (Fig. 24.4): Used to diagnose nTOS. Patients are asked to abduct the shoulder 90°, flex the elbows 90°, and open and close their hands for 3 min. A positive test will result in pain, paresthesias, heaviness, or weakness of the affected side.

Differential Diagnosis

- Several disease processes may mimic the symptoms of all three forms of TOS and should be considered during diagnosis.
  - Rotator cuff injuries.
  - Elbow or forearm overuse injuries.
  - Peripheral nerve entrapment.
  - Herniated cervical or thoracic disk.
  - Chronic pain syndromes.
  - Hypercoagulable states (aTOS, vTOS).
  - Atrial fibrillation.
  - Superior sulcus or Pancoast tumor.

Testing/Imaging

- Testing and imaging modalities are directed towards the suspected form of TOS.
- Chest radiographs may help in identifying cervical ribs or anomalous first ribs.

- For patients with suspected vTOS or aTOS, duplex ultrasound is an effective and noninvasive imaging modality and should be the initial imaging test of choice. For patients with equivocal ultrasounds, or for those undergoing surgical planning, CTA or MRA can be performed as well.
- Patients with suspected nTOS may undergo electromyography (EMG). A majority of patients will have negative results, but a positive result may aid in the diagnosis of nTOS.
- Patients with nTOS may also undergo a lidocaine anterior scalene muscle block which may produce relief of their symptoms for 4 h. Patients with successful lidocaine blocks are more likely to have symptom relief following decompressive surgery.
- Venography may be performed for suspected vTOS, commonly done at the time of initial procedure. This may be done with the arm in both the abducted and adducted position, with a positive test involving decreased or cessation of flow in the abducted position.

Treatment

The optimal treatment for TOS varies depending on the etiology.

nTOS

- Initial management is nonoperative. Conservative options include avoiding activities that precipitate symptoms, postural modifications, and TOS-focused physical therapy. Pharmacological options include NSAIDs for neuropathic pain and muscle relaxants, anticonvulsants, and antidepressants as adjuncts.
- Injections of local anesthetics, steroids, and botulinum toxin type A (Botox) have had varying degrees of success for nTOS.
- For those who have failed conservative management for at least 4–6 months, surgical decompression of the thoracic outlet can be considered.

aTOS

- Patients with acute limb ischemia may require emergent surgical intervention to remove embolus (embolectomy) or thrombus (thrombectomy).
- Patients with diagnosed aTOS are placed on anticoagulation.
- All patients with aTOS are indicated for surgical decompression.
- Depending on the degree of stenosis or aneurysm, arterial reconstruction may be needed. This may include direct arterial repair with patch angioplasty or resec-

tion and interposition bypass graft. Options for bypass conduit include prosthetic grafts, autologous vein (saphenous or superficial femoral), or cryopreserved artery/vein.

vTOS

- Patients with thrombosis are placed initially on anticoagulation to prevent further propagation and for dissolution of clot.
- For patients with severe thrombotic burden, thrombectomy and/or treatment with thrombolytics may be indicated.
- All patients with vTOS and evidence of thrombosis are indicated for surgical decompression, given the high likelihood of thrombosis recurrence.
- Patients may need venous reconstruction or venoplasty as an adjunct to surgery.

Surgical Options

- The surgical procedure for decompression of the thoracic outlet is a first-rib resection and anterior scalenectomy (FRRS). The three open surgical approaches to FRRS include transaxillary, supraclavicular, and infraclavicular. No significant difference in outcome has been noted between the three approaches, and selection usually is determined by surgeon preference and patient anatomy.
- Transaxillary approach.
  - The patient is placed in the lateral position, and the first rib is accessed between the pectoralis major and latissimus dorsi. Care must be taken to preserve the brachial plexus and the intercostal brachial nerve as it exists between the first and second ribs.
  - The subclavius muscle is first divided, followed by the division of the anterior scalene, with care to preserve the subclavian artery.
  - The first rib is then resected. This approach provides a more aesthetic incision as the incision is made in the axilla. However, visualization is decreased intraoperatively.
- Supraclavicular approach (Figs. 24.5 and 24.6).
  - The patient is placed in a supine position, and an incision is made 2 cm above the clavicle.
  - Care must be taken to preserve the phrenic nerve during the division of the anterior scalene, as it courses anterior to the muscle from lateral to medial.
  - The middle scalene is then divided, and the first rib/cervical rib is resected. This procedure has a greater exposure of the neurovascular structures than the transaxillary approach but has a worse cosmetic result.

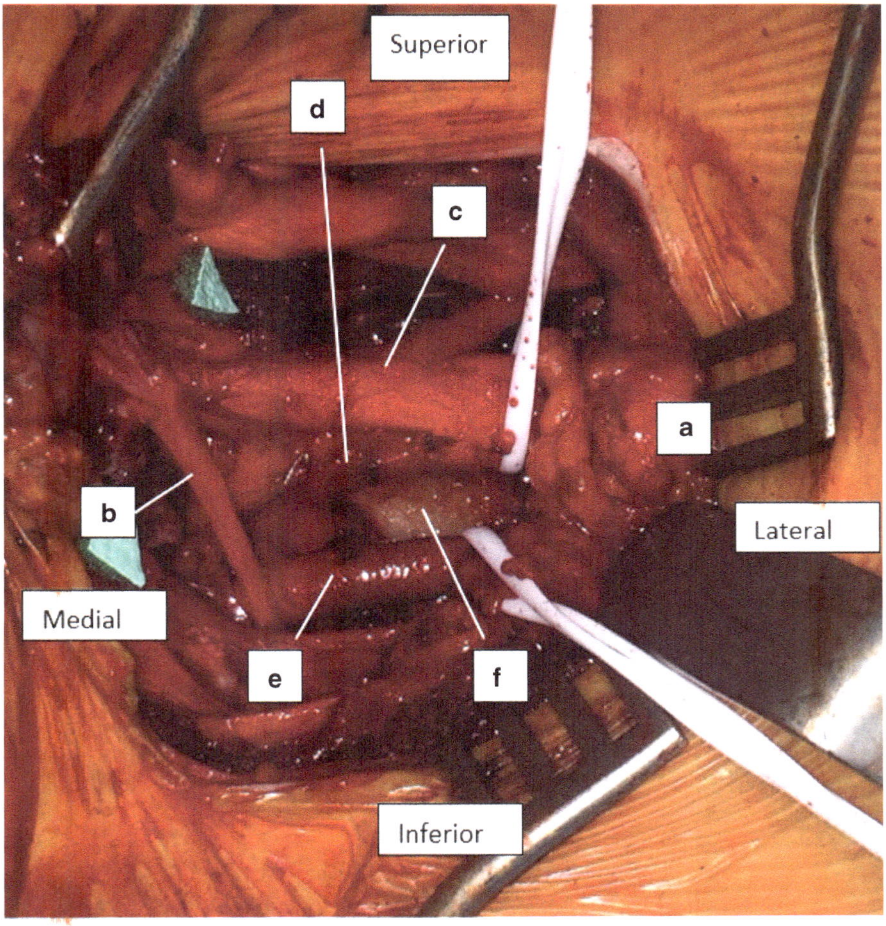

Fig. 24.5 Anatomy of supraclavicular approach. (**a**) Scalene fat pad. (**b**) Phrenic nerve. (**c**) Brachial plexus. (**d**) Subclavian artery. (**e**) Subclavian vein. (**f**) First-rib remnant (already resected). (Courtesy of author Michael E Barfield MD)

- Infraclavicular approach.
  - Most rarely used approach.
  - This approach provides the best exposure of the subclavian vein and may be used in conjunction with the supraclavicular approach if central venous exposure is needed.
- More recently, robotic- and thoracoscopic-assisted approaches have been utilized to minimize brachial plexus manipulation.

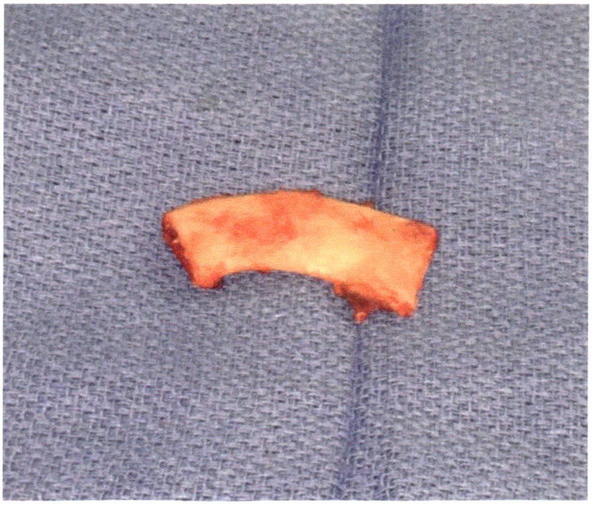

Fig. 24.6 The first rib after resection. (Courtesy of author Michael E Barfield MD)

Surgical Outcomes

Complications

- Several complications can be encountered during FRRS including:
  - Pneumothorax: Can happen in up to 10% of cases. If noted intraoperatively, a small chest tube can be placed.
  - Hemothorax.
  - Postoperative pain.
  - Bleeding.
  - Infection.
  - Injury to brachial plexus/phrenic nerve/long thoracic nerve.
  - Injury to vascular structures.
  - Injury to thoracic duct for left-sided procedures.

Prognosis

- Most patients with nTOS will have relief of their symptoms (56–89%) after surgery. Given that some patients do have recurrence or nonresponse after surgery, it is important to counsel patients that their symptoms may continue postoperatively.
- Functional outcomes after surgical treatment for aTOS and vTOS tend to be higher than for nTOS. A meta-analysis found that overall clinical success after surgery was >90% for vascular TOS and 60–80% for nTOS.
- For patients with recurrent symptoms after surgery, Botox injections, physical therapy, and repeat surgery may be considered.

Key Reference

- Jones MR, Prabhakar A, Viswanath O, et al. Thoracic outlet syndrome: a comprehensive review of pathophysiology, diagnosis, and treatment. Pain Ther. 2019;8(1):5–18.

Further Reading

Davoli F, Staffa G, Ciarrocchi AP, Stella F. Thoracic outlet syndrome: which surgical approach? Curr Chall Thorac Surg. 2021;3:3.

DiLosa KL, Humphries MD. Epidemiology of thoracic outlet syndrome. Semin Vasc Surg. 2021;34(1):65–70.

Freischlag J, Orion K. Understanding thoracic outlet syndrome. Scientifica (Cairo). 2014;2014:248163.

Peek J, Vos CG, Ünlü Ç, Schreve MA, van de Mortel RHW, de Vries JPM. Long-term functional outcome of surgical treatment for thoracic outlet syndrome. Diagnostics (Basel). 2018;8(1):7.

Peek J, Vos CG, Ünlü Ç, van de Pavoordt HDWM, van den Akker PJ, de Vries JPM. Outcome of surgical treatment for thoracic outlet syndrome: systematic review and meta-analysis. Ann Vasc Surg. 2017;40:303–26.

Povlsen S, Povlsen B. Diagnosing thoracic outlet syndrome: current approaches and future directions. Diagnostics (Basel). 2018;8(1):21.

Chapter 25
Hyperhidrosis

Melanie P. Subramanian and Stephanie H. Chang

Introduction

- Hyperhidrosis is excessive sweating that can lead to significant discomfort and anxiety for affected patients.
- Hyperhidrosis is relatively uncommon (1–3% of the population), affects men and women equally, and is present more frequently in hotter climates.
- Hyperhidrosis can be either primary or secondary. It is essential to differentiate these conditions, as the treatment algorithms differ.

Pathophysiology and Presentation

Primary Hyperhidrosis

- Primary hyperhidrosis is idiopathic and starts in childhood/puberty. It is secondary to a dysfunction in the sympathetic nervous system involving the thermoregulatory system.
- Primary hyperhidrosis often involves the hands (palmar surface), feet (plantar surface), or axilla, though can rarely present with facial sweating or blushing.

M. P. Subramanian
Division of Cardiothoracic Surgery, Department of Surgery, Washington University in St Louis, St Louis, MO, USA
e-mail: m.p.subramanian@wustl.edu

S. H. Chang (✉)
Division of Thoracic Surgery, Department of Cardiothoracic Surgery, New York University Langone Health, New York, NY, USA
e-mail: Stephanie.chang@nyulangone.org

T. Ng, T. Geraci (eds.), *Thoracic Surgery Clerkship*, Contemporary Surgical Clerkships, https://doi.org/10.1007/978-3-031-44645-0_25

- Patients with primary hyperhidrosis do not have sweating while asleep.
- Stress and heat can trigger episodes in hyperhidrosis.
- Familial history is present in 25–50% of patients.

Secondary Hyperhidrosis

- Secondary hyperhidrosis has generalized symptoms and is secondary to a different medical illness.
- Secondary hyperhidrosis often presents in adults, and sweating does occur while asleep.
- Common causes include infection, diabetes, certain malignancies, hyperthyroidism, menopause, obesity, and neurologic diseases.
- Treatment for secondary hyperhidrosis is management of the underlying disease.

Anatomy

- Typical sweat is from apocrine glands.
- Sweat from hyperhidrosis is from eccrine glands, with serous and non-odorous sweat.
- The important levels of the sympathetic chain for hyperhidrosis are:
  - T2 ganglia: facial blushing and hyperhidrosis.
  - T3 ganglia: palmar hyperhidrosis.
  - T4 ganglia: axillary hyperhidrosis.

Evaluation

- No tests exist to determine if hyperhidrosis is present.
- Qualitative metrics include:
  - Have they experienced ≥6 months of focal and visible excess sweat without cause.
  - If so, do they have two of the following:

    Bilateral and symmetric sweating.
    Sweating that impacts the patient's life.
    1+ episode per week
    Symptom onset prior to age 25.
    Sweating does not occur while asleep.
    Family history of similar symptoms.

Table 25.1 Hyperhidrosis disease severity scale

Score	Symptoms
1	My sweating is never noticeable and never interferes with my daily activities
2	My sweating is tolerable but sometimes interferes with my daily activities
3	My sweating is barely tolerable and frequently interferes with my daily activities
4	My sweating is intolerable and always interferes with my daily activities

- A different evaluation method includes the Hyperhidrosis Disease Severity Scale (Table 25.1). A score of 3 out of 4 is classified as severe hyperhidrosis.

Treatment for Primary Hyperhidrosis

Nonsurgical (First-Line Therapy)

- Aluminum chloride hexahydrate (common for axillary hyperhidrosis) is the most common and effective treatment for hyperhidrosis. This compound works by blocking the eccrine glands to prevent sweating. While effective, once the treatment is stopped, symptoms will recur.
- Iontophoresis (common for palmar and plantar hyperhidrosis) involves submerging the affected skin in water while an electric current is applied. Treatments are 3–4x per week until symptoms are controlled, with maintenance every 1–4 weeks.
- Botulinum toxin injections inhibit acetylcholine at the sympathetic cholinergic nerve endings. Symptoms are often controlled for greater than 6 months.
- Anticholinergic agents can be given topically or orally. Oral administration is associated with systemic side effects (blurry vision, dry mouth, urinary retention, constipation).

Surgery

- If nonsurgical treatments fail, patients should be placed on a trial of low-dose beta-blocker to mimic some possible postoperative effects of sympathicotomy.
- Surgery involves bilateral transection or clipping of the affected sympathetic fibers (T2, facial blushing; T3 ganglia, palmar; T4, axillary) (Fig. 25.1).
  - Surgery can be performed on minimally invasive platforms.
  - Patients may undergo a single side at initial surgery or choose to have both sides treated in one setting.

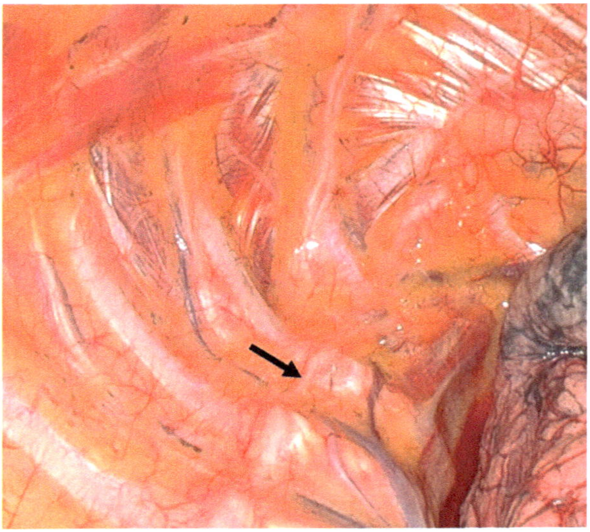

Fig. 25.1 Intraoperative visualization of the sympathetic nerve (black arrow)

- The ribs are identified, along with the intercostal spaces and sympathetic chain.
- At the appropriate level, the pleura lateral to the sympathetic chain is opened.
- The chain is then divided with cautery or clipped at the affected level.
- After closing on the first side, the same steps are performed on the opposite laterality.

Postoperative Complications

- After surgery, patients have compensatory sweating, which often involves sweating of the torso and legs.
  - Most patients tolerate this change in sweat distribution, but some patients regret having the procedure.
  - Risk factors for intolerable compensatory sweating involve multi-level transections or preoperative axillary hyperhidrosis.
- If the upper T1 nerve root is disrupted, the patient will have ipsilateral Horner's syndrome (miosis, ptosis, anhidrosis).

Key Reference

- Cerfolio RJ, De Campos JR, Bryant AS, et al. The Society of Thoracic Surgeons expert consensus for the surgical treatment of hyperhidrosis. Ann Thorac Surg. 2011;91(5):1642–48.

Further Reading

Compeau CG. Dorsal sympathicotomy for hyperhidrosis. In: Darling G, editor. Pearson's general thoracic surgery. Chicago, IL: Society of Thoracic Surgeons; 2021.

Henning MAS, Bouazzi D, Jemec GBE. Treatment of hyperhidrosis: an update. Am J Clin Dermatol. 2022;23(5):635–46.

Krause E, Burrows W. Thoracic sympathectomy. In: Watson J, Louis C, editors. TSRA clinical scenarios in cardiothoracic surgery. 2nd ed. Chicago: Thoracic Surgery Residents Association; 2020. p. 114–8.

Licht PB, Ladegaard L, Pilegaard HK. Thoracoscopic sympathectomy for isolated facial blushing. Ann Thorac Surg. 2006;81(5):1863–6.

Sugimora H, Spratt EH, Compeau CG, et al. Thoracoscopy sympathetic clipping for hyperhidrosis: long-term results and reversibility. J Thorac Cardiovasc Surg. 2009;137(6):1370–6.

Chapter 26
Lung Transplantation

Shair Ahmed and Lara Schaheen

History of Lung Transplantation

Lung transplantation is a life-saving treatment option for selected patients with end-stage lung disease. Although solid organ transplantation began in the 1950s, with kidney transplantation, it was not until a decade later that a human lung transplant would be attempted. In 1963, James Hardy and colleagues at the University of Mississippi performed the first successful human lung transplant with the recipient surviving 18 days. More than two decades later in 1986, Joel Cooper and his colleagues at the Toronto Lung Transplant Group published their experience with two patients who underwent single-lung transplantation. The field has grown exponentially over the past 20 years with the development of sophisticated immunosuppression medications, careful candidate selection, and advancements in surgical technique. To date, more than 2000 lung transplants are performed in the United States each year.

Indications for Lung Transplantation

General Guidelines

- Individuals with advanced lung disease.
- Limitations in functional status: classified as New York Heart Class III or IV.
- Less than a 50% 2-year predicted survival despite maximal medical therapy.
- No significant non-correctable comorbidity.

S. Ahmed (✉) · L. Schaheen
Norton Thoracic Institute, St. Joseph's Hospital and Medical Center, Phoenix, AZ, USA
e-mail: shair.ahmed@bswhealth.org; lara.schaheen@commonspirit.org

T. Ng, T. Geraci (eds.), *Thoracic Surgery Clerkship*, Contemporary Surgical Clerkships, https://doi.org/10.1007/978-3-031-44645-0_26

Risk Factors to Be Considered

- Age.
- Renal function.
- Coronary artery disease.
- Peripheral vascular disease.
- Heart failure.
- Connective tissue disease.
- Gastroesophageal reflux disease/esophageal dysmotility.
- Hematologic abnormalities.
- Body mass index (BMI) and nutritional status.
- Functional status/frailty.
- Infectious disease.
- Psychosocial factors.

Disease-Specific Criteria

- In addition to the general considerations and risk factors that affect an individual's lung transplant candidacy, there are important disease-specific considerations that should guide candidate selection.
- Cystic fibrosis.
  - Forced expiratory volume in 1 s (FEV1) <25% predicted.
  - Rapid decline in lung function (>30% relative decline in FEV1 over 12 months).
  - Frequent hospitalization, particularly if >28 days hospitalized in the preceding year.
  - Exacerbation requiring mechanical ventilation.
  - Chronic respiratory failure with hypoxemia or hypercapnia, particularly for those with increasing oxygen requirements or needing long-term noninvasive ventilation therapy.
  - Pulmonary hypertension (pulmonary arterial systolic pressure > 50 mmHg on echocardiogram or evidence of right ventricular dysfunction).
  - Worsening nutritional status as measured by a body mass index <18 kg/m^2 despite nutritional interventions.
  - Recurrent massive hemoptysis despite bronchial artery embolization.
- Chronic obstructive pulmonary disease (COPD).
  - BODE (BMI, airflow limitations: FEV1, dyspnea, 6 minute walk distance) score of 7–10.
  - Additional factors which may prompt listing:

    History of severe exacerbations.

    Moderate to severe pulmonary hypertension.
    FEV1 < 20% predicted.
    Chronic hypercapnia.

- Interstitial lung disease (ILD).
  - Desaturation to <88% on 6 min walk test or > 50 m decline in 6 min walk test distance in the past 6 months.
  - One of the following in the past 6 months despite appropriate treatment:

    Absolute decline in forced vital capacity (FVC) >10%, diffusing capacity of the lungs for carbon monoxide (DLCO) >10%, or FVC >5% with radiographic progression.

  - Pulmonary hypertension.
  - Hospitalization due to respiratory decline, pneumothorax, or acute exacerbation.
- Pulmonary arterial hypertension.
  - REVEAL Score > 10 on appropriate therapy (prostacyclin analogues).
  - Progressive signs of secondary organ dysfunction, not failure (liver, kidney).
  - Life-threatening hemoptysis.
- Acute respiratory distress syndrome (ARDS).
  - Persistent requirement for mechanical ventilation or ECMO with evidence of irreversible lung destruction and without expectation of clinical recovery.
- Post-COVID-19 pulmonary fibrosis.
  - Patients who have developed irreversible lung failure and pulmonary fibrosis after recovery from acute COVID infection.
  - Must fulfill standard requirements for lung transplant candidacy.
  - Failed a minimum of an 8–12 week trial of lung recovery by a high volume lung recovery center before consideration.
  - Negative COVID-19 virology with no evidence of active infection.

Contraindications to Lung Transplant

Absolute Contraindications

- Recent history of malignancy.
- Active extra pulmonary infection.
- Active HIV infection (detectable viral load).
- Medical noncompliance.
- Lack of social support system.

- Active or recent substance use.
- Advanced dysfunction of another organ system.
- Irreversible restrictive chest wall deformity.
- High-dose prednisone therapy (20 mg/day).

Relative Contraindications

- Age greater than 65.
- Severe coronary artery disease/cardiomyopathy.
- Critical condition/end-organ dysfunction.
- Limited functional status.
- Obesity or severe malnutrition (BMI < 16 or > 30).
- Severe osteoporosis.
- Mechanical ventilation or extracorporeal life support.
- Colonization with highly resistant organisms.

Evaluation Process and Candidate Selection

Initial candidate screening includes a complete history and review of pertinent studies, including radiology, pathology, and pulmonary function testing. Patients who meet medical criteria for consideration of lung transplantation and who are without obvious contraindication to lung transplantation at the time of their initial referral then begin the extensive assessment for lung transplant candidacy.

Preoperative Testing

Cardiac

- EKG.
- ECHO.
- Right and left heart catheterization.

Imaging

- Chest radiograph.
- CT scan chest, abdomen, and pelvis.
- Carotid and extremity ultrasound studies.

Lung Function

- Arterial blood gas (ABG).
- Pulmonary function tests.
- Spirometry.
- 6 min walk test

Other Organ Function

- Gastroesophageal testing.
- Bone mineral density.

Health Maintenance

- Colonoscopy.
- Mammogram.
- Pap smear.
- Dental exam.

Laboratory

- Complete blood count (CBC with differential), complete metabolic panel, coagulation panel, hepatic panel, and lipid panel.
- Infectious disease: hepatitis, HIV, CMV, EBV, HSV, VZV, toxoplasma, and coccidioides.
- Blood type and antibodies.

Once patients have completed all components of the clinical, psychosocial, and financial assessment, they are discussed at a multidisciplinary patient selection committee, and candidacy and timing for activation on the national transplant waiting list are determined. Members of the Transplant Patient Selection Committee often include, but are not limited to, pulmonary transplant physicians, cardiothoracic transplant surgeons, psychiatrists, infectious disease physicians, pharmacists, transplant coordinators, social workers, nutritionists, and financial coordinators.

Waiting List and Lung Allocation

- The “Lung Allocation Score” (LAS) System was designed to maximize allocation of organs to individuals with the highest risk of death on the waiting list and the greatest likelihood of post-transplant survival and benefit. The individual patient score is determined by an algorithm that incorporates the following measurements:

- Age.
- Body mass index (BMI).
- Diagnosis.
- Pulmonary artery pressure (PAP).
- Pulmonary capillary wedge pressure (PCWP).
- Functional status: 6 min walk test.
- Supplemental oxygen.
- Forced vital capacity (FVC).
- Partial pressure of carbon dioxide (pCO2).
- Ventilator use.
- Creatinine.
- Diabetes mellitus.
- Total bilirubin.

- Scores range between 0 and 100. The higher the score, the higher the priority for transplantation. As a result, patients with longer waiting times alone no longer receive a higher priority in this new system and may be bypassed by newly listed patients with higher LAS scores.
- Organs are also matched to recipients based on blood type and height compatibility depending on the disease process. The measurements of the chest between donor and recipient are secondarily important for matching.

Donor Evaluation

- ABO compatibility.
- < 55 years of age
- $PO_2 > 300$ mmHg on 100% FiO_2, PEEP of 5.
- Normal radiographic imaging.
- Normal bronchoscopic examination.
- Lung vertical sizing match (as measured on CXR).

Surgical Technique

- Bilateral lung transplant versus single-lung transplant: determined by disease etiology, recipient age, presence of pulmonary hypertension, and preference of transplant center.
- Bilateral lung transplant.

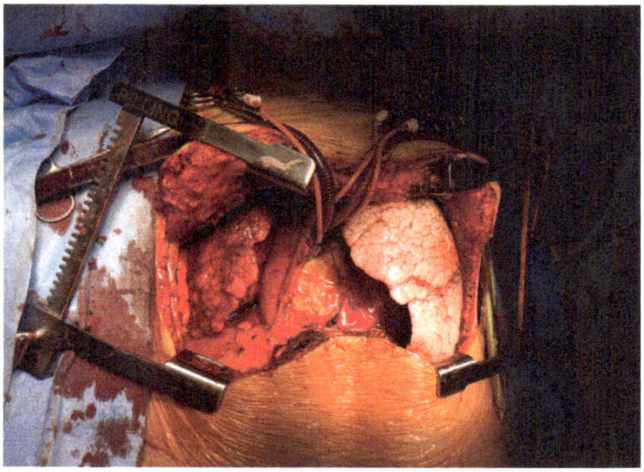

Fig. 26.1 Bilateral lung transplant via clamshell incision. Note the diseased right recipient lung, and the left implanted donor lung. In this case, the patient is centrally cannulated for venoarterial extracorporeal membrane oxygenation (VA-ECMO)

- Clamshell incision (Fig. 26.1).

  Bilateral anterior thoracotomies with transverse sternotomy.
  Offers access to bilateral pleural spaces and mediastinum, optimal for central cannulation if cardiopulmonary support is needed.

- Sternal sparing bilateral anterior thoracotomy or bilateral posterolateral thoracotomy.

  Right thoracotomy offers access for central cannulation.
  Left thoracotomy will require groin cannulation if mechanical support is needed (ECMO or CPB).

• Single-lung transplant.

  - Anterior versus posterolateral thoracotomy.

• Intraoperative mechanical circulatory support.

  - Options include cardiopulmonary bypass (CPB) or extracorporeal membrane oxygenation (ECMO).
  - Required in the setting of pulmonary hypertension (pre- or intraoperatively), RV dysfunction, or inability to tolerate single-lung ventilation.

Outcomes

• Lung transplant complications.

  - Wound complications.

Affects 15% of patients.
Risk factors particular to transplant patients include high doses of immunosuppression, contamination from the airway, extensive surgical trauma, and use of mechanical support.

- Primary graft dysfunction (PGD) (2016 ISHLT definition).

  The most common cause of early morbidity and mortality.
  Risk factors present in the donor and recipient.
  PGD grading is shown in Table 26.1.

- Airway ischemia.

  Incidence of 15–35%.
  Etiology is limited blood supply to the bronchial anastomosis.
  Recipient associated risk factors include graft dysfunction and prolonged mechanical ventilation.
  Donor-derived risk factors include prolonged ischemic time.

- Vascular complications.

  Incidence of 1–3%.
  Pulmonary embolism is the most common complication.

    Up to 45% mortality.

  Also include anastomotic complications and lung torsion.

- Bleeding complications.

  Intraoperative and postoperative.

- Pleural space complications.

  Effusions can result from graft reperfusion, recipient volume overload, bleeding, and interruption of lymphatics during donor lung procurement.
  Late effusions (>2 weeks) may be a consequence from infection, rejection, or trapped lung from pleural fibrosis or malignancy.

- Donor lung and recipient size mismatch.

  Undersized donor lungs may lead to bronchial dehiscence or persistent airspace complications.
  Oversized donor lungs can lead to atelectasis and pulmonary shunting.
  Oversized allograft may require volume reduction, wedge resections, or formal lobectomy.

Table 26.1 Primary graft dysfunction grading

PGD grade	Pulmonary edema on CXR	P/F ratio
0	No	Any
1	Yes	>300
2	Yes	200–300
3	Yes	<200

Recipient Survival

- Survival of lung transplant recipients is less than that seen with solid-organ transplant recipients for a variety of factors including the lungs' constant exposure to the outside environment and susceptibility to infection and injury.
- Acute cellular rejection (ACR) and antibody-mediated rejection (AMR).
  - ACR mediated by T cell antibodies.

    Affects vasculature and small airways.
  - AMR, humoral mediated.

    Hyper acute rejection from preformed antibodies.
    Also related to donor-specific antibodies (DSA).
- Chronic lung allograft dysfunction (CLAD).
  - Remains the major barrier for long-term survival.
  - Bronchiolitis obliterans syndrome (BOS).

    The most common cause of CLAD.
    The major risk factor is the development of ACR.
    50% of patients at 5 years develop BOS.
    Leading cause of morbidity and mortality.
- Survival after transplantation.
  - Median survival is 5.8 years in adults.
  - Median survival is 5.4 years in the pediatric population.
  - Survival is better for bilateral lung transplant than single-lung transplant.
  - Patients with cystic fibrosis have better overall outcomes.

Emerging Technology/Techniques

- Use of extracorporeal membrane oxygenation (ECMO) as bridge to transplant.
  - In appropriately selected patients, veno-venous or venoarterial ECMO can be used as a bridge to transplant.
  - Allows for hemodynamic and pulmonary support while awaiting transplantation.
- Ex vivo lung perfusion (EVLP).
  - A method to assess and potentially recover donor lungs that were not felt to be suitable for transplant at the time of organ offer. Important advancement designed to decrease the gap between organ availability and organ need.
  - Three current protocols.

Lund Protocol.
Toronto Protocol.
Organ Care System.

- Normothermic perfusion system.

  Utilizing acellular versus cellular perfusate solution.
  Pulsatile flow of perfusate through the pulmonary vasculature.
  Perfusate recirculates in a closed versus open system (depending on protocol/system used).

- Allows assessment of ventilation, oxygenation, and perfusion.

  Lung compliance and vascular resistance can be measured.

- Potential for lung reconditioning and therapeutic intervention for marginal donors.

Key Reference

- Costa J, Benvenuto L and Sonett J. Long-term outcomes and management of lung transplant recipients. Best Pract Res Clin Anaesthesiol. 2017;31(2):285–97.

Further Reading

Leard L, Holm A, Valapour M, Glanville A, Attawar S, Aversa M, Campos S, Christon L, Cypel M, Dellgren G, Hartwig M, Kapnadak S, Kolaitis N, Kotloff R, Patterson C, Shlobin O, Smith P, Solé A, Solomon M, Weill D, Wijsenbeek M, Willemse B, Arcasoy S, Ramos K. Consensus document for the selection of lung transplant candidates: an update from the International Society for Heart and Lung Transplantation. J Heart Lung Transplant. 2021;40(11):1349–79.

Lease ED, Budev MM. Infectious complications in lung transplant recipients. Thorac Surg Clin. 2022;32(2):211–20.

Panchabhai T, Chaddha U, McCurry K, Bremner R, Mehta A. Historical perspectives of lung transplantation: connecting the dots. J Thorac Dis. 2018;10(7):4516–31.

Schaheen L, Bremner R, Walia R, Smith M. Lung transplantation for coronavirus disease 2019 (COVID-19): the who, what, where, when, and why. J Thorac Cardiovasc Surg. 2022;163(3):865–8.

Snell G, Yusen R, Weill D, Strueber M, Garrity E, Reed A, Pelaez A, Whelan T, Perch M, Bag R, Budev M, Corris P, Crespo M, Witt C, Cantu E, Christie J. Report of the ISHLT working group on primary lung graft dysfunction, part I: definition and grading—a 2016 consensus group statement of the International Society for Heart and Lung Transplantation. J Heart Lung Transplant. 2017;36(10):1097–103.

Todd EM, Biswas Roy S, Hashimi AS, Serrone R, Panchanathan R, Kang P, Varsch KE, Steinbock BE, Huang J, Omar A, Patel V, Walia R, Smith MA, Bremner RM. Extracorporeal membrane oxygenation as a bridge to lung transplantation: a single-center experience in the present era. J Thorac Cardiovasc Surg. 2017;154(5):1798–809.

Chapter 27
Esophageal Reflux and Barrett's Esophagus

Andrew Hawkins and Philip Carrott

Overview

- Gastroesophageal reflux disease (GERD) is the most common abdominal complaint during outpatient clinic visits and affects 18–28% of people living in North America.
- GERD is characterized by persistent symptoms of heartburn and regurgitation, and complications include esophagitis, strictures, and Barrett's esophagus that can progress to cancer.
- Lifestyle changes (weight loss and smoking cessation), proton pump inhibitors, and surgery are the mainstay in management.

Pathogenesis

The esophagogastric junction consists of the lower esophageal sphincter (LES) and the crural diaphragm.

- The LES is a physiologic location denoted as the location with the highest intraluminal pressure generated by the musculature of the esophagus (Fig. 27.1).
- Four structures contribute to the LES function.
  - Smooth musculature of the distal esophagus.
  - Sling fibers of the gastric cardia.

A. Hawkins · P. Carrott (✉)
Division of Thoracic and Cardiovascular Surgery, University of Virginia, Charlottesville, VA, USA
e-mail: pc3sf@virginia.edu; ADH2TP@hscmail.mcc.virginia.edu

T. Ng, T. Geraci (eds.), *Thoracic Surgery Clerkship*, Contemporary Surgical Clerkships, https://doi.org/10.1007/978-3-031-44645-0_27

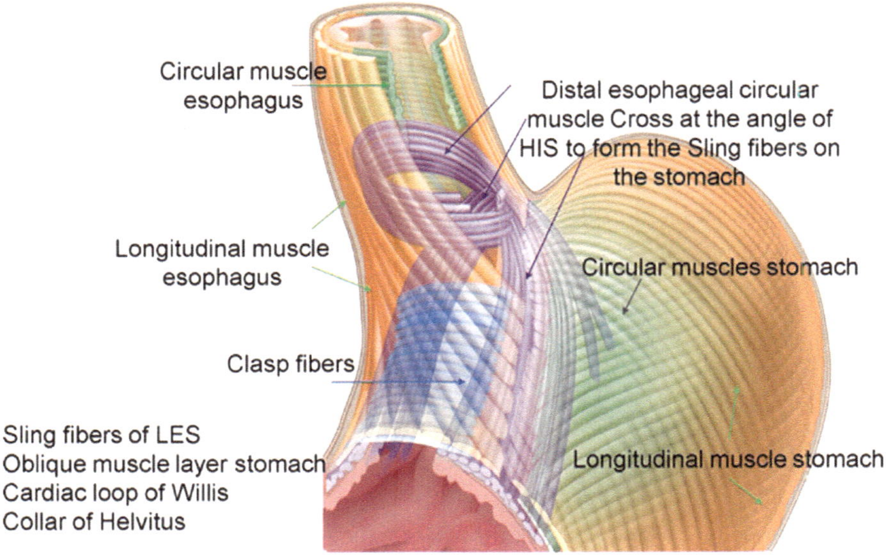

Fig. 27.1 The lower esophageal sphincter consists of both intrinsic and extrinsic sphincters. (Adapted from Mittal and Lipham 2023)

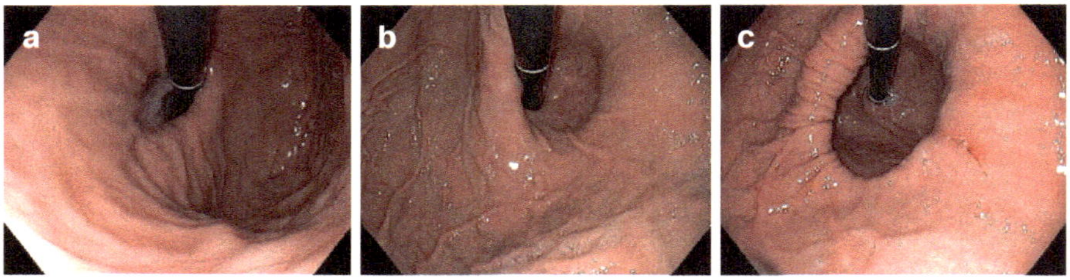

Fig. 27.2 Endoscopic view of paraesophageal hiatal hernia will demonstrate a portion of fundus located above the visualized diaphragmatic rim. Examples ranging from small (**a**), to medium (**b**), to large (**c**). (Adapted from Weitzendorfer et al. 2017)

  - Crural diaphragm.
  - Intra-abdominal anchoring of the gastroesophageal junction.

- Inspiration produces a "pinching effect" by the diaphragm on the LES that augments its function. If the anatomy becomes distorted such as with hiatal hernia, the combined effect of the external and internal components of the gastroesophageal junction can become dissociated, which increases risk for reflux (Fig. 27.2).
- Gastric reflux occurs via three mechanisms and results from dysfunction of the esophagogastric junction barrier against acidic stomach contents.

  - Frequent or prolonged relaxation of the lower esophageal sphincter.
  - Low pressure of the lower esophageal sphincter (ineffective barrier against acidic gastric contents).

  - Hiatal hernia (portion of stomach herniation through diaphragm).
- Additional factors that contribute to GERD.
  - Ineffective esophageal motility can result in prolonged exposure of the esophageal mucosa to acid and diminishes the protective process of swallowing salivary bicarbonate.
  - Delayed gastric emptying can increase pressure gradient between the stomach and the esophagus.
  - Carbonated beverages and overeating contribute to gastric fullness and dilation of the esophageal sphincter.
- Risk factors for GERD include obesity, tobacco use, and genetic predisposition.
  - Obesity is associated with increased intra-abdominal pressures, which results in a higher pressure gradient between the abdominal and thoracic cavity. During transient relaxation of the esophageal sphincter, this gradient causes more gastric contents to reflux. A higher body mass index (BMI) also correlates with a higher prevalence of hiatal hernia.
  - Tobacco use results in reduced pressure of the lower esophageal sphincter and can provoke acid reflux via increases in intra-abdominal pressure caused by coughing or deep inspiration.
- Hiatal hernias are often associated with GERD due to the displacement of the LES relative to the diaphragm and loss of intra-abdominal position.
  - Since the chest is under negative pressure, this stents the lower esophagus open and allows for reflux that may not be controlled with medical therapy alone.
- Barrett's esophagus is a sequela of GERD and is caused by intestinal metaplasia of the native squamous epithelium of the esophagus (Fig. 27.3).

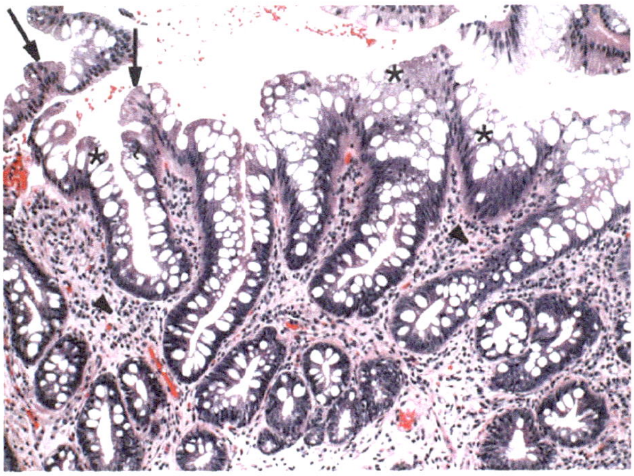

Fig. 27.3 Biopsy specimen of Barrett's esophagus shows intestinal metaplasia with characteristic goblet cells (asterisk). (Adapted from Odze 2009)

– Metaplasia can progress from low-grade dysplasia to high-grade dysplasia before becoming in situ carcinoma and, ultimately, invasive esophageal adenocarcinoma.

Evaluation

History

- Cardinal symptoms of GERD include acid regurgitation and heartburn and less often chest pain. Less common symptoms are dysphagia (difficulty swallowing), cough, hoarseness, and teeth erosions.
- The differential diagnosis for abdominal pain is broad, and it is important to consider diseases of the heart, esophagus, stomach, liver, and pancreas (Table 27.1).
- Warning signs for cancer ("alarm symptoms") include progressive dysphagia, involuntary weight loss, or bleeding.
- Duration, intensity, and frequency of symptoms should be determined.
- A validated symptom questionnaire such as GerdQ can assist in screening patients (Table 27.2).

Physical Examination

- Physical exam may reveal extraesophageal manifestations of reflux including voice hoarseness, otitis media, expiratory wheezing, and enamel decay.
- Both symptoms and exam findings of reflux, particularly laryngeal and pulmonary manifestations, can be nonspecific.

Table 27.1 Differential diagnosis for gastric reflux including characteristic symptoms and diagnostic testing. (Adapted from Maret-Ouda et al. 2020)

Diagnosis	Symptoms	Diagnostic test
Coronary heart disease	Chest pain, especially if exertional	ECG, stress test, troponin level
Peptic ulcer disease	Epigastric pain, nausea, vomiting	Endoscopy
Biliary tract disease (gallstones, cholecystitis)	Abdominal pain (fatty foods), jaundice	Ultrasound, bilirubin, lipase
Pancreatitis	Epigastric pain, nausea, vomiting	Lipase level, CT scan
Gastrointestinal cancer	Unintentional weight loss, eating difficulties, abdominal pain	Endoscopy, CT scan
Esophageal motility disorder	Dysphagia, regurgitation	Esophageal manometry
Eosinophilic esophagitis	Difficulty swallowing	Endoscopy

Table 27.2 GerdQ self-assessment questionnaire. (Adapted from Tielemans and van Oijen 2013)

		Symptom presence			
	Symptoms in the previous week	0 days	1 day	2–3 days	4–7 days
	Question:				
1.	How often did you have a burning feeling behind your breastbone (heartburn)?	0	1	2	3
2.	How often did you have stomach contents (liquid or food) moving upwards to your throat or mouth (regurgitation)?	0	1	2	3
3.	How often did you have a pain in the center of the upper stomach?	3	2	1	0
4.	How often did you have nausea?	3	2	1	0
5.	How often did you have difficulty getting a good night's sleep because of your heartburn and/or regurgitation?	0	1	2	3
6.	How often did you take additional medication for your heartburn and/or regurgitation other than what the physician told you to take (such as Maalox)?	0	1	2	3

- Physical exam alone is often not helpful in confirming or excluding the diagnosis of GERD but can assist in identification of other disease processes.

Proton Pump Inhibitor Trial

- For patients with classic symptoms (heartburn/regurgitation) and no warning signs, a short course (4–8 weeks) of a proton pump inhibitor (PPI) such as pantoprazole is recommended by the American College of Gastroenterology.
- Symptom relief from PPI therapy has a sensitivity of 78% and specificity of 54% for the diagnosis of reflux when compared to 24 h pH monitoring as reference standard.
  - A favorable response to PPI does not confirm the diagnosis as patients with other conditions such as esophageal acid hypersensitivity or functional disorders can experience symptom relief.
- Given concerns for potential side effects of long-term PPI therapy (drug interactions, osteoporotic fractures, and infections), further testing including endoscopy and pH testing is warranted to establish diagnosis even if a patient responds to therapy.

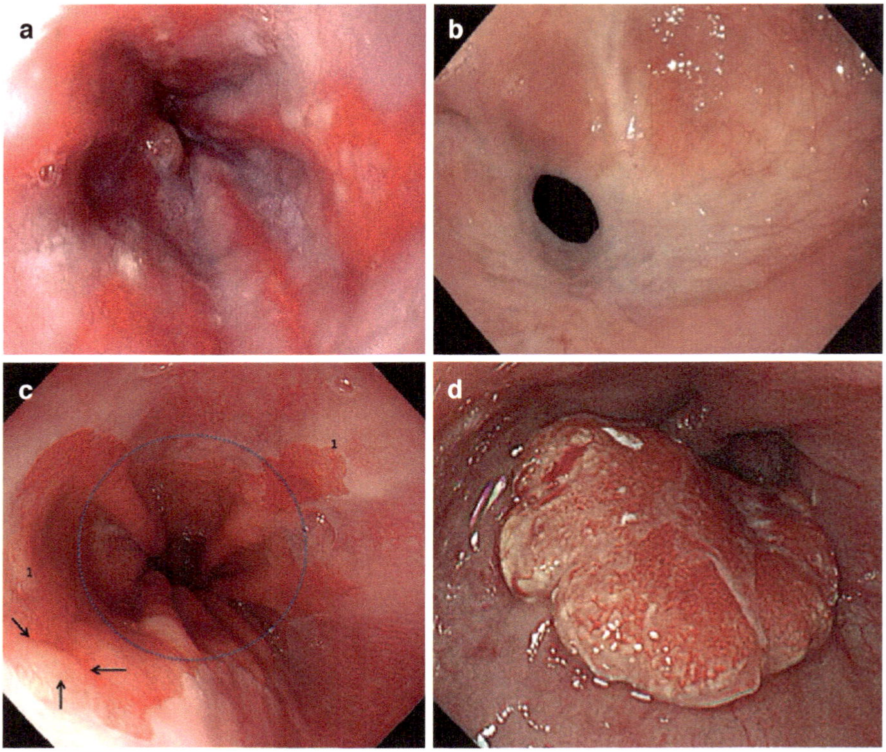

Fig. 27.4 Endoscopic findings associated with reflux. (**a**) Linear esophageal erosions. (**b**) Esophageal stricture. (**c**) Barrett's esophagus with characteristic red velvet appearance. (**d**) Esophageal adenocarcinoma. (Adapted from Wangrattanapranee et al. 2022; van Boeckel and Siersema 2015; Barrie et al. 2021; Kuwayama et al. 2021)

Endoscopy

- Patients with GERD symptoms who do not respond to an 8 week trial of PPI or have alarm symptoms should have an upper endoscopy.
- Gastroesophageal reflux can result in esophagitis with distal erosions of the esophageal mucosa, luminal narrowing due to stricture, Barrett's esophagus with a salmon pink color compared to a normal pale appearance of the mucosa, and esophageal adenocarcinoma with the presence of a luminal mass (Fig. 27.4).
- The presence of severe esophagitis or Barrett's esophagus confirmed on biopsy is pathognomonic for GERD.
  - Normal endoscopy or mild esophagitis does not exclude significant reflux.

- Endoscopy should include a retroflexed view of the gastroesophageal junction to confirm the presence of hiatal hernia.
- In cases of Barrett's esophagus, four quadrant biopsies should be taken along every 2 cm of metaplastic mucosa to screen for dysplasia.

Ambulatory pH and Impedance Monitoring

- pH monitoring is the "gold standard" test for GERD and allows calculation of the DeMeester score, which is derived from the following parameters in a 24 h period.
  - Total number of episodes of reflux.
  - Total time during which pH < 4 (%).
  - Number of reflux episodes ≥5 min.
  - Longest reflux episode (min).
- 24-h pH monitoring is performed by passing a catheter through the patient's nose into the distal esophagus 5 cm proximal to the LES or by leaving an endoscopic-placed remote monitor (Fig. 27.5).
- Ambulatory pH monitoring can be coupled with symptom reporting and impedance monitoring (electrical flow between two electrodes) that can detect retrograde liquid reflux (Fig. 27.6).
- pH-impedance monitoring should be performed while off PPI therapy.
- Acid exposure time and symptom association with reflux events detected by impedance best predict response to medical and surgical anti-reflux therapy.

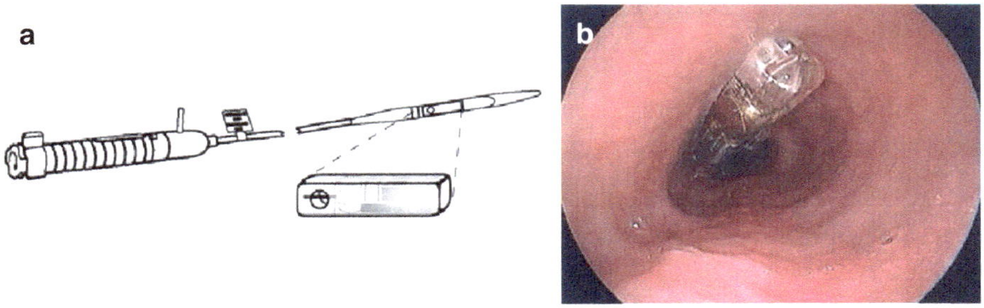

Fig. 27.5 Remote pH monitor. (**a**) Endoscopic delivery system and implantable capsule with electrode. (**b**) Endoscopic view of capsule fixed to esophageal mucosa 5 cm above the lower esophageal sphincter. (Adapted from Schneider et al. 2007)

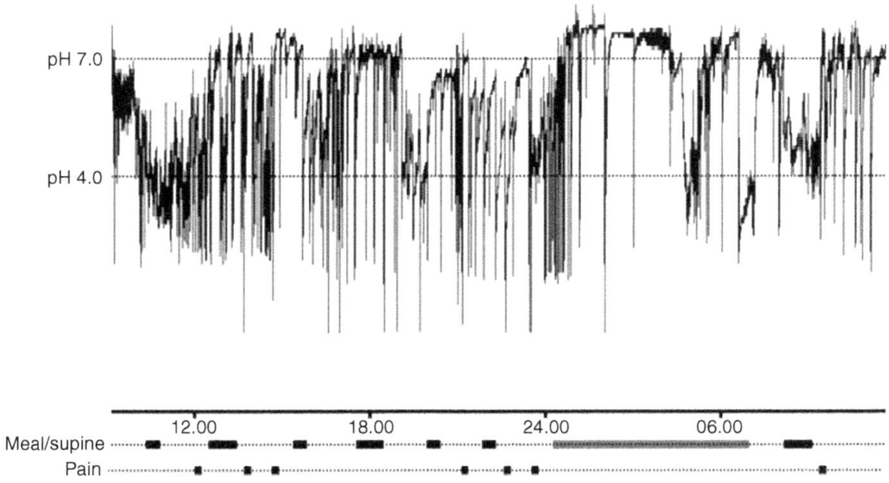

Fig. 27.6 Ambulatory pH monitoring with temporal reporting of patient symptoms. (Adapted from Bredenoord et al. 2005)

Esophageal Manometry

- High-resolution esophageal manometry collects pressure tracings over time along the esophageal body and lower esophageal sphincter (Fig. 27.7).
- The Chicago classification of esophageal motility disorders is identified using manometry results.
  - Incomplete LES relaxation – achalasia or esophagogastric junction obstruction.
  - Impaired motility – esophageal spasm, hypercontractile esophagus, or absent contractility.
  - Peristaltic abnormalities – minor disorders.
- Severe GERD can be characterized by a lower than normal LES pressure. Prolonged exposure of the esophagus to acid can also alter motility.
- Motility disorders may result in symptoms of chest pain or regurgitation, which can mimic GERD. This must be considered during surgical planning as Nissen fundoplication (360° wrap of the fundus) in the setting of disordered motility can produce postoperative dysphagia.

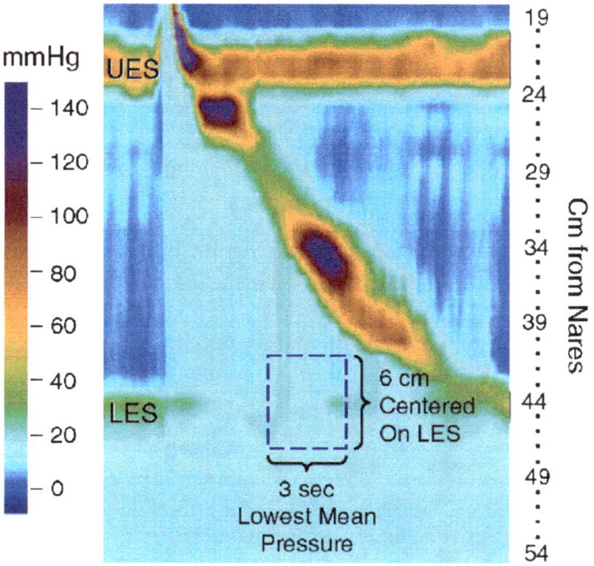

Fig. 27.7 Esophageal manometry is typically performed with a flexible catheter with spaced pressure sensors along the length of the device. High-resolution manometry typically involves up to 36 sensors. A normal manometry study is depicted with a swallow demonstrating propagation of the peristaltic pressure wave with appropriately timed relaxation of the esophagogastric junction. Modern manometry presents data as a topographic plot or heat map with time on x-axis and depth on y-axis. (Adapted from Conklin et al. 2009)

Treatment

Medical Management

- Weight loss, avoidance of meals within 2–3 h of bedtime, and cessation of tobacco/alcohol use are lifestyle modifications that are recommended to reduce reflux symptoms.
- PPIs are the first-line treatment for erosive esophagitis and symptom relief. For patients with severe erosive esophagitis, Barrett's esophagus should be maintained on PPIs indefinitely.
- In observational studies, long-term PPI use has been associated with reduced bone density, vitamin/mineral deficiencies (iron, calcium, B-12, magnesium), and bacterial overgrowth in the small intestine, but the quality of this evidence is low. Nonetheless, the indication for PPI therapy should be well established.

Endoscopic Surveillance and Treatment of Barrett's Esophagus

- Intestinal dysplasia of the esophagus is associated with a 0.5% per year risk of developing esophageal adenocarcinoma.
  - Proton pump inhibitors are effective in preventing neoplastic progression.
  - Anti-reflux surgery does not reduce cancer risk of progression.
- Scheduled regular surveillance endoscopy with biopsies should be pursued in patients with Barrett's esophagus with normal mucosa or low-grade dysplasia (Table 27.3).
- High-grade dysplasia is treated with endoscopic mucosal resection and/or radio-frequency ablation (Fig. 27.8).
- Esophagectomy can be considered in patients who do not respond to endoscopic intervention.

Table 27.3 Recommended endoscopic surveillance for categories of dysplasia associated with Barrett's esophagus. (Adapted from Booth and Thompson 2012)

Histology	Follow-up
Normal	Repeat EGD within 1 year, EGD every 3 year
Low-grade dysplasia (cytologic atypia extending to mucosal surface)	Repeat EGD within 6 months, yearly EGD after
High-grade dysplasia (architectural distortion, enlarged nuclei)	Repeat EGD within 3 months, consider endoscopic mucosal resection

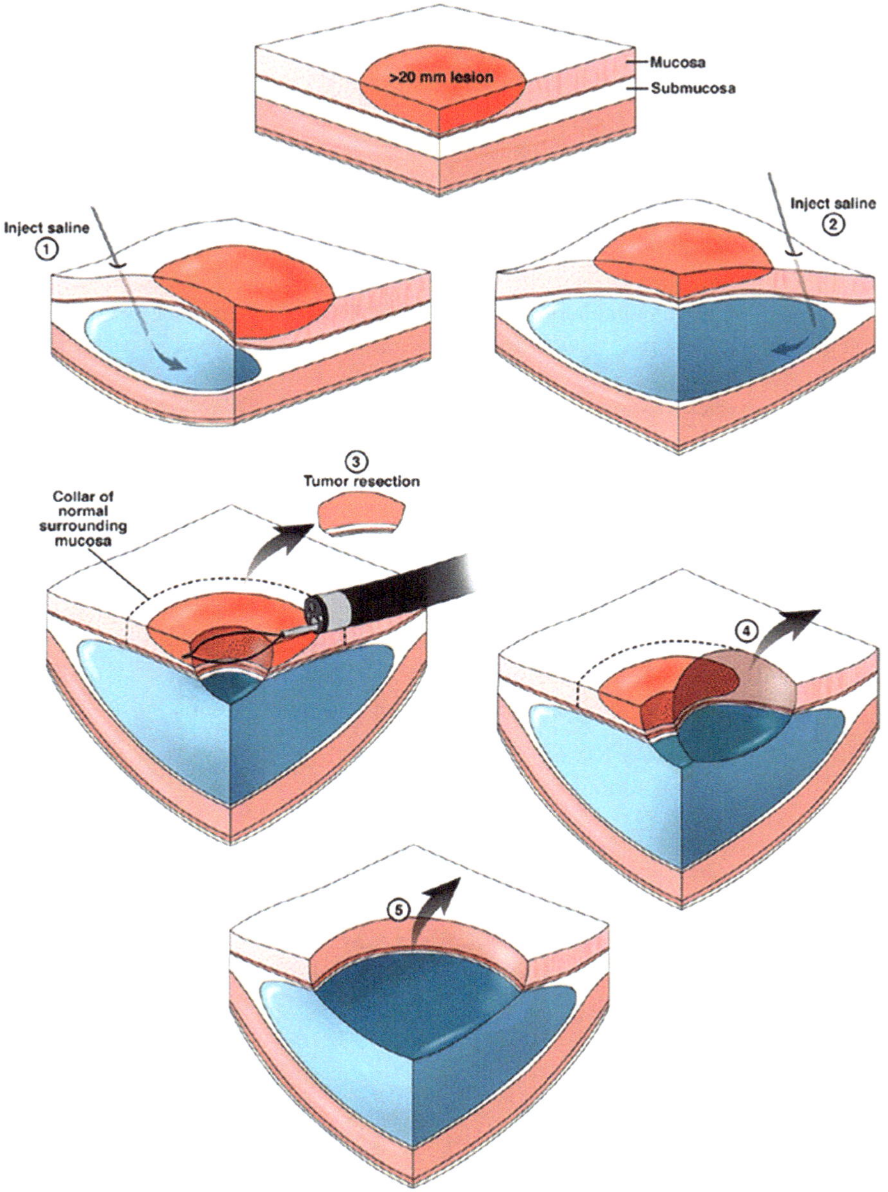

Fig. 27.8 Endoscopic mucosal resection involves targeted submucosal saline injection, endoscopic grasping techniques, and suction to resect dysplastic mucosa. (Adapted from Ladhani et al. 2017)

Surgical Treatment

- Between 32 and 45% of patients treated with PPIs report persistent symptoms of heartburn and regurgitation.
- Medication compliance and timing with meals should be discussed with patients with incomplete symptom resolution.
  - Trial of twice-daily PPI can be offered.
- Anti-reflux surgery should be recommended for patients with severe reflux esophagitis, large hiatal hernias, and persistent GERD symptoms.
- Patients who respond well to PPIs often have symptomatic improvement with surgery.
- Preoperative evaluation involves confirmation of GERD diagnosis, exclusion of esophageal dysmotility, and characterization of the gastroesophageal junction anatomy.
  - Barium esophogram is useful to detect hiatal hernia and length of intra-abdominal esophagus for operative planning.
- The Nissen fundoplication is the "gold standard" in anti-reflux surgery (Fig. 27.9).
  - Involves restoration of 3–4 cm of the esophagus below the diaphragmatic hiatus.
  - A Toupet fundoplication is a 270° wrap of the fundus around the esophagus.

    Equivalent to a Nissen fundoplication with regard to symptom relief and incidence of complications.

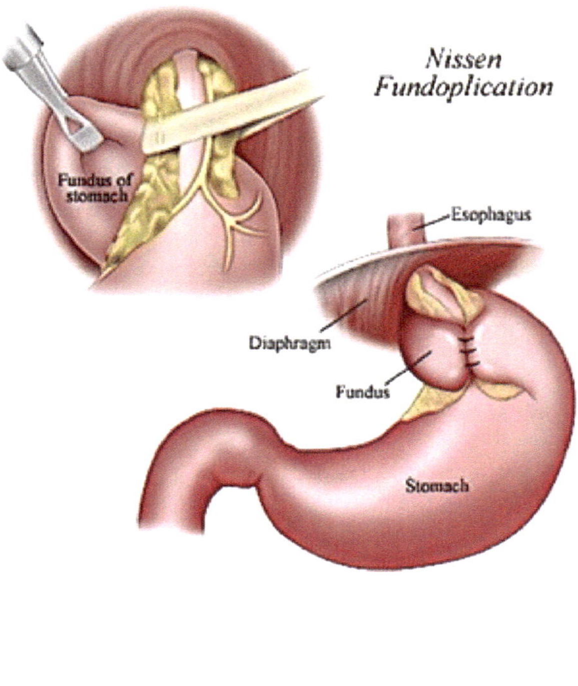

Fig. 27.9 Nissen fundoplication involves a 360° wrap of the stomach fundus immediately above the esophagogastric junction. This involves placement of 3–4 sutures between the posterior and anterior portion of the stomach. The fundoplication functionally reconstitutes the lower esophageal sphincter. (Adapted from Min and Ganz 2014)

A 180° partial fundoplication (Dor) can be performed in patients with abnormal esophageal peristalsis but is considered a less durable repair.

- Patients receiving surgical treatment report less frequent heartburn/regurgitation compared to medical therapy alone and are overall satisfied.
- Roux-en-Y gastric bypass (RYGB) should be considered for obese patients.
  - Elevated intra-abdominal pressure increases risk of fundoplication disruption and herniation.
  - Gastric bypass is a highly effective weight loss operation and is associated with reduction in reflux symptoms.

Key Reference

- Spechler SJ. Barrett esophagus and risk of esophageal cancer: a clinical review. JAMA. 2013;310(6):627–36.

Further Reading

Barrett C, Choksi Y, Vaezi MF. Mucosal impedance: a new approach to diagnosing gastroesophageal reflux disease and eosinophilic esophagitis. Curr Gastroenterol Rep. 2018;20(7):1–7.

Barrie J, Yanni F, Sherif M, Dube AK, Tamhankar AP. Length of Barrett's esophagus in the presence of low-grade dysplasia, high-grade dysplasia, and adenocarcinoma. Surg Endosc. 2021;35(8):4756–62.

Becher A, El-Serag H. Systematic review: the association between symptomatic response to proton pump inhibitors and health-related quality of life in patients with gastro-oesophageal reflux disease. Aliment Pharmacol Ther. 2011;34(6):618–27.

Booth CL, Thompson KS. Barrett's esophagus: a review of diagnostic criteria, clinical surveillance practices and new developments. J Gastrointest Oncol. 2012;3(3):232.

Bredenoord AJ, Weusten BL, Smout AJ. Symptom association analysis in ambulatory gastro-oesophageal reflux monitoring. Gut. 2005;54(12):1810–7.

Conklin J, Pimentel M, Soffer E, editors. Color atlas of high resolution manometry. Cham: Springer; 2009.

Du X, Hu Z, Yan C, Zhang C, Wang Z, Wu J. A meta-analysis of long follow-up outcomes of laparoscopic Nissen (total) versus Toupet (270) fundoplication for gastro-esophageal reflux disease based on randomized controlled trials in adults. BMC Gastroenterol. 2016;16(1):1–1.

El-Serag HB, Sweet S, Winchester CC, Dent J. Update on the epidemiology of gastro-oesophageal reflux disease: a systematic review. Gut. 2014;63(6):871–80.

Herbella FA, Patti MG. Gastroesophageal reflux disease: from pathophysiology to treatment. World J Gastroenterol: WJG. 2010;16(30):3745.

Hom C, Vaezi MF. Extra-esophageal manifestations of gastroesophageal reflux disease: diagnosis and treatment. Drugs. 2013;73(12):1281–95.

Johnson LF, DeMeester TR. Development of the 24-hour intraesophageal pH monitoring composite scoring system. J Clin Gastroenterol. 1986;8(Suppl 1):52–8.

Kahrilas PJ, Bredenoord AJ, Fox M, Gyawali CP, Roman S, Smout AJ, Pandolfino JE. International High Resolution Manometry Working Group. The Chicago Classification of esophageal motility disorders, v3. 0. Neurogastroenterol Motil. 2015;27(2):160–74.

Katz PO, Gerson LB, Vela MF. Guidelines for the diagnosis and management of gastroesophageal reflux disease. Am Coll Gastroenterol. 2013;108(3):308–28.

Kim M, Navarro F, Eruchalu CN, Augenstein VA, Heniford BT, Stefanidis D. Minimally invasive Roux-en-Y gastric bypass for fundoplication failure offers excellent gastroesophageal reflux control. Am Surg. 2014;80(7):696–703.

Kuwayama N, Hoshino I, Gunji H, Kurosaki T, Tonooka T, Soda H, Sonoda I, Eto R, Takiguchi N, Nabeya Y, Itami M. CA19-9-producing esophageal adenocarcinoma originating from the esophageal cardia of the mid-thoracic esophagus: a case report. Surg Case Rep. 2021;7(1):1–5.

Ladhani H, Khadra H, Marks J. Endoscopic mucosal resection (EMR). In: Advanced colonoscopy and endoluminal surgery. Cham: Springer; 2017. p. 149–57.

Laine L, Nagar A. Long-term PPI use: balancing potential harms and documented benefits. Am Coll Gastroenterol. 2016;111(7):913–5.

Lehault LW, Hughes DM. Review of the long-term effects of proton pump inhibitors. Fed Pract. 2017;34(2):19.

Maret-Ouda J, Markar SR, Lagergren J. Gastroesophageal reflux disease: a review. JAMA. 2020;324(24):2536–47.

Martinucci I, De Bortoli N, Giacchino M, Bodini G, Marabotto E, Marchi S, Savarino V, Savarino E. Esophageal motility abnormalities in gastroesophageal reflux disease. World J Gastrointest Pharmacol Ther. 2014;5(2):86.

Min MX, Ganz RA. Update in procedural therapy for GERD–magnetic sphincter augmentation, endoscopic transoral incisionless fundoplication vs laparoscopic Nissen fundoplication. Curr Gastroenterol Rep. 2014;16(2):1–5.

Mittal RK, Balaban DH. The esophagogastric junction. N Engl J Med. 1997;336(13):924–32.

Mittal RK, Lipham JC. GERD pathophysiology: the role of the sphincter and crural diaphragm. In: The AFS textbook of foregut disease. Cham: Springer; 2023. p. 229–18.

Odze RD. Barrett esophagus: histology and pathology for the clinician. Nat Rev Gastroenterol Hepatol. 2009;6(8):478–90.

Patel A, Sayuk GS, Gyawali CP. Parameters on esophageal pH-impedance monitoring that predict outcomes of patients with gastroesophageal reflux disease. Clin Gastroenterol Hepatol. 2015;13(5):884–91.

Pennathur A, Gibson MK, Jobe BA, Luketich JD. Oesophageal carcinoma. Lancet. 2013;381(9864):400–12.

Rickenbacher N, Kötter T, Kochen MM, Scherer M, Blozik E. Fundoplication versus medical management of gastroesophageal reflux disease: systematic review and meta-analysis. Surg Endosc. 2014;28(1):143–55.

Schneider JH, Kramer KM, Königsrainer A, Granderath FA. Ambulatory pH: monitoring with a wireless system. Surg Endosc. 2007;21(11):2076–80.

Shaheen NJ, Hansen RA, Morgan DR, Gangarosa LM, Ringel Y, Thiny MT, Russo MW, Sandler RS. The burden of gastrointestinal and liver diseases, 2006. Am Coll Gastroenterol. 2006;101(9):2128–38.

Shaheen N, Provenzale D. The epidemiology of gastroesophageal reflux disease. Am J Med Sci. 2003;326(5):264–73.

Tielemans MM, van Oijen MG. Online follow-up of individuals with gastroesophageal reflux disease using a patient-reported outcomes instrument: results of an observational study. BMC Gastroenterol. 2013;13(1):1–7.

van Boeckel PG, Siersema PD. Refractory esophageal strictures: what to do when dilation fails. Curr Treat Options Gastroenterol. 2015;13(1):47–58.

Wangrattanapranee P, Khrucharoen U, Jensen DM, Wongpongsalee T, Jensen ME. Severe upper gastrointestinal hemorrhage caused by reflux esophagitis. Dig Dis Sci. 2022;67(1):159–69.

Weitzendorfer M, Köhler G, Antoniou SA, Pallwein-Prettner L, Manzenreiter L, Schredl P, Emmanuel K, Koch OO. Preoperative diagnosis of hiatal hernia: barium swallow X-ray, high-resolution manometry, or endoscopy? Eur Surg. 2017;49(5):210–7.

Zheng Z, Nordenstedt H, Pedersen NL, Lagergren J, Ye W. Lifestyle factors and risk for symptomatic gastroesophageal reflux in monozygotic twins. Gastroenterology. 2007;132(1):87–95.

Chapter 28
Hiatal Hernias

Ashley J. McCormack, Costas Bizekis, and Travis Geraci

Anatomy and Physiology

- The distal esophagus is anchored to the diaphragm by the phrenoesophageal membrane.
- Normally approximately 2 cm of the esophagus is within the abdomen.
- Herniation of the stomach and/or other abdominal tissues through the hiatus results from the weakening of the muscular apparatus of the hiatus, loss of strength and elasticity of the connective tissues of the phrenoesophageal membrane, and conditions that increase intra-abdominal pressure (obesity).
- With each swallow, the esophagus shortens as the longitudinal muscle contracts and the phrenoesophageal membrane is stretched; its elastic recoil then pulls the gastroesophageal junction (GEJ) back to its normal position following each swallow. The repetitive stress of swallowing, in addition to abdominal straining and episodes of vomiting, causes degeneration of the phrenoesophageal membrane over time.

A. J. McCormack · C. Bizekis · T. Geraci (✉)
Division of Thoracic Surgery, Department of Cardiothoracic Surgery, New York University Langone Health, New York, NY, USA
e-mail: ashley.lamparello@nyulangone.org; costas.bizekis@nyulangone.org
travis.geraci@nyulangone.org

T. Ng, T. Geraci (eds.), *Thoracic Surgery Clerkship*, Contemporary Surgical Clerkships, https://doi.org/10.1007/978-3-031-44645-0_28

Classification (Fig. 28.1)

- Hiatal hernia: general umbrella term referring to all types of herniation of the stomach through the diaphragmatic hiatus. Hiatal hernias are classified into Types I–IV.
- Paraesophageal hernia: herniation of the stomach into the chest, anterior or lateral to the esophagus. Types II–IV as a group are referred to as paraesophageal hernias.

Type I

- Sliding hiatal hernia.
- Weakening of the hiatal muscles, resulting in upward thoracic displacement of the GE junction above the diaphragm.
- The gastric fundus remains below the GEJ.
- Most common type, accounting for 95% of all hiatal hernias.

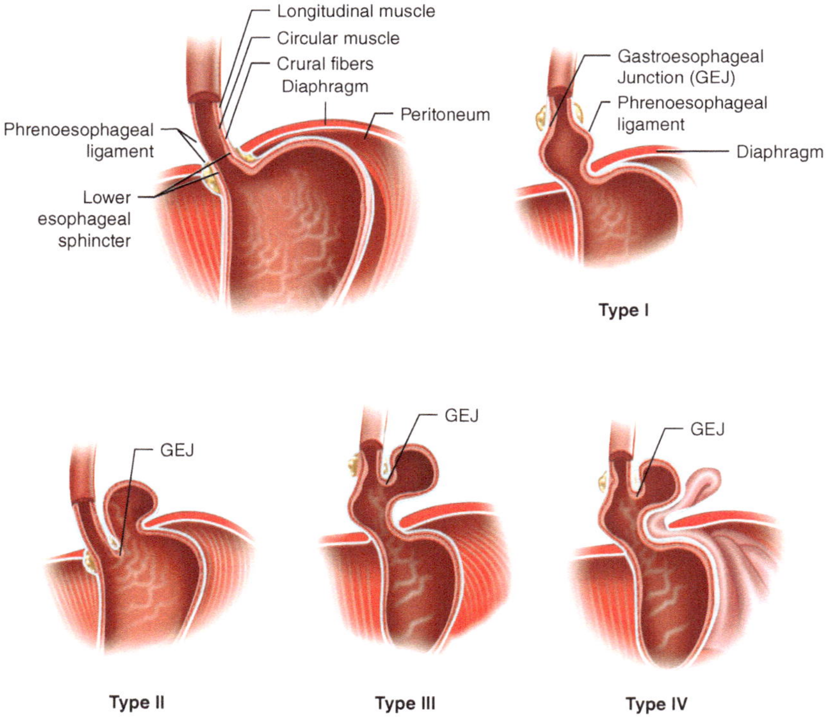

Fig. 28.1 Anatomy of the distal esophagus and the classification of hiatal hernias

Type II

- A "true" paraesophageal hernia, where the gastric fundus herniates above the diaphragm and the GEJ remains in the abdomen.
- Rare, least common type.

Type III

- "Mixed" paraesophageal hernia involving elements of Types I and II.
- Both the GEJ and fundus herniate through the hiatus.
- Includes "giant" hernias where more than half of the stomach herniates into the chest.
- May be associated with gastric volvulus, of which there are two types:
  - Organo-axial (most common): twisting of the stomach along its axis, resulting in the "inverted" or "upside down" stomach (Fig. 28.2).
  - Meso-axial: the stomach folding onto itself.
- Accounts for more than 90% of paraesophageal hernias.

Type IV

- Paraesophageal hernia with a large defect in the phrenoesophageal membrane.
- The hernia sac contains organs other than the stomach, such as the colon, spleen, or small intestine.

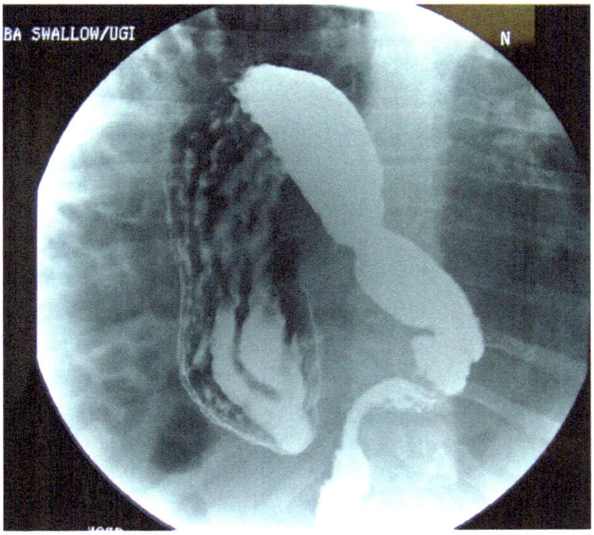

Fig. 28.2 Type III paraesophageal repair with organo-axial volvulus, resulting in the "inverted" or "upside down" stomach seen on barium esophagram

Presentation

- Type I.
  - Usually asymptomatic (found incidentally on chest/ abdomen imaging) or minimally symptomatic with vague intermittent complaints.
  - May have symptoms of gastroesophageal reflux disease (GERD), substernal pain, regurgitation, dysphagia, nausea, cough, or hoarseness.
- Types II–IV.
  - May have vague symptoms (similar to type 1).
  - May have more severe symptoms of progressive gastric volvulus: postprandial pain, regurgitation or vomiting, or reflux.
  - Rarely, large hernias may affect pulmonary function causing cough or dyspnea.
  - Fatigue from anemia due to congestion and ulcer of the stomach.
- "Complicated" hernias.
  - Gastric volvulus (organo-axial most common) with obstruction: twisting of the stomach in the chest may result in closure of the distal esophagus and/or difficulty in emptying of the stomach. May progress to gastric ischemia, necrosis, and perforation.
  - Cameron's ulcer: bleeding from a marginal pressure ulcer in the herniated gastric mucosa may cause recurrent low-grade bleeding with iron-deficiency anemia.
  - Incarceration: the herniated stomach may become trapped and pressed in the chest, leading to tissue ischemia and potentially necrosis leading to perforation.

Diagnosis

- Chest radiograph.
  - Air-fluid level in the chest suggesting a portion of intrathoracic stomach (Fig. 28.3a, b).
- Barium swallow (Figs. 28.4a, b).
  - Gold standard diagnostic test.
  - Can demonstrate the anatomy, size of herniation, orientation of the stomach, and location of the GEJ.
  - Will also show the transit of contrast through the esophagus to the stomach.
  - Type I: demonstration of at least three rugal folds traversing the diaphragm.
  - Types II–IV: portion of the gastric fundus visualized herniating along the distal esophagus.

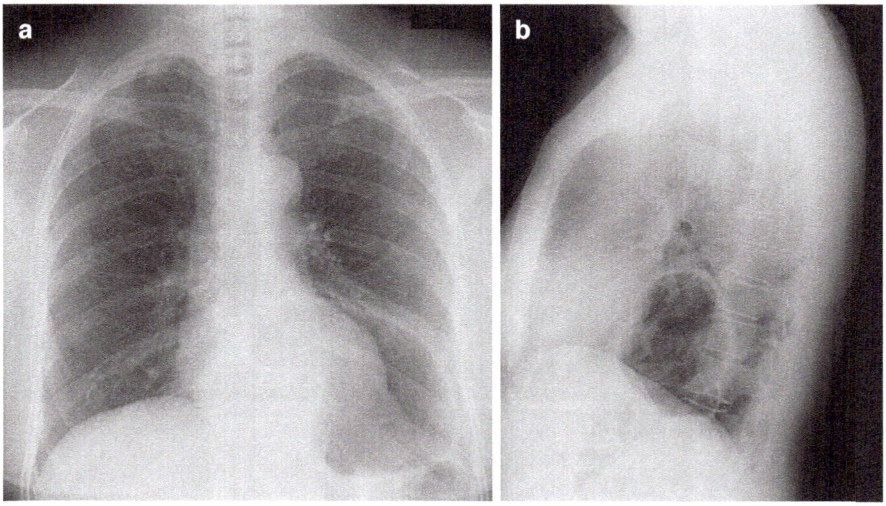

Fig. 28.3 Chest radiograph of paraesophageal hernia, showing gastric air above the diaphragm and behind the cardiac silhouette. (**a**) Posterior-anterior view; (**b**) lateral view

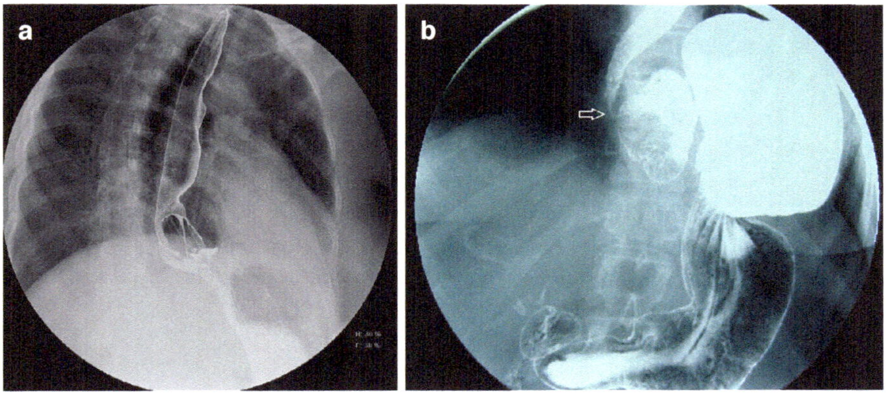

Fig. 28.4 Barium swallow showing paraesophageal hernia. (**a**) Type I sliding hiatal hernia; (**b**) Type III paraesophageal hernia with herniation of the gastric fundus and gastroesophageal junction (arrow) above the diaphragm

- Computed tomography scan (CT) (Figs. 28.5a–c).
  - Demonstrates herniation and orientation of the stomach (volvulus) and identifies whether other organs or tissues have herniated through the hiatus.
- Upper endoscopy.
  - Precisely identifies the GEJ.
  - In cases of significant volvulus, it may be difficult if not impossible to pass the endoscope into the stomach.
  - A retroflexed view shows a portion of the stomach herniating upward through the diaphragm.

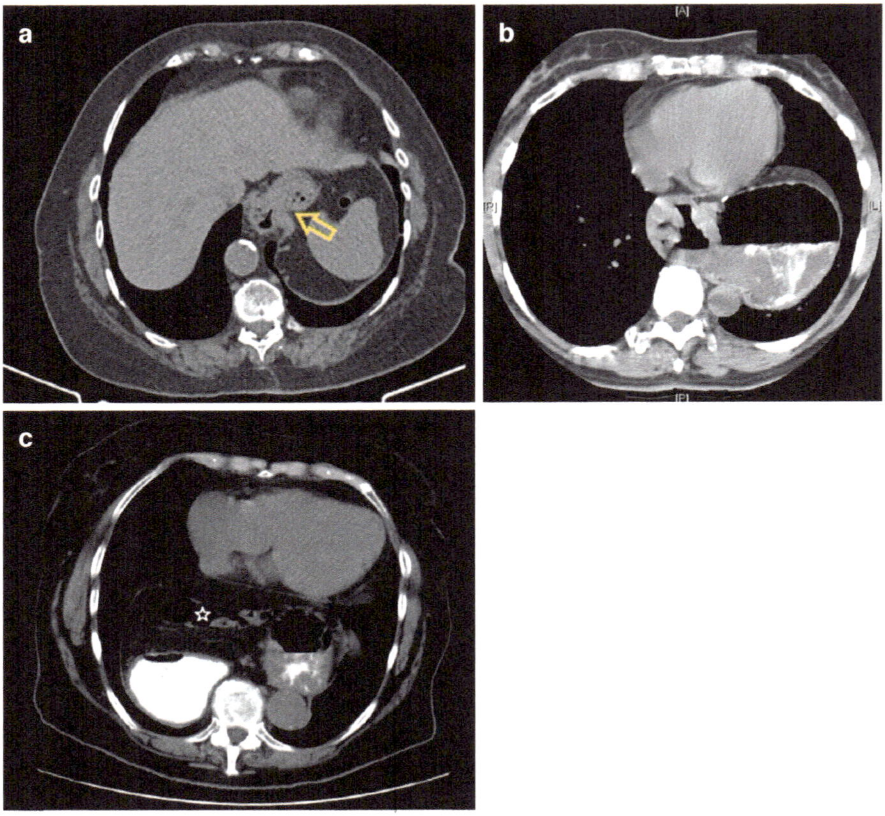

Fig. 28.5 Axial view computer tomography scan of paraesophageal hernia. (**a**) Type I sliding hiatal hernia with the stomach above and below the hiatus (arrow); (**b**) Type III paraesophageal hernia; (**c**) Type IV with the colon (star) herniating adjacent to the stomach

- High-resolution manometry.
  - Permits real-time localization of the GEJ.
  - Hernia characterized by separation of the crural diaphragm from LES by a pressure trough.

Treatment

- Symptomatic Type I: management of GERD symptoms beginning with lifestyle modifications (weight loss, dietary modifications, tobacco and alcohol cessation, elevation of bed), to medical therapy with proton pump inhibitor, to intervention with antireflux procedure (see Chap. 28).
- Asymptomatic Types II–IV.

  - Prophylactic surgical repair may be recommended, but controversial; observation is also an option in asymptomatic patients. Patient's baseline health status may play a role in deciding.
  - Surgery favored in young, healthy patients.
  - Surgery is recommended in Type IV hernias.
- Symptomatic or complicated Types II–IV: surgical repair indicated.

Surgical Technique: Fundoplication

- Approaches.
  - Transabdominal: open, laparoscopic, or robotic.
  - Transthoracic: left posterolateral thoracotomy, video-assisted thoracoscopic surgery (VATS).
- Approach chosen may depend on physician preference, hernia size, risk of recurrence, previous attempts at repair, prior surgery, and patient comorbidities.
- Principles of surgery.
  - Complete dissection and removal of the hernia sac from the mediastinum with reduction of all hernia contents.
  - Resection of the hernia sac.
  - Sufficient mobilization of the lower esophagus in the mediastinum to return GEJ into the abdomen and obtain adequate length of intra-abdominal esophagus, $\geq$ 3 cm without tension.
  - Tension-free closure of hiatal defect with primary suture repair, with controversy regarding the utility of mesh reinforcement.
  - Fundoplication.

    Complete or partial fundoplication to restore competency of the GEJ, especially in patients with symptomatic GERD.
    Esophageal motility is assessed preoperatively to help decide on the degree of wrap. If there is impaired motility a partial wrap is preferred.
    Types of fundoplication (Fig. 28.6).

      Dor: 180-degree anterior esophageal wrap.
      Toupet: 270-degree posterior esophageal wrap.
      Nissen: 360-degree, "complete" esophageal wrap.
      Belsey: 270-degree, transthoracic fundoplication.

    Fundoplication can be sutured to the diaphragm (gastropexy) to further help prevent recurrence.

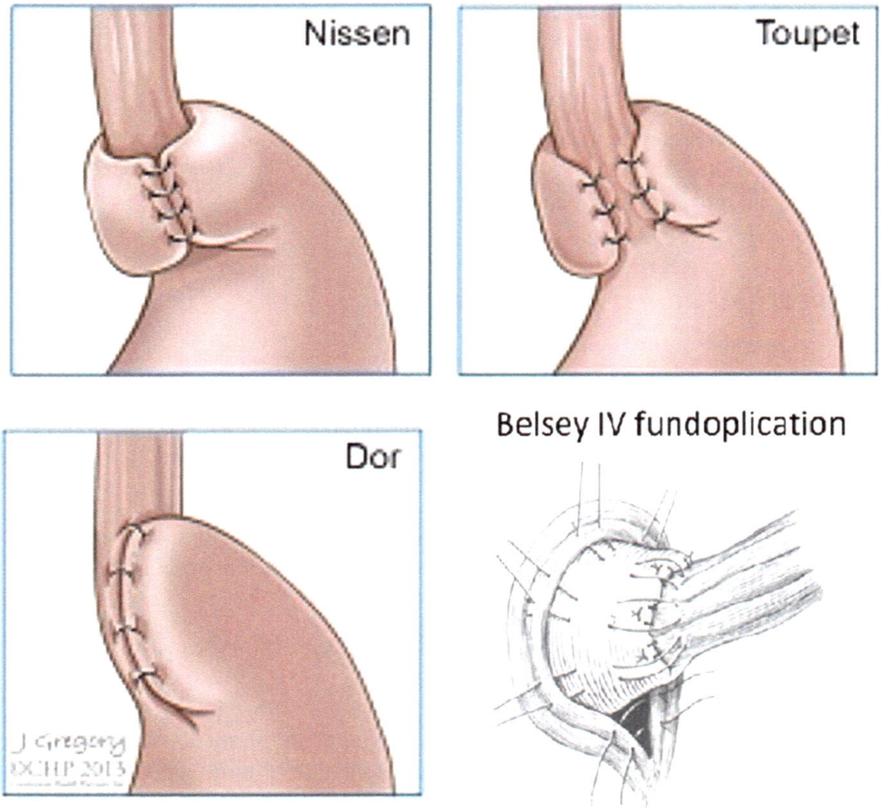

Fig. 28.6 Types of surgical fundoplication

Operative Technique

Transabdominal Approach

- Division of the gastrohepatic ligament with dissection of the hiatus.
- Observe and preserve the anterior and posterior vagal nerves.
- Reduction of the hernia sac contents with eversion and resection of the hernia sac.
- Avoid entry into the bilateral pleural spaces to prevent pneumothorax.
- Mobilization of the esophagus up the mediastinum to obtain length of the intra-abdominal esophagus with the goal of greater than ≥3 cm.
- Divide the short gastric vessels along the upper greater curvature.
- Hiatus is closed with crural sutures. An esophageal bougie (54–56 Fr) can be placed to assure appropriate sizing of the hiatus. If tension is significant, the patient may benefit from biologic mesh reinforcement or relaxing diaphragm counter incision with patch closure.

- Fundoplication.
- The stomach may be sutured (gastropexy) to the diaphragm to reduce displacement and reduce the risk of recurrence.

Transthoracic: Belsey Mark IV

- Access via the left chest; thoracotomy or VATS/robotic.
- Mobilize the hernia sac from the pericardium and posterior mediastinum.
- Excise the hernia sac from the stomach, and reduce the contents into the abdomen.
- Partial 270 degree fundoplication is created in two tiers, with the final tier stitches passed through the diaphragm to secure the repair below the diaphragm.
- Hiatus is closed with crural sutures. An esophageal bougie (54–56 Fr) can be placed to assure appropriate sizing of the hiatus. If tension is significant, the patient may benefit from biologic mesh reinforcement or relaxing diaphragm counter incision with patch closure.

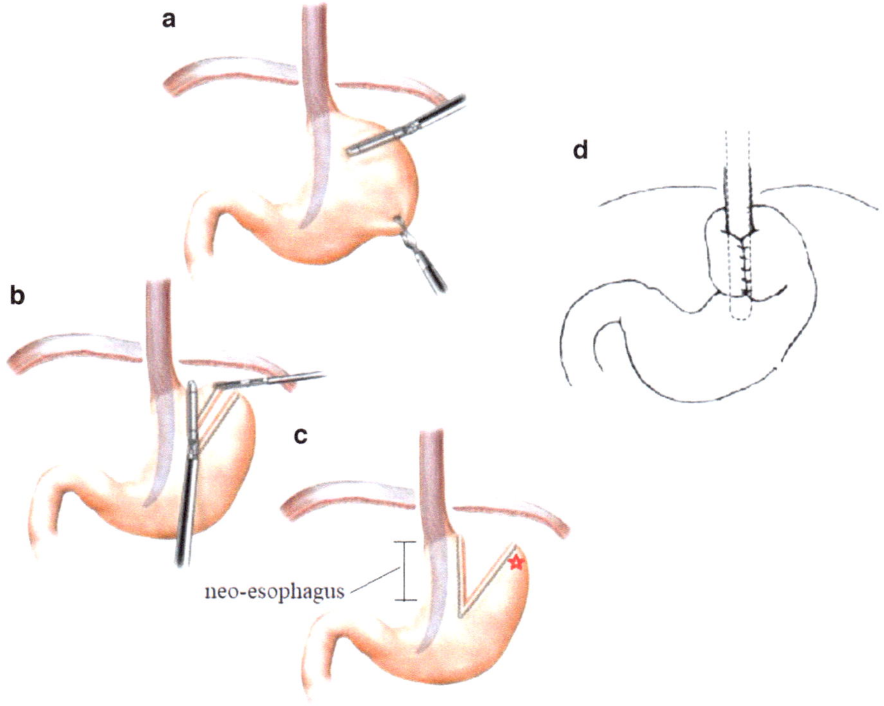

Fig. 28.7 Collis gastroplasty. (**a**) initial staple; (**b**) vertical staple over bougie to create a neo-esophagus from the proximal stomach; (**c**) the neo-esophagus is wrapped with the remaining gastric fundus (star); (**d**) completed Collis-Nissen fundoplication

Shortened Esophagus

- If less than 2 cm of intra-abdominal esophagus can be mobilized, then the esophagus is shortened and is at a higher risk for recurrence.
- Collis gastroplasty is utilized to gain intra-abdominal esophageal length by creating a neo-esophagus from the proximal stomach (Fig. 28.7). The gastroplasty is created by vertical stapling of the proximal greater curvature of the stomach, thereby creating a neo-esophagus. The remaining gastric fundus is then wrapped by Nissen fundoplication or Belsey fundoplication (Pearson transthoracic procedure) techniques.

Gastropexy to the Anterior Abdominal Wall

- Fixation of the stomach to the anterior abdominal wall (anterior gastropexy) can be done to reduce risk of re-herniation.
- In select patients, a gastropexy can be performed alone (without fundoplication), specifically in emergent situations, with an unstable patient or a patient with significant comorbidities.

Emergency Surgical Intervention

- Patients with signs and symptoms of gastric ischemia, unrelenting symptoms with failure to decompress the stomach, should undergo immediate surgical repair before progression to necrosis and perforation.

Postoperative Care

- An esophagram study may be obtained postoperatively to exclude the possibility of an esophageal leak and to evaluate esophageal transit through the hiatus.
- Diet is advanced slowly and stepwise, starting with liquids and advancing to more solid foods over a period of days or weeks.
- A majority of patients experience excellent, long-term relief of symptoms after surgery in 85–99% of patients, regardless of approach.

Postoperative Complications

- Esophageal leak.
  - Results from a defect in the esophagus or stomach during dissection or suturing.
  - Presents with signs and symptoms of sepsis: fever, tachycardia, and leukocytosis.
  - Diagnosed clinically or on postoperative esophagram or CT scan with oral contrast.
  - A small contained leak may be managed conservatively with NPO and antibiotics until resolution on repeat imaging.
  - A larger leak may require surgical reintervention to close an esophageal tear.
- Failed fundoplication.
  - A rare complication that may manifest in a number of different ways. A failed fundoplication often requires reoperation to take down the previous repair and create a new one.
  - A wrap that is too tight or too long may cause dysphagia or food intolerance/obstruction.
  - A wrap that is too loose or disrupted may result in regurgitation or reflux.
  - Slipped fundoplication: the stomach herniates through the fundoplication and is trapped above the repair.
- Recurrence of hiatal hernia.
  - Acutely in the immediate postoperative period, this is due to technical failure. This can result in incarceration, ischemia, and perforation of the re-herniated portion of the stomach, in which case emergent surgical intervention is indicated.
  - With long-term follow-up, recurrence rates are high with laparoscopic repair. Symptomatic recurrence occurs in <10–15% and may require redo surgery. Asymptomatic, radiologic recurrence is detected in 25–40% and may be observed.
  - Transthoracic repair, although viewed as more morbid than the laparoscopic approach, may have the lowest recurrence rates, setting a standard of comparison at 2%.

Key Reference

- Kohn GP, Price RR, DeMeester SR, et al. Guidelines for the management of hiatal hernia. Surg Endosc. 2013;27(12):4409–28.

Further Reading

Bredenoord AJ, Weusten BL, Timmer R, et al. Intermittent spatial separation of diaphragm and lower esophageal sphincter favors acidic and weakly acidic reflux. Gastroenterology. 2006;130(2):334–40.
Kahrilas PJ, Kim HC, Pandolfino JE. Approaches to the diagnosis and grading of hiatal hernia. Best Pract Res Clin Gastroenterol. 2008;22(4):601–16.
Lerut T, Deschamps C. Techniques for repair of paraesophageal hiatal hernia. In: Sugarbaker DJ, Bueno R, Burt BM, Groth SS, Loor G, Wolf AS, Williams M, Adams A, editors. Sugarbaker's adult chest surgery. 3rd ed. New York, NY: McGraw Hill; 2020.
Lidor AO, Steele KE, Stem M, et al. Long-term quality of life and risk factors for recurrence after laparoscopic repair of paraesophageal hernia. JAMA Surg. 2015;150(5):424–31.
Mattar SG, Bowers SP, Galloway KD, et al. Long-term outcome of laparoscopic repair of paraesophageal hernia. Surg Endosc. 2002;16(5):745–9.
Maziak DE, Todd TR, Pearson FG. Massive hiatus hernia: evaluation and surgical management. J Thorac Cardiovasc Surg. 1998;115(1):53–60.
Rathore MA, Andrabi SI, Bhatti MI, et al. Meta analysis of recurrence after laparoscopic repair of paraesophageal hernia. JSLS. 2007;11(4):456–60.

Chapter 29
Esophageal Motility Disorders

Travis Geraci and Thomas Ng

Esophageal Dysmotility

Esophageal motility disorders are disease states that cause abnormal esophageal peristalsis and/or contractions, leading to impaired transit of food that results in dysphagia, chest pain, or regurgitation.

- Primary esophageal disorders are those that cannot be attributed to another disease state, such as scleroderma, amyloidosis, diabetes mellitus, or neuromuscular disorders (these are considered "secondary").
  - The cause of the majority of primary esophageal motility disorders is unknown.
  - Disorders are classified according to esophageal manometry patterns.
  - Approaches to treatment include observation, medications, endoscopic interventions, and surgery.
- The esophagus has two muscular sphincters (upper and lower) that control the entrance and egress of food, aiding in transit and preventing reflux of gastric contents.

T. Geraci
Division of Thoracic Surgery, Department of Cardiothoracic Surgery, New York University Langone Health, New York, NY, USA
e-mail: travis.geraci@nyulangone.org

T. Ng (✉)
Division of Thoracic Surgery, University of Tennessee Health Science Center, College of Medicine, Memphis, TN, USA
e-mail: tng4@uthsc.edu

T. Ng, T. Geraci (eds.), *Thoracic Surgery Clerkship*, Contemporary Surgical Clerkships, https://doi.org/10.1007/978-3-031-44645-0_29

- The lower esophageal sphincter (LES), which is the most distal portion of the esophagus, acting as a barrier from the stomach, is commonly abnormal in esophageal motility disorders.
- At rest, the LES maintains a contracted state with an elevated pressure around 15–25 mmHg.
- In a normal swallow, as food travels down the esophagus, the LES relaxes allowing passage into the stomach. The LES then returns to a contracted state until the next bolus of food.
- The esophagus is controlled by the central and enteric nervous systems.

Achalasia

Achalasia is an esophageal motility disorder in which the LES fails to relax, maintaining a constantly contracted state.

- The term achalasia derives from Greek for "does not relax."
- Pathogenesis is thought to be a result from loss of inhibitory neuronal drive from degeneration of ganglion cells in the myenteric plexus.
- Associated with a loss of esophageal peristalsis with progressive dilation of the mid to distal esophagus.

Presentation

- Relatively rare disease (1–100,000/year) affecting men and women equally, which typically presents between the ages of 30–60.
- The classic clinical presentation is insidious (over months to years) but progressive dysphagia to solid food and liquids.
- Patients may also present with early satiety, regurgitation, retrosternal chest pain, heartburn, or weight loss attributed to poor intake.
- Associated with a risk of developing esophageal squamous cell carcinoma.

Diagnosis

- Barium esophagram/swallow is the initial study for patients with a clinical presentation consistent with achalasia.
  - The esophagus fills with contrast, demonstrating a distal narrowing at the contracted LES referred to as a "bird's beak" appearance, with or without proximal esophageal dilation (Fig. 29.1).
  - May be accompanied by a false (pulsion) epiphrenic diverticulum.

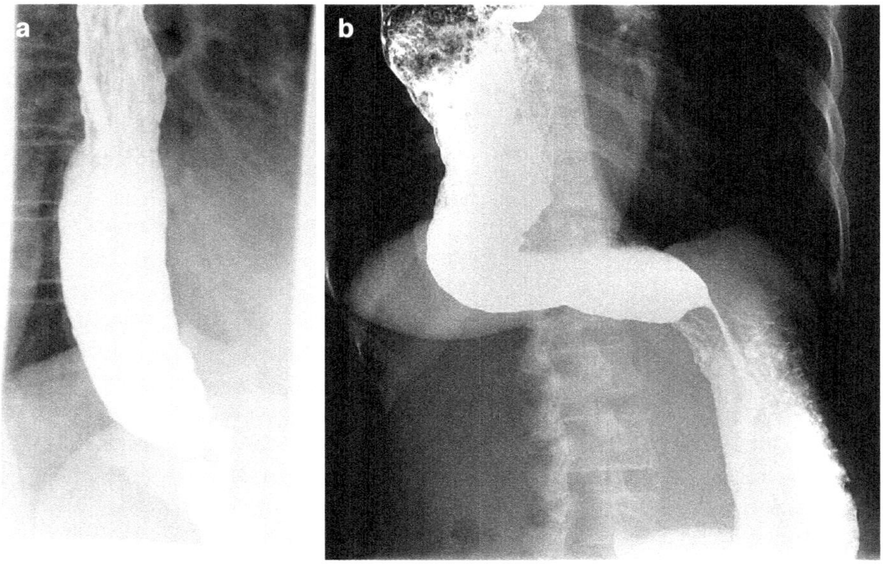

Fig. 29.1 Barium esophagrams of two different patients, each consistent with achalasia with distal narrowing of the distal esophagus at the lower esophageal sphincter and proximal dilation

- A timed esophagram defines the rate and effectiveness of esophageal emptying, which may be delayed in patients with achalasia.
- A distal esophageal malignancy may produce a similar narrowing to achalasia (termed pseudoachalasia) but is more often asymmetric. Therefore, while a barium esophagram is highly sensitive for achalasia, other pathologies must be evaluated via endoscopy.

• High-resolution manometry.

- An esophageal catheter with sensors is placed, and pressure tracings are generated during resting and swallowing states.
- Classic findings of achalasia include incomplete relaxation of the LES with esophageal aperistalsis.
- Chicago Classification is a system that subclassifies achalasia based on intraluminal pressure patterns of the esophageal body:

  Type I: normal esophageal pressure.
  Type II: panesophageal pressurization (greater than 30 mmHg).

    Most responsive to therapy.

  Type III (spastic): premature, simultaneous, abnormal contractions or spasm.

    Lower overall treatment response.

- Endoscopy.
  - Upper endoscopy, with biopsy, is utilized to examine the esophageal mucosa, gastroesophageal junction, and stomach to rule out other disease states or malignant lesions (pseudoachalasia).
  - In achalasia, the esophageal mucosa may appear inflamed or ulcerated secondary to stasis of food.
  - Biopsy is obtained for mass/abnormal lesions and to rule out secondary causes of esophageal dysmotility.

Treatment

- The primary aim of all treatment modalities is to decrease LES pressure.
- There is no medication or procedure that restores the loss of esophageal peristalsis.
- Treatment overview:
  - Medical therapy has a limited duration of activity and is indicated for patients with mild symptoms or those unable to undergo invasive procedures.
  - Botox injection is most useful in older patients (over age 50) who are at a higher risk for mechanical dilation or myotomy.
  - Patients with type I or II achalasia with acceptable surgical risk should undergo pneumatic dilation or myotomy (surgical or peroral), as these interventions provide the best and most durable results.
  - Myotomy should be considered as initial therapy for patients with acceptable surgical risk with type III achalasia.
- Medical therapy.
  - Calcium channel blockers and/or nitrates.

    Relaxes smooth muscle of the LES.
    Medication is taken at mealtimes and has a short duration of action.
    Effectiveness diminishes over time, and adherence is variable due to adverse side effects such as headache, tachyphylaxis, and hypotension.
- Endoscopic therapy.
- Dilation of the LES.
  - Mechanical stretching/weakening of the muscles of the LES.
  - Post-dilation emptying time of contrast on post-procedure esophagram is the best indicator of treatment success.
  - Esophageal perforation rate is reported between 2 and 6%.
  - Bougie dilation.

    Temporal measure given limited duration of effect of weeks to months.

Endoscopic pneumatic dilation.

Achieves good clinical results in the majority of patients that are comparable to surgical myotomy.
Symptom relief is often durable over years, although patients may require repeat dilations.
Predictors of treatment failure include persistent chest pain, esophageal diameter less than 4 cm, age, and type III achalasia.

- Botulinum (Botox) injection.
  - Endoscopic injection of botox in the region of the LES inhibits the release of acetylcholine from neurons.
  - Good immediate symptom relief, but limited median duration of 6 months.
  - More effective in older patients (over 50 years of age).
- Peroral endoscopic myotomy (POEM).
  - An esophageal myotomy is made via endoscopic instrumentation.
  - POEM has a similar resolution of dysphagia and similar rates of perioperative complications as a surgical myotomy, but with a higher rate of reflux (40–60% of patients) and esophagitis.
  - For type III achalasia, POEM is superior to surgical myotomy, in terms of resolution of dysphagia and fewer adverse events.
  - Can be an effective option in cases of incomplete surgical myotomy.
- Surgical myotomy with partial fundoplication.
  - Commonly performed by laparoscopy.
  - A surgical myotomy (modified Heller myotomy) involves division of the longitudinal and circular muscle fibers (exposing the mucosa) at the level of the LES, often performed by laparoscopy but can also be by thoracoscopy.
  - Partial fundoplication.

    Provides symptomatic relief of the reflux that results after myotomy.
    Can be anterior (Dor) or posterior (Toupet) for laparoscopic approach or Belsey for transthoracic approach.
    Due to a lack of peristalsis of the lower esophagus, partial fundoplication is preferred over complete (Nissen).

  - Technique (Fig. 29.2a, b).

    The myotomy should extend 5 cm into the intrathoracic esophagus and at least 3 cm onto the anterior fundus of the stomach.
    Most commonly, an anterior 180 degree fundoplication (Dor) is performed, covering the mucosa of the LES.
    Endoscopy is performed at the end of the procedure to assure a complete myotomy and evaluate for mucosal defects.

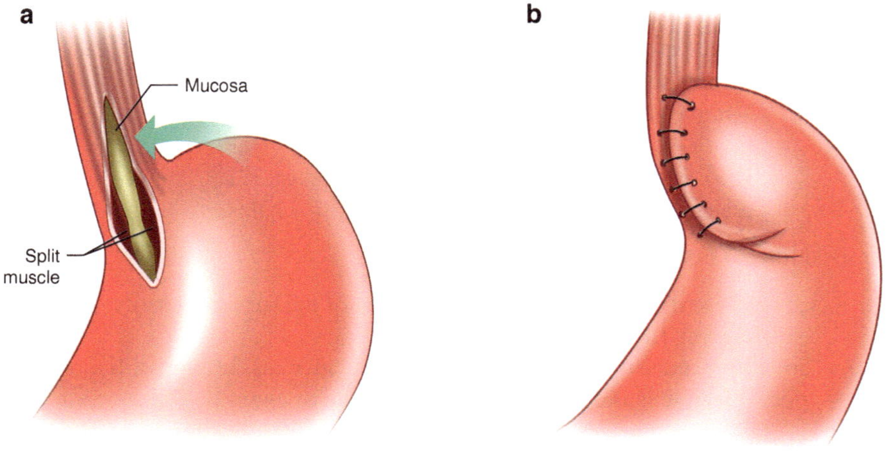

Fig. 29.2 Technique for laparoscopic myotomy with partial fundoplication. (**a**) Division of the longitudinal and circular muscles of the esophagus (**b**) and fundoplication (in this depiction an anterior wrap)

  - Recurrence is treated with repeat myotomy, with extension of the myotomy to 10–12 cm above the LES and 3 cm additional on the gastric cardia.

- Recurrent dysphagia after therapy.
  - Incomplete myotomy.
  - Reflux stricture.
  - Development of squamous cell carcinoma of the esophagus.
  - Fundoplication too tight.
  - Progression to end-stage achalasia.

Diffuse Esophageal Spasm

- The pathogenesis is not completely understood, but is theorized to involve defective nitric oxide synthesis, thereby affecting esophageal smooth muscle.
- Symptoms include dysphagia and chest pain.
- Barium esophagram (Fig. 29.3).
  - Demonstrates contractions throughout the esophagus creating a "corkscrew" appearance.
  - May be accompanied by a false diverticulum.

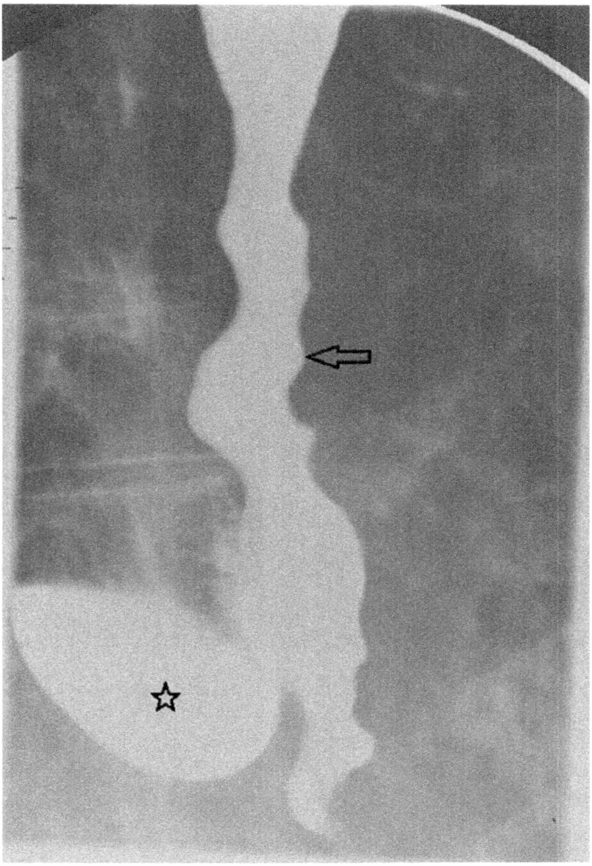

Fig. 29.3 Barium swallow of diffuse esophageal spasm, showing the esophagus with corkscrew appearance (arrow) and a false diverticulum (star)

- Esophageal manometry reveals spontaneous, repetitive contractions of prolonged duration.
  - Diagnostic criteria: simultaneous contractions of at least 30 mmHg for more than 20% of measured swallows.
  - Associated with abnormal LES pressure, either with a high resting pressure or failure of complete relaxation.
- Treatment.
  - Medical therapy with calcium channel blockers and/or nitrates.
  - Surgical therapy by transthoracic approach.

    Long surgical myotomy (Fig. 29.4a): the division of the esophageal muscle fibers is performed on the entire length of the dysfunctional esophagus. Diverticulum, if present, is resected (Fig. 29.4b, c).

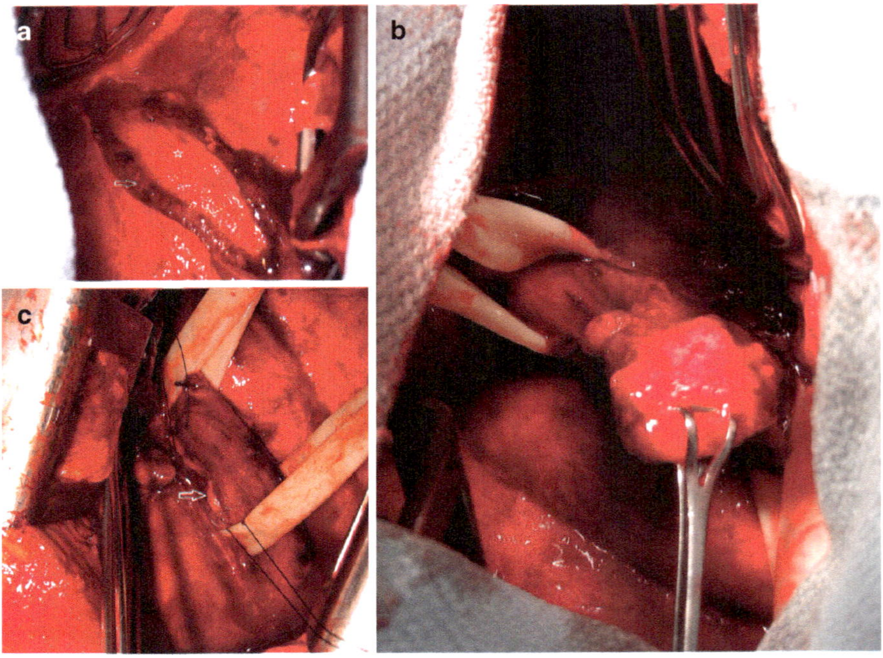

Fig. 29.4 Surgical therapy for diffuse esophageal spasm. (**a**) Long esophageal myotomy (arrow) with the exposed underlying mucosa (star); (**b**) presence of false esophageal diverticulum; (**c**) staple line (arrow) after stapled diverticulectomy, which will subsequently be covered over with a layer of muscle closure; also note the long myotomy will be 180 degrees on the opposite side of the esophagus

Esophagectomy for End-Stage Motility Disorders

- For select patients with end-stage esophageal motility disorders, an esophagectomy is considered as a last treatment option.
- Patients often have persistent and debilitating symptoms of dysphagia and/or esophageal reflux and may have undergone repeat procedures or several interventions prior to considering esophagectomy.
- All indications are relative and must be considered in the setting of patient health and anticipate perioperative outcomes:
  - Advanced stage esophageal motility disorder with refractory symptoms.
  - Recurrent aspiration due to regurgitation.
  - Malnutrition from an inability to eat (regurgitation, obstruction, pain).
- Perioperative complications remain a significant source of morbidity, similar to an esophagectomy for cancer (35–60% of patients), most commonly cardiopulmonary complications.
- Functional results vary based on disease process, patient health, and operative course.

Zenker's Diverticulum

Epidemiology and Pathophysiology

- Usually found in elderly patients, in their seventh decade of life or beyond.
- Uncommon, with a reported prevalence of 0.01–0.11%, but this may be an underestimate as it may not account for asymptomatic patients.
- During normal swallowing, the pharyngeal constrictor muscles contract to push the food bolus through a relaxed cricopharyngeus muscle (or upper esophageal sphincter) and into the esophagus.
- If the cricopharyngeus muscle fails to relax upon swallowing, the high pressure created by the contraction of the pharyngeal constrictors against a closed upper esophageal sphincter will result in the development of a false diverticulum (Zenker's) through Kilian's triangle, directed posteriorly and inferiorly (Fig. 29.5).
- The borders of Kilian's triangle consist of the two parts of the inferior pharyngeal constrictor muscles above and the cricopharyngeal muscle below.
- As with any false or pulsion diverticulum, Zenker's diverticulum contains only the mucosa and submucosa layers, lacking the muscularis layer.

Fig. 29.5 Anatomy of Zenker's diverticulum

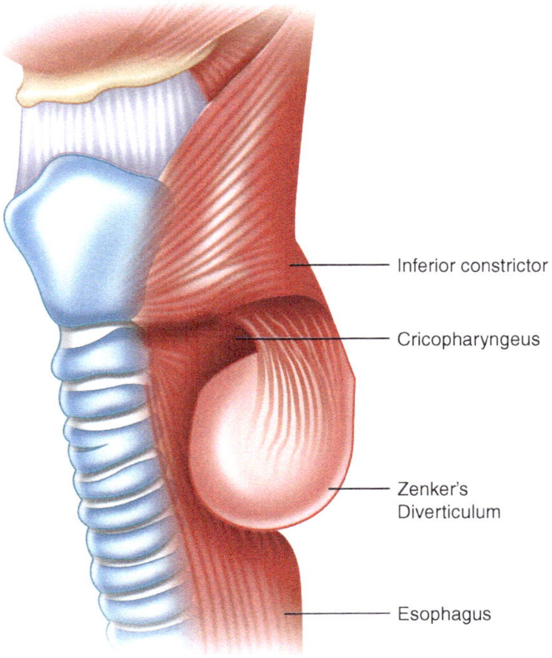

Presentation

- Dysphagia.
- Halitosis.
- Regurgitation of undigested food.
- Choking.
- Recurrent pneumonia form repeated aspiration.
- Minimal to no weight loss.
- Rarely, malignancy within the diverticulum.
- Perforation from instrumentation such as EGD or transesophageal echocardiography, commonly without awareness of its presence.

Workup

- Barium swallow: a cervical esophageal diverticulum is diagnostic (Fig. 29.6).
- Manometry: it may show failure of the cricopharyngeus to relax with swallowing, but this study is not necessary and often inaccurate for evaluating the cervical esophagus.

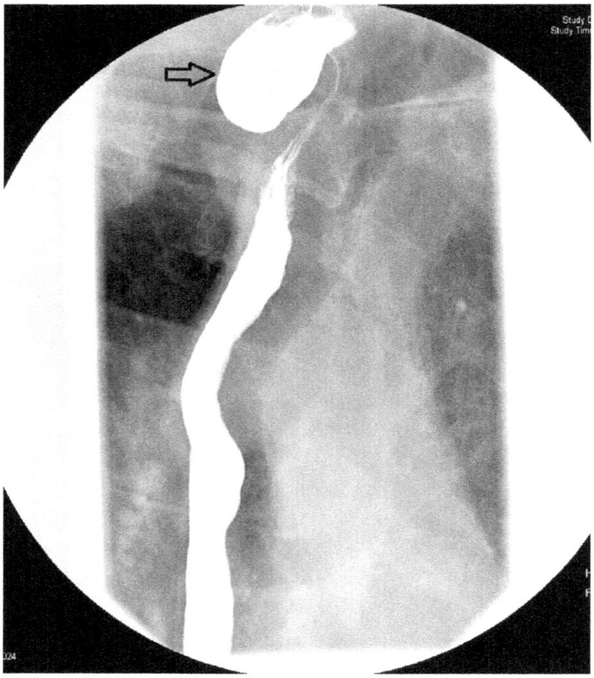

Fig. 29.6 Barium swallow showing cervical esophageal (Zenker's) diverticulum (arrow)

- EGD: it is not necessary and risks perforation if the existence of diverticulum is not known, and the discovery of malignancy within the diverticulum is exceedingly rare.

Treatment

- Symptoms are unlikely to improve without intervention and can slowly worsen with time.
- Indications for treatment include:
  - Presence of debilitating symptoms, as perceived by the patient.
  - Recurrent pneumonia due to aspiration.
- Treatment options.
  - Surgical (Fig. 29.7a, b).

General anesthesia.
Left cervical incision.
Cricopharyngeal myotomy extending down the esophagus 4–5 cm.
Handling of the diverticulum.

No intervention for the diverticulum if small (< 2–3 cm).
Diverticulectomy, commonly performed using linear cutting stapler over a bougie.
Cephalad pexy of the diverticulum to prevertebral fascia or posterior pharynx, performed if avoiding an esophageal staple line is desired, especially in cases where wound healing is of concern (such as patients on steroids).

Risks of surgery.

Overall risk of surgery is low.
Injury to major vessels – carotid artery, jugular vein.
Injury to nerves – recurrent laryngeal, vagus.
Injury to the trachea.
Diverticulectomy staple line leak.

- Endoscopic transoral stapling (Fig. 29.8).

General anesthesia.
Requires adequate neck extension and mouth opening.
Linear cutting stapler is fired to both cut the cricopharyngeus muscle and open up the diverticulum together with the esophagus so that food will not get hung up.

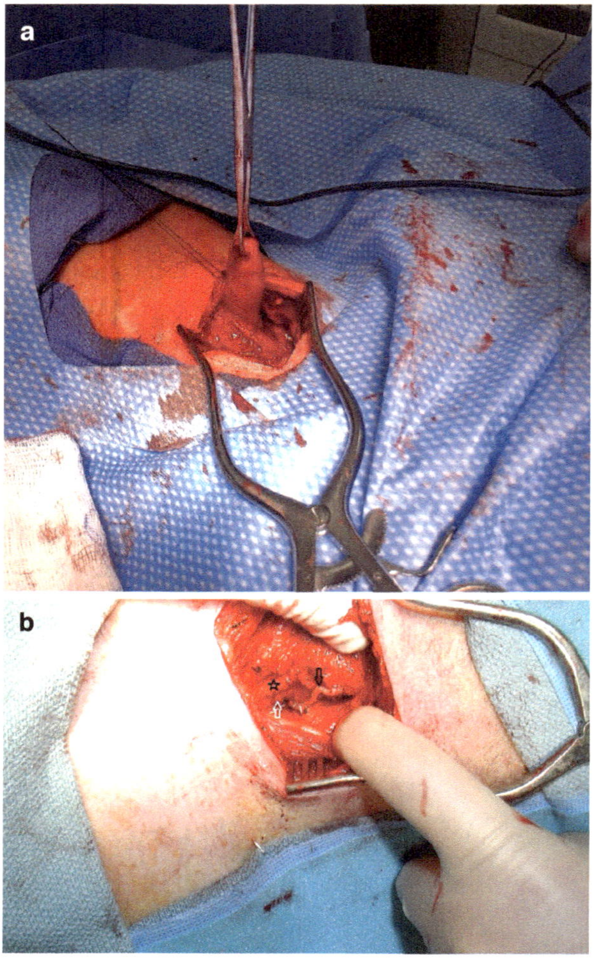

Fig. 29.7 Surgical treatment for Zenker's diverticulum. (**a**) Left neck incision with dissection of the diverticulum; (**b**) completion of surgery showing the diverticulectomy staple line (black arrow), myotomized muscle edge (star), and exposed esophageal mucosa (white arrow)

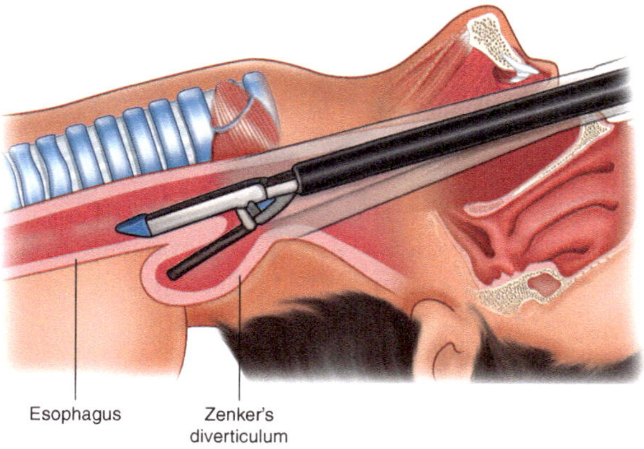

Fig. 29.8 Endoscopic transoral stapling

Not ideal for a large diverticulum, as the stapler will not have inadequate length to open the entire diverticulum; thus, the hang up of food will persist.
Not ideal for a small diverticulum, as this would not allow the stapler to be inserted far enough to achieve complete cricopharyngeal myotomy, resulting in persistent symptoms.
Avoids an incision and the risk of injury to major vessels and nerves.
Complications – staple line leak, damage to the teeth.
Surgical intervention after previous transoral stapling, if required, will now be more difficult.

Outcomes

- No randomized comparisons available to determine the optimal therapy for Zenker's diverticulum.
- All treatment techniques have been shown to be safe and successful in relieving symptoms, with meta-analyses suggesting that the surgical approach has the highest success of complete symptom resolution and the lowest re-intervention rate, but with a slightly higher morbidity and length of hospital stay as compared with endoscopic approaches.

Key Reference
- Schlottmann F, Herbella FAM, Patti MG. The evolution of the treatment of esophageal Achalasia: from the open to the minimally invasive approach. World J Surg. 2022;46(7):1522–26.

Further Reading

Albers DV, Kondo A, Bernardo WM, Sakai P, Moura RN, Silva GL, Ide E, Tomishige T, de Moura EG. Endoscopic versus surgical approach in the treatment of Zenker's diverticulum: systematic review and meta-analysis. Endosc Int Open. 2016;4(6):E678–86.

Bhatt NK, Mendoza J, Kallogjeri D, Hardi AC, Bradley JP. Comparison of surgical treatments for Zenker diverticulum: a systematic review and network meta-analysis. JAMA Otolaryngol Head Neck Surg. 2021;147(2):190–6.

Howell RJ, Giliberto JP, Harmon J, Masch J, Khosla S, Postma GN, Meinzen-Derr J. Open versus endoscopic surgery of Zenker's diverticula: a systematic review and meta-analysis. Dysphagia. 2019;34(6):930–8.

Mittal R, Vaezi MF. Esophageal motility disorders and gastroesophageal reflux disease. N Engl J Med. 2020;383(20):1961–72.

Patel DA, Yadlapati R, Vaezi MF. Esophageal motility disorders: current approach to diagnostics and therapeutics. Gastroenterology. 2022;162(6):1617–34.

Rohof WOA, Bredenoord AJ. Chicago classification of esophageal motility disorders: lessons learned. Curr Gastroenterol Rep. 2017;19(8):37.

Sato H, Takahashi K, Mizuno KI, Hashimoto S, Yokoyama J, Hasegawa G, Terai S. Esophageal motility disorders: new perspectives from high-resolution manometry and histopathology. J Gastroenterol. 2018;53(4):484–93.

Schlottmann F, Luckett DJ, Fine J, Shaheen NJ, Patti MG. Laparoscopic heller myotomy versus peroral endoscopic myotomy (POEM) for achalasia: a systematic review and meta-analysis. Ann Surg. 2018;267(3):451–60.

Verdonck J, Morton RP. Systematic review on treatment of Zenker's diverticulum. Eur Arch Otorhinolaryngol. 2015;272(11):3095–107.

Watson TJ, DeMeester TR, Kauer WK, Peters JH, Hagen JA. Esophageal replacement for end-stage benign esophageal disease. J Thorac Cardiovasc Surg. 1998;115(6):1241–7; discussion 1247–9.

Chapter 30
Benign Esophageal Tumors

Mohammad Abdallat and John S. Young

Introduction

Benign esophageal neoplasms have an incidence of less than 1% on autopsy series and are significantly less common than malignant esophageal carcinomas. The majority only require diagnosis or surveillance given their slow rate of growth and rarity of symptoms. Surgical resection is sometimes required for symptoms, for select pathologies, and in cases of an uncertain diagnosis. Outcomes are typically excellent with surgery.

Anatomy

- The esophageal wall is composed of mucosa, submucosa, and muscularis propria layers.
  - Mucosa (innermost) has three layers:

    Epithelium: stratified, nonkeratinizing squamous epithelium
    Lamina propria: collagen and elastic fibers, as well as lymphatics
    Muscularis mucosa: smooth muscle

  - Submucosa

    Connective tissue with the vascular arcade, nerve bundles, and lymphatics
    Strength layer of the esophageal wall

M. Abdallat · J. S. Young (✉)
Division of Thoracic Surgery, Brigham and Women's Hospital, Boston, MA, USA
e-mail: mabdallat@bwh.harvard.edu; jyoung0@bwh.harvard.edu

T. Ng, T. Geraci (eds.), *Thoracic Surgery Clerkship*, Contemporary Surgical Clerkships, https://doi.org/10.1007/978-3-031-44645-0_30

- Muscularis propria has an inner circular and outer longitudinal layer

  Proximal esophagus striated
  Gradual transition to smooth muscle distally

- Periesophageal tissue made up of fibrofatty tissue.

Clinical Presentation

While carcinoma is a disease of the older patients, the mean age for benign esophageal tumors is 30–50 years. Esophageal duplications on the other hand are far more common in children and comprise 12% of mediastinal tumors in the pediatric population.

Most patients are asymptomatic, and the tumors are incidentally found. However, they may develop symptoms due to obstruction from intraluminal growth, compression of adjacent tissue by extraluminal tumor, regurgitation of a pedunculated tumor, and ulceration with bleeding.

- Dysphagia is the most common symptom.
- Retrosternal or epigastric pain is next most common.
- May also have respiratory symptoms (cough, dyspnea, or pneumonia) from compression of the airways.
- Reflux and hiccups may also be seen.

Diagnosis

- Benign esophageal tumors are frequently incidentally found on imaging or endoscopy.
- A contrast swallow study is a helpful first test in the workup of a benign esophageal tumor – benign tumors are typically smooth bordered and mobile.
- Cross-sectional imaging with a CT chest helps delineate anatomical relationships and evaluate for other pathology and aids in preoperative planning.
- Esophagogastroscopy (EGD; also referred to as upper endoscopy) and endoscopic ultrasound (EUS) are mandatory in the workup:
  - Endoscopy allows for inspection of the mucosa to evaluate and biopsy intraluminal tumors and rule out malignancy.
  - Endoscopic biopsy of tumors should be avoided if the overlying mucosa appears normal as this may make future enucleation challenging.
  - Intramural lesions are not well seen on endoscopy, but if suspected, confirmation of an intact mucosa should be obtained.
  - EUS allows for visualization of the esophageal wall and periesophageal tissue as five distinct alternating hyperechoic and hypoechoic layers:

Superficial mucosa (inner layer, hyperechoic)
Deep mucosa (second layer, hypoechoic)
Submucosa (third layer, hyperechoic)
Muscularis propria (fourth layer, hypoechoic)
Periesophageal tissue (fifth layer, hyperechoic)

- EUS helps in the diagnosis based on sonographic properties and location of the tumor and can aid in preoperative planning and surveillance.
- Benign lesions are typically homogenous anechoic, hypoechoic, or of intermediate echogenicity, are smaller, have smooth borders, and have no associated enlarged lymph nodes.
- Heterogeneous lesions may be either benign or malignant.
- EUS-directed fine-needle aspiration (FNA) should be performed on suspicious lesions or lymph nodes.

Intraluminal Tumors

Endoluminal biopsy of these lesions is appropriate to confirm the diagnosis.

Squamous Papilloma

- Solitary, small (<1 cm), pink projections in the distal esophagus, linked with human papilloma virus (HPV) and GERD, endoscopic resection for symptomatic lesions.

Fibrovascular Polyps

- Most common benign intraluminal tumor of the esophagus.
- Usually located in the cervical esophagus, fleshy sausage-like lesion, may present with regurgitation or sudden death from asphyxia.
- Either endoscopic or surgical resection is recommended due to the risk of airway obstruction.

Hemangioma

- Benign vascular tumor arising from submucosa.

- Found in the distal esophagus, appear as blue polypoid compressible lesions, can be diagnosed with CT with contrast, MRI, or EUS.
- These should not be biopsied due to risk of hemorrhage.
- Can be treated endoscopically or surgically if symptomatic.

Adenoma

- Polyps from benign neoplastic process of columnar cells.
- May harbor high-grade dysphagia.
- Should be removed endoscopically or ablated if proven to be benign.

Inflammatory Pseudotumor

- Distal esophageal masses made of fibroblasts and inflammatory cells.
- Linked with chronic reflux and Epstein-Barr virus (EBV).
- These should be biopsied as they can be confused with malignancy.

Granular Cell Tumor

- Distal esophageal tumor arising from neural cells in the submucosa.
- 1–3% risk of malignancy.
- Pale yellow wide-based polypoid lesions with thin intact mucosa.
- Resection is indicated if there is concern for malignancy, if symptomatic, if rapidly growing, or if tumor is greater than 1 cm.

Intramural Tumors

Leiomyoma

- Leiomyomas are the most common benign esophageal tumor (more than 70%) and typically arise from the inner circular layer, or less commonly the muscularis mucosa, in the bottom half of the esophagus.
- Frequently asymptomatic and slow growing, 2:1 male-to-female ratio, peak presentation between 30 and 50 years old.
- Contrast swallow study (Fig. 30.1a) shows a smooth filling defect that is mobile and nonobstructing.

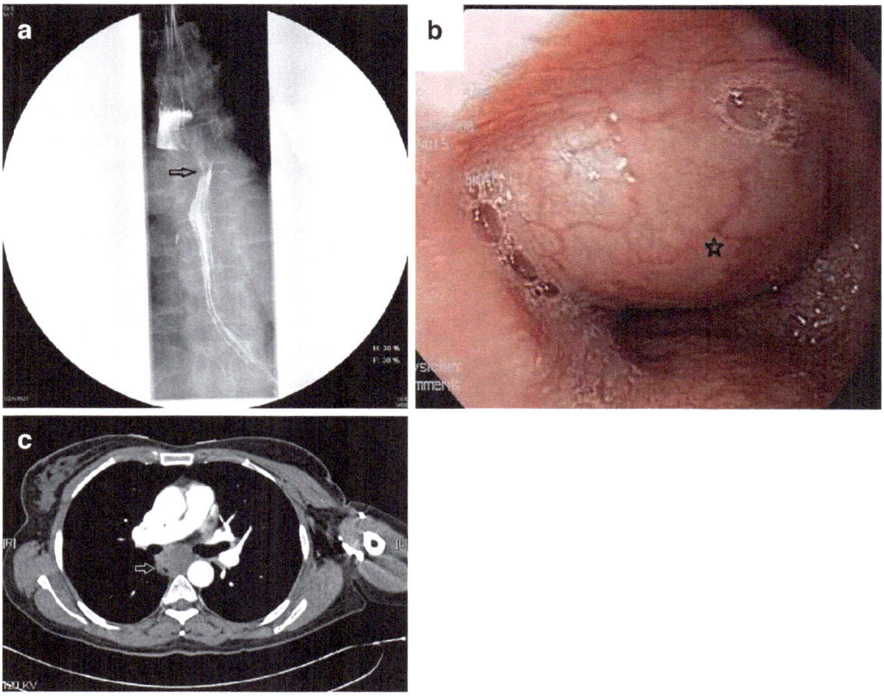

Fig. 30.1 Esophageal leiomyoma. (**a**) Barium swallow showing smooth indentation of the esophagus by a submucosal lesion (arrow); (**b**) endoscopic view showing mass lesion with normal overlying mucosa (star); (**c**) CT scan showing mass narrowing the esophageal lumen (arrow)

- On EGD (Fig. 30.1b), they are firm, rubbery, well-encapsulated masses with intact mucosa on EGD, blind endoscopic biopsy not recommended.
- Homogenous, hypoechoic, smooth bordered lesion from the fourth layer on EUS.
- Biopsy with EUS-FNA only indicated if diagnosis is in question.
- Will appears as a smooth, homogenous mass on CT scan (Fig. 30.1c).
- Indications for resection: symptomatic, size greater than 4 cm, or concern for malignancy.
- Resection typically involves surgical enucleation (Fig. 30.2), either in an open or a minimally invasive fashion (thoracoscopy or robotic approach).
  - Longitudinal myotomy over the tumor.
  - Leiomyoma is bluntly freed from surrounding tissue, taking care not to injure the mucosa.
  - Myotomy is closed after enucleation of tumor.
- Esophagectomy indicated in tumors greater than 8 cm, diffuse involvement, ulceration or damage of mucosa, or concern for leiomyosarcoma.
- Endoscopic mucosal resection (EMR) is an option in leiomyomas arising from the muscularis mucosa.

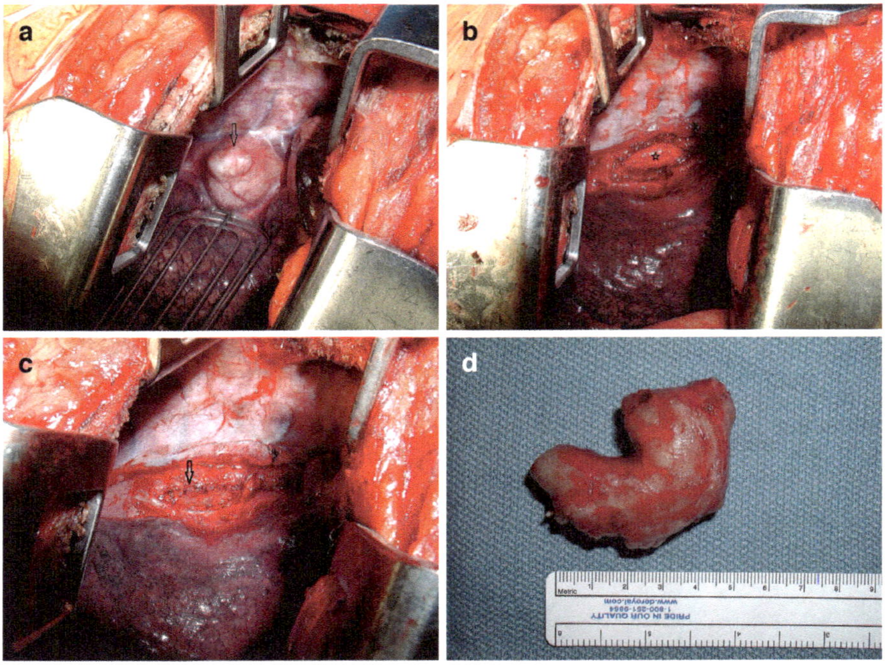

Fig. 30.2 Leiomyoma enucleation. (**a**) View of tumor prior to resection (arrow); (**b**) after enucleation showing intact mucosa (star); (**c**) closure of myotomy (arrow); (**d**) resected specimen

Gastrointestinal Stromal Tumor (GIST)

- Can be found in the distal esophagus and arise from the interstitial cells of Cajal.
- Much less common than leiomyomas but can be very difficult to distinguish from with similar findings on contrast swallow, endoscopy, and EUS.
- PET can be useful as GISTs are PET-avid in contrast to leiomyomas.
- EUS-FNA can be helpful as well as GISTs expressing *c-kit* uniformly on immunohistochemistry.
- While the majority have a low risk of metastasis, there is heterogeneity of GISTs, and esophageal GISTs are more aggressive than GISTs located in other areas.
- Management of GISTs includes imatinib as well as surgical resection with either enucleation or esophagectomy.

Periesophageal

Esophageal cysts, while not tumors, are the second most common benign tumorlike condition. The majority are congenital foregut cysts but also include inclusion cysts and neuroenteric cysts.

- Esophageal duplication cysts have epithelial, submucosal, and muscular layers and are part intramural.
- Inclusion cysts have epithelial lining, but no muscular elements.
- May be associated with vertebral/spinal cord abnormalities.
- Symptoms include dysphagia, dyspnea, and stridor.
- Patients may also present with infection of the cyst.
- EGD (Fig. 30.3a) shows lesion with normal overlying mucosa.
- EUS can clearly show the location and cystic nature.
- CT scan (Fig. 30.3b) helps delineate characteristics and relevant anatomy for preoperative planning.
- These should not be biopsied as they may become infected, and it may make surgical resection more challenging.
- Resection (Fig. 30.3c, d) by enucleation is performed with open or minimally invasive techniques (thoracoscopy or robotic approach), indicated for symptomatic patients.

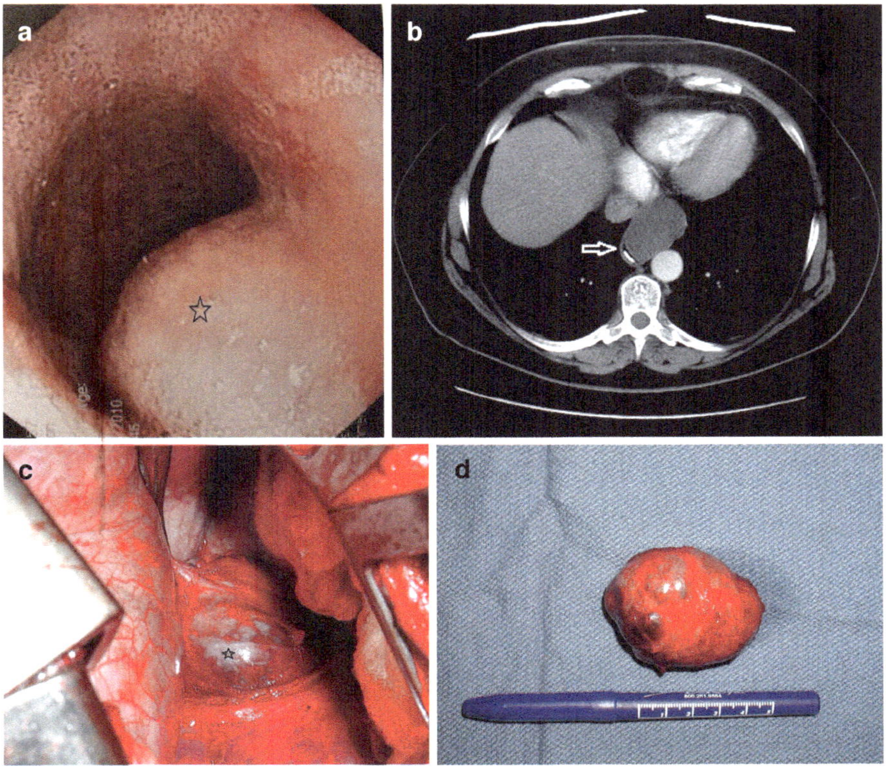

Fig. 30.3 Esophageal duplication cyst. (**a**) Endoscopic view showing lesion with normal overlying mucosa (star); (**b**) CT scan showing low-density lesion narrowing the esophageal lumen (arrow); (**c**) intraoperative view of cyst prior to resection (star); (**d**) resected specimen after enucleation

Key Reference

- Rice TW. Benign esophageal tumors: esophagoscopy and endoscopic esophageal ultrasound. Semin Thorac Cardiovasc Surg. 2003;15(1):20–6.

Further Reading

Choong CK, Meyers BF. Benign esophageal tumors: introduction, incidence, classification, and clinical features. Semin Thorac Cardiovasc Surg. 2003;15(1):3–8.

Ha C, Regan J, Cetindag IB, Ali A, Mellinger JD. Benign esophageal tumors. Surg Clin North Am. 2015;95(3):491–514.

Samphire J, Nafteux P, Luketich J. Minimally invasive techniques for resection of benign esophageal tumors. Semin Thorac Cardiovasc Surg. 2003;15(1):35–43.

Shin S, Choi YS, Shim YM, Kim HK, Kim K, Kim J. Enucleation of esophageal submucosal tumors: a single institution's experience. Ann Thorac Surg. 2014;97(2):454–9.

Chapter 31
Esophageal Perforation and Caustic Injury

Dana Ferrari-Light and Oliver S. Chow

Anatomy (Fig. 31.1)

- **Cervical esophagus**
  - Begins at cricopharyngeus muscle, ends at sternal notch.
  - Lies just behind trachea, attached to cervical spine via prevertebral fascia.
  - Carotid sheath and inferior pole of thyroid gland lie laterally to esophagus.
  - Killian's triangle: space immediately above cricopharyngeus muscle and below inferior pharyngeal constrictor (thyropharyngeus muscle), triangle-shaped area of weakness.
- **Thoracic esophagus**
  - Lies between vertebral column and trachea in superior mediastinum, extends from suprasternal notch to diaphragm
  - Passes behind aortic arch (T4–T5) and enters posterior mediastinum
- **Abdominal esophagus**
  - Between diaphragm and fundus of stomach
  - Passes through right crus of diaphragm (T10) and into cardia of stomach (T11)

D. Ferrari-Light (✉)
Department of Surgery, New York Presbyterian-Queens, Weill Cornell Medicine, New York, NY, USA

O. S. Chow
Department of Cardiothoracic Surgery, New York Presbyterian-Queens, Weill Cornell Medicine, New York, NY, USA
e-mail: osc4001@med.cornell.edu

T. Ng, T. Geraci (eds.), *Thoracic Surgery Clerkship*, Contemporary Surgical Clerkships, https://doi.org/10.1007/978-3-031-44645-0_31

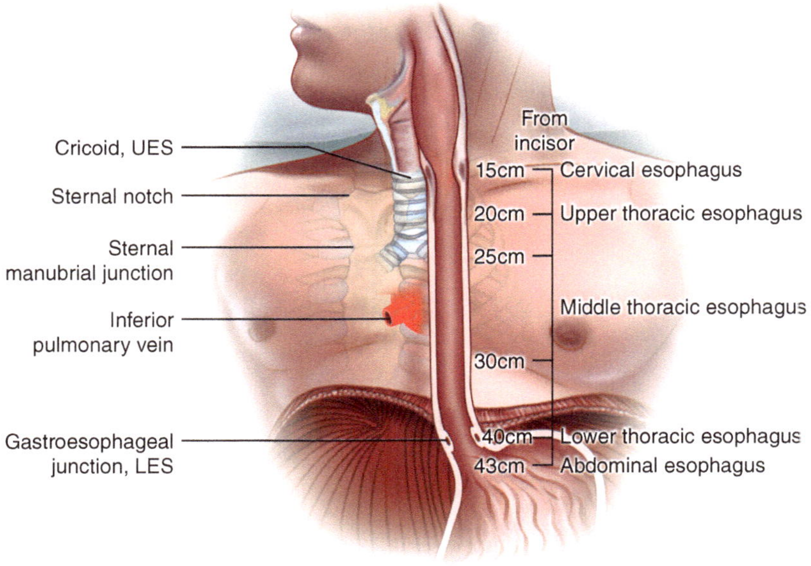

Fig. 31.1 Anatomy of the esophagus, with measurements as referenced from the incisors, along with the corresponding anatomical landmarks (arrows). *UES* upper esophageal sphincter, *LES* lower esophageal sphincter

Esophageal Perforation

Pathogenesis

- Iatrogenic
  - Major cause (50–70%) of esophageal perforations
  - Most common site of perforation: cervical esophagus, in Killian's triangle, perforation during rigid endoscopy and flexible endoscopy
  - During endoscopic procedures such as dilation
  - Can also be caused by traumatic intubation, nasogastric tube placement, esophageal operations (Heller myotomy, hiatal hernia repair, fundoplication), thoracic aneurysm repair, head and neck surgery (tracheostomy, thyroidectomy), or any surgery near the esophagus
- Boerhaave syndrome (spontaneous perforation)
  - Caused by forceful retching or vomiting, weightlifting, childbirth, straining during defecation, fits of coughing/laughing, seizures

  - Most common site of perforation: left posterior wall of the lower third of esophagus, just proximal to GE junction
  - Risk greatest with alcoholism and food overindulgence
  - Worse outcomes when compared with iatrogenic as diagnosis may be delayed
- Foreign body ingestion
  - Direct perforation
  - Lodge at site of esophageal narrowing causing pressure necrosis leading to defects
  - Coins and pills most common
- Trauma
  - Penetrating trauma

    Need to consider injury to surrounding structures:

    - Neck: trachea, internal jugular vein, carotid artery, spinal cord
    - Chest: great vessels, heart, lungs, spinal cord, diaphragm, abdominal viscera
  - Blunt trauma (rare)

    Diagnosis often delayed due to concomitant injuries
- Malignancy
  - Rare, usually advanced esophageal cancer paired with forceful vomiting
  - Also caused by mediastinal invasion of para-esophageal cancers or lung cancer
- Caustic ingestion
  - Alkaline substances

    Produces liquefactive necrosis and transmural deep tissue injury
    Typically ingestion of household cleaning agents, detergents
  - Acidic substances

    Reacts with tissue to form acid proteins, injury spreads more superficially

Evaluation

- **History**
  - Recent ingestion of foreign body or caustic substances, esophageal instrumentation, forceful vomiting, trauma.
  - Risk increases with the presence of preexisting esophageal pathology (GERD, hiatal hernia, malignancy, Barrett esophagus, radiation, strictures, achalasia).

- Time duration since the onset of the inciting incident (the longer the delay, the worse the outcome will be).

- **Physical examination**
  - Neck pain, chest pain, abdominal pain.
  - Subcutaneous emphysema in neck or chest

    Mackler triad: vomiting, chest pain, subcutaneous emphysema

    - Only present in 50% of spontaneous perforation

  - Tachycardia and tachypnea are present before fever develops.
  - Hypotension, confusion, fever.
  - Hamman sign: crunching sound over precordium caused by mediastinal emphysema.
  - Hematemesis is rare and should direct examiner to other pathology (Mallory-Weiss tear).

- **Laboratory tests**
  - Limited utility in diagnosis.
  - May see leukocytosis and lactic acidosis in critically ill patients.
  - Thoracentesis may reveal food particles or elevated amylase in pleural fluid.

- **Imaging**
  - Chest radiograph (Fig. 31.2a, b)

    May show pneumomediastinum, widening of mediastinal shadow, pneumothorax, or pleural effusion

  - Lateral neck radiograph

    Not commonly used due to more sensitive imaging modalities
    More useful when cervical esophageal perforation is suspected

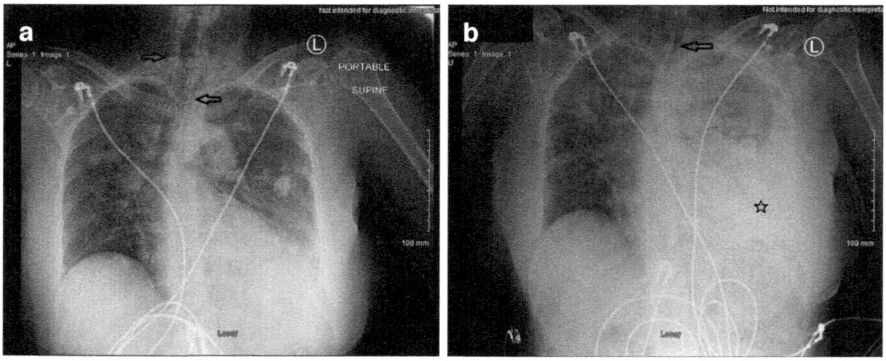

Fig. 31.2 Chest radiograph of esophageal perforation after emesis. (**a**) Pneumomediastinum (arrows) on presentation; (**b**) pneumomediastinum (arrow) and large left effusion (star) 4 h after presentation

Can show air in, or widening of, the prevertebral space

- Contrast esophagram (Fig. 31.3)

  Look for esophageal mucosal irregularity or extravasation of oral contrast.
  As it is a real-time study, it is better than CT in identifying the location of leak, which is of importance when determining the approach for repair.
  Avoid water-soluble agent (diatrizoate/Gastrografin) if there is a risk for aspiration, such as decrease mental status or delayed gastric emptying, as aspiration of such contrast can lead to life-threatening pneumonitis.
  Barium or thin barium (editors' choice of contrast) is a better contrast agent for imaging, is inert, and will not cause pneumonitis, mediastinitis, or pneumonitis, but extravasated barium remains long term or is difficult to clean out during surgery.

- CT scan (Fig. 31.4)

  Used if contrast esophagram is unavailable, or is equivocal and suspicion remains high, or patient is unable to perform esophagram (such as an intubated patient).
  Can see extraluminal gas or fluid collection in neck, mediastinum, pleural space, or abdominal cavity.
  Can use oral contrast to demonstrate leak and IV contrast to delineate esophageal wall; however, despite revealing extravasation of contrast, the precise location of leak may still be unclear.

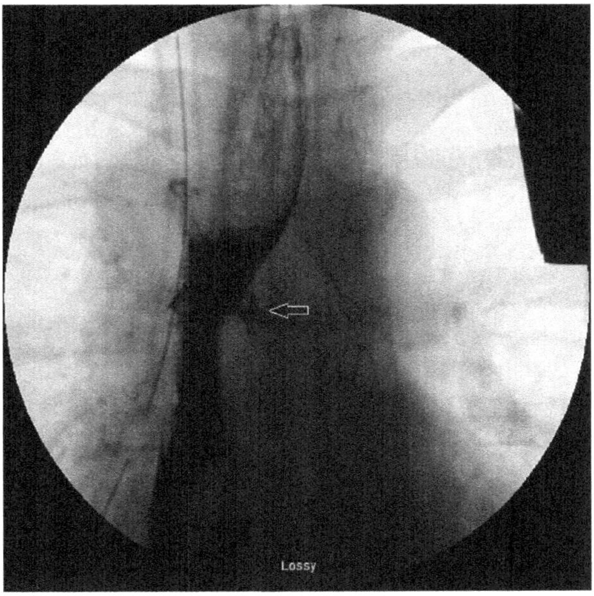

Fig. 31.3 Barium esophagram showing contained small esophageal leak (arrow)

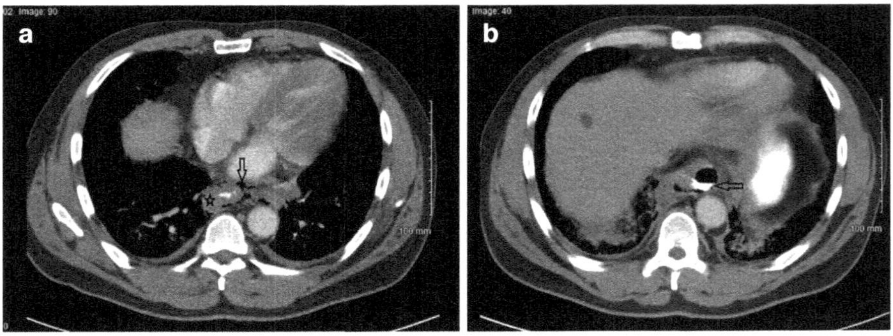

Fig. 31.4 CT scan of esophageal perforation after emesis. (**a**) Showing thickened esophagus (star) and pneumomediastinum (arrow); (**b**) lower axial images showing the free contrast extravasation in the mediastinum (arrow)

- Esophagoscopy

  Can be utilized to help further rule out perforation when imaging is negative
  Not as sensitive as other modalities – small tears can be missed
  Can be performed prior to surgical repair to confirm the precise location of perforation/tear and to rule out other pathologies (tumor, stricture, retained foreign body)

Treatment

- **Initial management**
  - Immediate resuscitation and stabilization should be initiated.
  - Large-bore IV access for fluid resuscitation.
  - Hemodynamic monitoring in an intensive care unit, urinary catheter.
  - NPO, avoid nasogastric tube placement unless this can be performed during esophagram to ensure proper placement.
  - Broad-spectrum IV antibiotics.
  - Tube thoracostomy to gain some degree of source control if there is moderate to large effusion/pneumothorax due to leakage into pleural cavity.
- **Conservative treatment**
  - Best utilized in perforations with small contained leak (a leak that drains back into esophagus on esophagram), not involving neoplasm or obstruction, no signs of sepsis, with immediately available contrast imaging and thoracic surgeon if needed
  - NPO for 7–10 days, proton-pump inhibitor (PPI), broad-spectrum antibiotics, consider total parenteral nutrition (TPN)
  - Then repeat esophagram to ensure successful treatment prior to initiating oral intake

- **Surgical treatment**
  - Cervical esophagus

    Neck incision on the side of contrast extravasation, if midline then left, as this decreases the risk of injury to the recurrent laryngeal nerve.
    A wide drainage is the primary goal; as perforation may not be completely accessible in this confined space, drainage will convert the situation into a controlled fistula which will eventually heal with time.
    If perforation is accessible, then repair and buttress with local flap such as strap muscle or sternocleidomastoid muscle, followed by a wide drainage (which remains the primary goal).

  - Thoracic or abdominal esophagus

    Primary repair (Fig. 31.5)

    - Best for early (<24 h) esophageal perforations, as longer delays will likely result in an esophagus that cannot be repaired.
    - Preferred treatment in both stable and unstable patients if the esophagus deemed repairable.
    - Right thoracotomy for mid to upper, left thoracotomy for lower, and laparotomy for abdominal esophageal perforations.
    - Thoroughly evacuate all contamination in the pleural space and decorticate the lung.
    - Debride laceration to healthy tissue, extend myotomy/muscularis defect to visualize full extent of mucosal defect as the mucosa/submucosa is the most important layer for primary repair.

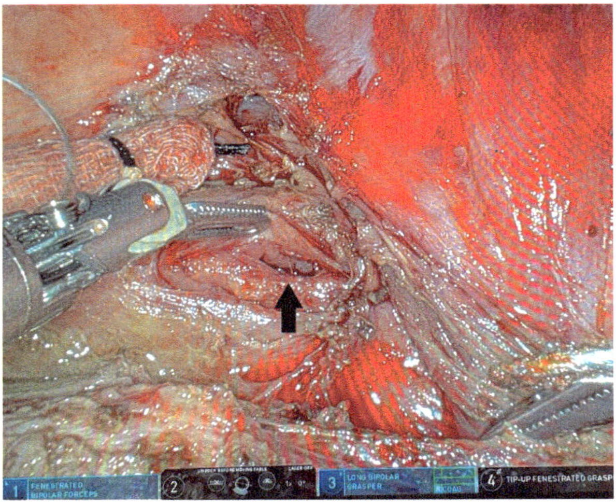

Fig. 31.5 Robotic approach to a perforation of the distal esophagus from the left chest. Note the exposure of the full thickness esophageal perforation (black arrow)

    - Close in two layers, mucosa/submucosa and muscularis, followed by buttressing with local tissue flap (chest: intercostal muscle flap (preferred), pericardial fat flap, pleural flap; abdomen: gastric fundus, omentum).
    - Place chest tubes for drainage.

    Exclusion and diversion

    - Reserved for hemodynamically unstable patients with severe esophageal perforation that is deemed unrepairable.
    - Several variations: one such is staple esophagus above and below perforation, wide drainage, gastric tube, and nasal-esophageal tube.
    - Will require return to operating room when more stable to consider a more formal diversion with resection and cervical esophagostomy (see below).

    Esophageal resection and cervical esophagostomy

    - For hemodynamically stable patients with esophageal perforation that is deemed unrepairable/unsalvageable.
    - The severely damaged esophagus is resected, the cervical esophagus is brought out of the neck as a cervical esophagostomy (spit fistula), and gastric/jejunal tubes are placed.
    - After full recovery, many months later, reconstruction may be considered; this may be by substernal gastric pull-up for anastomosis to the cervical esophagus.

- **Endoscopic stenting**
  - Placement of a covered stent placed via endoscopy to exclude the leak site.
  - If iatrogenic perforation is recognized immediately at the time of endoscopy, clip closure can also be utilized.
  - Not appropriate for cervical esophageal perforation as stent at high this level is not well tolerated by the patient.
  - Due to tendency to migrate, especially if esophagus is normal/without structure, it is ideal to clip or endoscopically suture the stent in place.
  - Ideal for perforated malignancies, as workup may not have been completed or the tumor may not be unresectable.
  - Less ideal for unstable patients as there is little room for failure in such a critical situation.
  - Less ideal for Boerhaave syndrome as stent is more likely to migrate with normal esophagus, and failure will result in the delay of leak control, which may convert a repairable situation to an unrepairable/unsalvageable esophagus.
  - Must be accompanied by drainage of any concomitant fluid collections, either by interventional radiology or thoracoscopy/thoracotomy, for complete source control.
  - Esophagram immediately after stenting to ensure resolution of leak.

Caustic Esophageal Injury

Introduction

- By accidental ingestion or by suicide; thus, prevention/education and psychiatric evaluation are key.
- Acid ingestion (batteries, paint thinners, industrial cleaning agents, metal cleaners)
  - Coagulative necrosis
  - Eschar formation
  - Less depth of esophageal penetration than alkalis
- Alkali ingestion (drain cleaners, oven cleaners, washing powders)
  - Liquefactive necrosis
  - Longer contact time and deeper penetration than acid and thus more destructive

Presentation

- Symptoms
  - Pain: mouth, throat, chest, abdomen
  - Shortness of breath
  - Dysphagia
  - Odynophagia
- Signs
  - Oral/pharyngeal burns
  - Stridor, tachypnea
  - Tachycardia
  - Subcutaneous emphysema
  - Peritonitis

Initial Management

- If airway is threatened, then secure with endotracheal intubation or tracheostomy.
- IV access, fluid resuscitation.
- Antibiotics and antiacid medications are of questionable benefit.
- Steroids are of no benefit.

- Avoid gastric lavage, emesis, and pH neutralization as these can cause more harm.
- Nasogastric tube
  - Should be placed during endoscopy rather than blindly
  - Helps keep stomach decompressed to avoid emesis
  - Nutrition
  - Helps maintain a path for future dilation if necessary
- Imaging
  - Chest radiograph: look for signs of perforation:

    Pneumomediastinum
    Pneumothorax
    Pleural effusion
    Free intra-abdominal air

  - CT scan

    Assess the extent of esophageal, stomach, and intestinal injury/necrosis:

    - Wall thickening
    - Wall enhancement with IV contrast
    - Surrounding fluid and edema

    Assess for perforation:

    - Extraluminal air in the mediastinum, pleural space, or abdomen
    - Oral contrast extravasation

  - Esophagram
    Utilized if there continues to be a suspicion for perforation after other testing
- Endoscopy
  - Evaluate the extent of injury to the esophagus, stomach, and duodenum.
  - Grading

    0: normal
    1: superficial mucosal edema/erythema
    2A: superficial ulcerations/erosions
    2B: deep or circumferential ulcerations
    3A: focal necrosis
    3B: extensive necrosis
    4: perforation

- Bronchoscopy
  - Assess for airway involvement.

Management

- Grade 1 to 2A
  - Initiate oral intake as tolerated; discharge after short period of observation.
- Grade 2b to 3B
  - Close observation in monitored unit for the development of transmural necrosis, ischemia, or perforation.
  - Nasogastric or nasoduodenal/jejunal tube left in place after endoscopy for nutrition and to maintain path for future dilation if necessary.
  - May require exploration (especially if condition unstable or worsening) to rule out transmural gastrointestinal necrosis, ischemia, or perforation; at the same time, gastrostomy or jejunostomy tube can be placed.
- Grade 4
  - Antibiotics
  - Surgical resection (high mortality, reported from 15% to 80%)

    Esophagectomy
    Gastrectomy (partial or total)
    Cervical esophagostomy
    Gastrostomy tube, jejunostomy tube

  - Reconstruction many months later

    Substernal gastric pull-up (if stomach was initially free of injury)
    Substernal colon interposition

Long-Term Sequelae

- Esophageal dysmotility
- Ineffective lower esophageal sphincter leading to reflux
- Esophageal stricture
  - Grade 2b: 71% incidence of stricture development
  - Grade 3: 100% incidence of stricture development
  - Management:

    Requiring frequent dilation: antegrade or retrograde (via gastrostomy tube), guided by nasogastric "string" if necessary
    Trial of stenting
    Refractory stricture, consider:

    - Resection:

    - Esophagectomy
    - Gastric pull-up if free of injury or colon interposition
  - Bypass (leaving diseased esophagus, if deemed not possible to remove):
    - Substernal gastric pull-up if free of injury or colon interposition
    - Less optimal as the retained esophagus may develop mucocele or malignancy
- Risk for esophageal squamous cell carcinoma

Key Reference
- Carrott PW Jr., Low DE. Advances in the management of esophageal perforation. Thorac Surg Clin. 2011;21(4):541–55.

Further Reading

Altorjay A, Kiss J, Vörös A, Bohák A. Nonoperative management of esophageal perforations. Is it justified? Ann Surg. 1997;225(4):415–21.

Blasberg JD, Wright CD. Management of Esophageal Perforation. In: Sugarbaker DJ, Bueno R, Burt BM, Groth SS, Loor G, Wolf AS, Williams M, Adams A, editors. Sugarbaker's adult chest surgery, 3e. McGraw Hill; 2020. Accessed May 18, 2022. https://accesssurgery.mhmedical.com/content.aspx?bookid=2781&sectionid=239709180.

Chirica M, Bonavina L, Kelly MD, Sarfati E, Cattan P. Caustic ingestion. Lancet. 2017;389(10083):2041–52. https://doi.org/10.1016/S0140-6736(16)30313-0. Epub 2016 Oct 26

Contini S, Scarpignato C. Caustic injury of the upper gastrointestinal tract: a comprehensive review. World J Gastroenterol. 2013;19(25):3918–30. https://doi.org/10.3748/wjg.v19.i25.3918. PMID: 23840136; PMCID: PMC3703178

Herrera A, Freeman RK. The evolution and current utility of esophageal stent placement for the treatment of acute esophageal perforation. Thorac Surg Clin. 2016;26(3):305–14. https://doi.org/10.1016/j.thorsurg.2016.04.012.

Chapter 32
Esophageal Cancer

Jacques P. Fontaine and Jose M. Pimiento

Epidemiology

- Represents 1% of all new cancers diagnosed annually in the United States.
- It is the 12th most frequently diagnosed cancer and the 11th leading cause of cancer-related deaths in the United States.
- An estimated 21,560 are diagnosed, and 16,120 die of this disease in the United States.
- Men are four times more likely to develop esophageal cancer than women.
- The highest incidence in the United States is in Caucasian males and the least in Asian women.
- Certain regions in the world have a much higher incidence: Iran, Northern China, India, and Southeast Africa.
- The most common histology worldwide is squamous cell carcinoma; in the United States, it is adenocarcinoma (75%) followed by squamous cell carcinoma (25%); and gastrointestinal stromal tumors (GIST), melanoma, and lymphoma are the least common (<1%).

J. P. Fontaine (✉)
Department of Thoracic Oncology, Moffitt Cancer Center, Tampa, FL, USA
e-mail: Jacques.fontaine@moffitt.org

J. M. Pimiento
Department of Gastrointestinal Oncology, Moffitt Cancer Center, Tampa, FL, USA
e-mail: Jose.pimiento@moffitt.org

T. Ng, T. Geraci (eds.), *Thoracic Surgery Clerkship*, Contemporary Surgical Clerkships, https://doi.org/10.1007/978-3-031-44645-0_32

Risk Factors

Squamous Cell Carcinoma

- Age > 55
- Male sex predominance
- Tobacco and alcohol (synergistic risk factors)
- Remote history of injury to esophageal mucosa (lye ingestion)
- Repeated esophageal mucosa injury (intake of very hot beverages)
- Achalasia
- Tylosis
- Bloom syndrome
- Fanconi anemia
- Human papillomavirus (HPV) infection (for cervical esophageal squamous cell carcinoma)

Adenocarcinoma

- Age > 55
- Male sex predominance
- Tobacco and alcohol (to a lesser degree than in squamous cell carcinoma)
- Gastroesophageal reflux disease (GERD) and its associated risk factors: obesity, high-fat diet, and hiatal hernia
- Barrett's esophagus (the more dysplasia, the higher the risk)

Barrett's Esophagus

- Chronic exposure of the normal esophageal mucosa to gastric acid can lead over time to its transformation from a normal stratified squamous epithelium to a specialized columnar epithelium.
- On endoscopy, Barrett's esophagus presents as salmon-colored "tongues" emanating into the lower esophagus from the gastroesophageal (GE) junction (Fig. 32.1).
- Histologically, Barrett's esophagus is characterized by intestinal metaplasia with goblet cells.
- With persistent injury from the gastric acid exposure, genetic mutations may accrue within this abnormal esophageal mucosa and lead to histologic dysplasia. Dysplasia can be classified into low-grade dysplasia and high-grade dysplasia depending on the degree of cellular abnormalities.

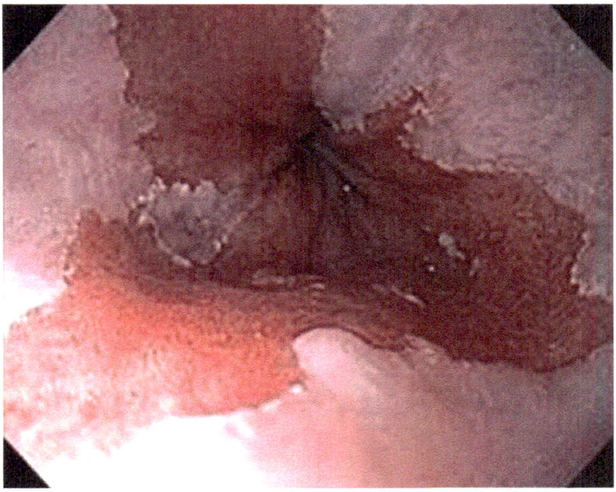

Fig. 32.1 Salmon-colored "tongues" of Barrett's esophagus

- Barrett's esophagus occurs in 10–15% of individuals suffering from GERD. Although a risk factor for adenocarcinoma of the esophagus, only 0.5% of all patients with Barrett's esophagus develop cancer. However, the subgroup of patients with Barrett's esophagus with high-grade dysplasia can have up to a 40% risk of developing adenocarcinoma of the esophagus.

Clinical Presentation

- Most patients with early-stage disease have no symptoms or mild symptoms associated with GERD.
- Patients with locally advanced disease usually present with dysphagia (initially to solids progressing to liquids), weight loss, and possible chest/epigastric discomfort.
- Patients with metastatic disease have additional symptoms of fatigue, failure to thrive, or symptoms related to specific site of metastases.

Workup

- Barium swallow
  - Commonly obtained for a patient with a history of dysphagia (Fig. 32.2)
  - Historically used, but without current clear indication
  - Will demonstrate a filling defect in the esophagus

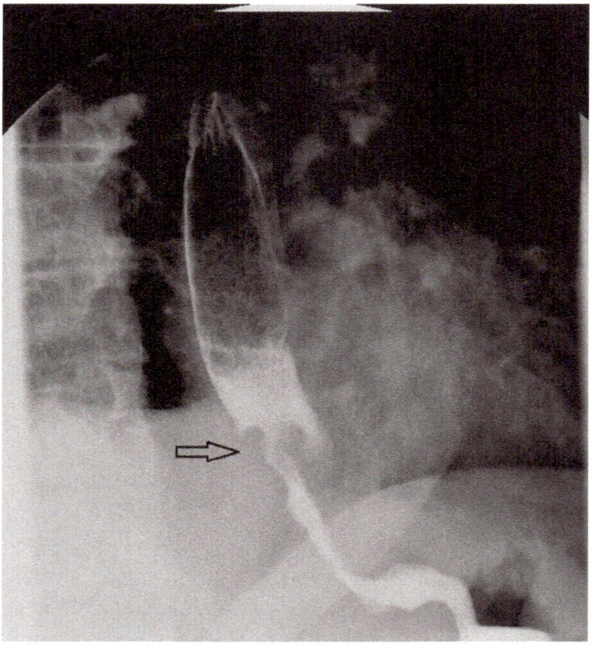

Fig. 32.2 Barium swallow showing classic malignant stricture of esophageal cancer (arrow)

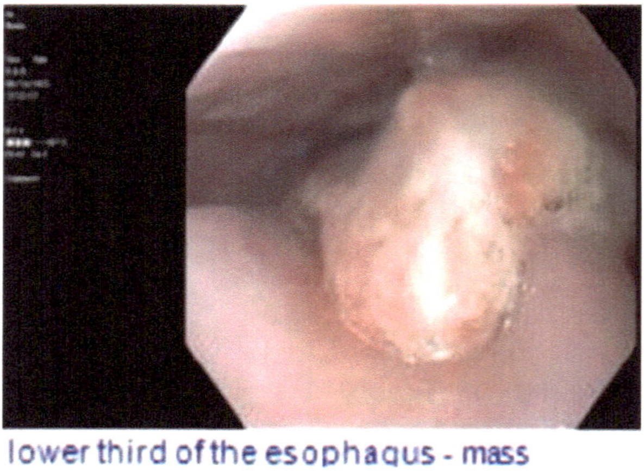

Fig. 32.3 Upper endoscopy revealing mass in the distal esophagus

- Endoscopy
  - Initial diagnosis is always made by endoscopy with a biopsy of the lesion (Fig. 32.3).
  - Biopsy material must be in sufficient quantity not only to determine histologic type but also to perform biomarker testing (important in unresectable locally advanced, recurrent or metastatic disease, when considering targeted therapy).

    Human epidermal growth factor receptor 2 (HER2) expression by immunohistochemistry (IHC), in adenocarcinoma, is of prime importance.

- Score 0 or 1+ considered negative.
- Score 2+ considered equivocal, examination by FISH is indicated.
- Score 3+ or 2+ /FISH+ is considered positive: candidate monoclonal anti-HER2 antibody trastuzumab.

Microsatellite instability (MSI) by PCR/next-generation sequencing (NGS) or mismatch repair (MMR) by IHC; MSI high or deficient MMR are candidates for programmed cell death protein 1 (PD-1) monoclonal antibody nivolumab or pembrolizumab.
Programmed death ligand-1 (PDL-1) testing by IHC for tumor combined positive score (CPS).
NGS testing for which there is targeted therapy including HER2 amplification, NTRK gene fusion, RET gene fusion, BRAF V600E mutation, and tumor mutation burden (TMB).

  - Important endoscopic findings to note: appearance of lesion, location measured in cm from the incisors, extension into the cardia of the stomach, and the presence and extent of other mucosal abnormalities such as Barrett's esophagus.

- Endoscopic ultrasound (EUS)
  - Used for locoregional staging (Fig. 32.4).
  - To determine the depth of invasion (T stage) and presence of suspicious lymph nodes (N stage) and to perform needle biopsy (FNA/fine-needle aspiration) of suspicious lymph nodes.
  - Peritumoral lymph nodes cannot be biopsied as the biopsy needle would need to traverse the malignant tumor to reach the lymph node and result in a false positive and cause oncologic contamination.
  - EUS may be used to place radio-opaque fiducials at the level of the tumor to track its movement during radiation therapy treatments (image-guided respiratory gating).

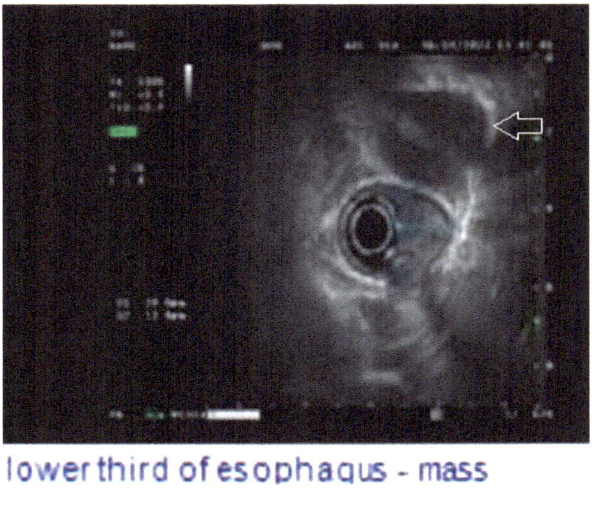

Fig. 32.4 Endoscopic ultrasound showing mass (arrow) to invade the muscularis propria but not beyond, stage T2N0

- CT scan chest/abdomen/pelvis with IV contrast
  - To determine the presence of distant disease and anatomic relationship between tumor and surrounding structures (Fig. 32.5)
- FDG PET scan
  - To determine the presence of locoregional lymph node metastasis and distant metastatic disease (Fig. 32.6)

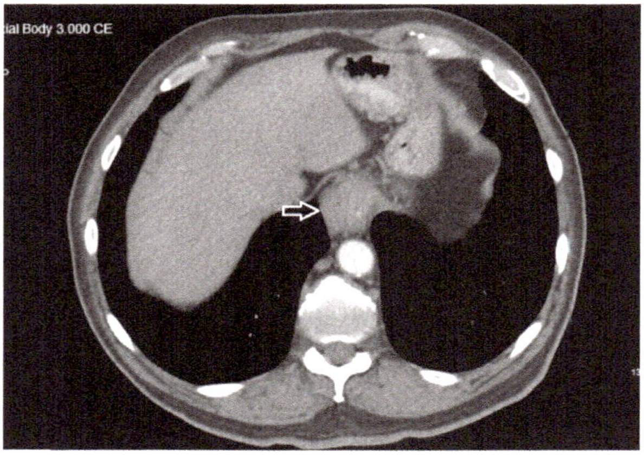

Fig. 32.5 CT scan showing mass in the lower esophagus (arrow)

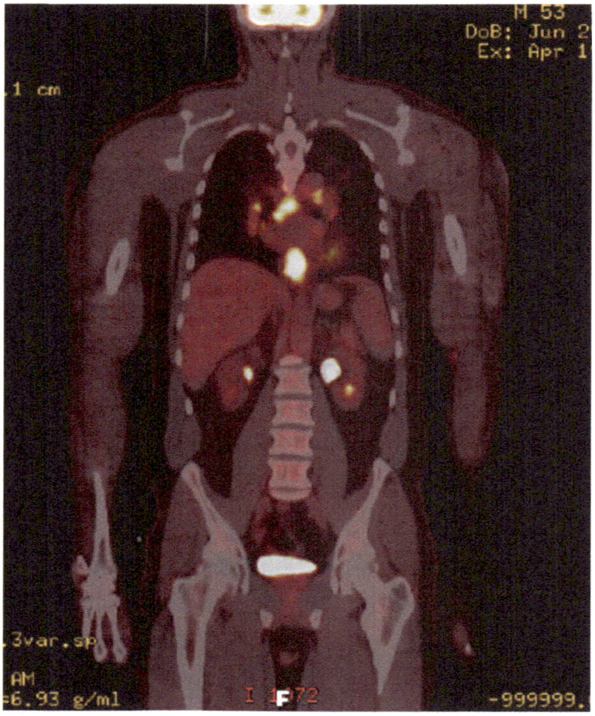

Fig. 32.6 PET scan of thoracic esophageal cancer with mediastinal lymph node involvement

- Bronchoscopy
  - For tumors at or above the level of the carina, to rule out airway involvement which would be T4b stage, unresectable disease

Classification

Cervical Esophageal Cancer

- Predominantly squamous cell carcinoma.
- Treated with definitive chemoradiation.
- Surgical resection is for salvage (residual or locally recurrent disease after chemoradiation), as there is a higher rate of complete pathological response with chemoradiation, and surgery may involve laryngectomy which is more morbid.

Thoracic Esophageal Cancer

- Squamous cell carcinoma (upper/mid) or adenocarcinoma (lower).
- Usually found on endoscopy between 20 and 38 cm from the incisors.
- May present with invasion of the posterior wall of the trachea (for mid esophageal cancer, bronchoscopy is indicated to assess) and/or major vascular structures, factors that make tumor unresectable (T4b stage).
- Treatment varies based on stage.

Gastroesophageal Junction (GEJ) Cancer

- Increasing incidence of this type of cancer in the United States.
- Predominantly adenocarcinoma.
- Usually found 38–42 cm from the incisors (i.e., located at GE junction).
- Treatment varies based on stage and Siewert classification. Siewert I and II tumors are treated as thoracic esophageal cancer. Siewert III tumors are treated as gastric cancers.

Siewert Classification (Fig. 32.7)

- Siewert I: epicenter of tumor located in the distal esophagus, 1–5 cm above the GE junction (Z-line).

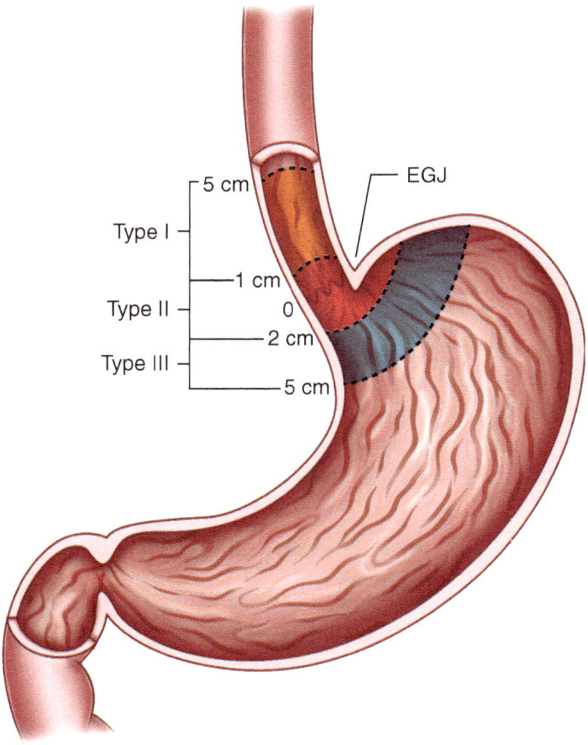

Fig. 32.7 Siewert classification

- Siewert II: epicenter of tumor located 1 cm above to 2 cm below the GE junction.
- Siewert III: epicenter of tumor located in the stomach, 2–5 cm below the GE junction; these tumors are classified as gastric cancers.

Staging

The staging of esophageal and gastroesophageal junction cancers is by the American Joint Committee on Cancer (AJCC) system. This AJCC system is updated periodically; since 2018, the eighth edition of the AJCC has been utilized (Tables 32.1, 32.2, and 32.3 and Fig. 32.8).

Table 32.1 The American Joint Committee on Cancer eighth edition staging for adenocarcinoma and squamous cell carcinoma of the esophagus and esophagogastric junction: TMN, grade, and location definitions

T	Primary tumor
TX	Primary tumor cannot be assessed
T0	No evidence of primary tumor
Tis	High-grade dysplasia, defined as malignant cells confined to the epithelium by the basement membrane
T1	Tumor invades the lamina propria, muscularis mucosae, or submucosa
T1a	Tumor invades the lamina propria or muscularis mucosae
T1b	Tumor invades the submucosa
T2	Tumor invades the muscularis propria
T3	Tumor invades adventitia
T4	Tumor invades adjacent structures
T4a	Tumor invades the pleura, pericardium, azygos vein, diaphragm, or peritoneum
T4b	Tumor invades other adjacent structures, such as the aorta, vertebral body, or airway
N	**Regional lymph nodes**
NX	Regional lymph nodes cannot be assessed
N0	No regional lymph node metastasis
N1	Metastasis in one or two regional lymph nodes
N2	Metastasis in three to six regional lymph nodes
N3	Metastasis in seven or more regional lymph nodes
M	**Distant metastasis**
M0	No distant metastasis
M1	Distant metastasis
G	**Histologic grade**
GX	Grade cannot be assessed
G1	Well differentiated
G2	Moderately differentiated
G3	Poorly differentiated, undifferentiated
Squamous cell carcinoma	
Location	**Location criteria**
X	Location unknown
Upper	Cervical esophagus to lower border of azygos vein
Middle	Lower border of azygos vein to lower border of inferior pulmonary vein
Lower	Lower border of inferior pulmonary vein to stomach, including gastroesophageal junction

Note: Location is defined by the position of the epicenter of the tumor in the esophagus

Table 32.2 The American Joint Committee on Cancer eighth edition staging for adenocarcinoma and squamous cell carcinoma of the esophagus and esophagogastric junction: groupings for adenocarcinoma

Clinical staging (cTNM)				Pathological (pTNM)					Post-neoadjuvant therapy (ypTNM)			
	cT	cN	M		pT	pN	M	G		ypT	ypN	M
Stage 0	Tis	N0	M0	**Stage 0**	Tis	N0	M0	N/A	**Stage I**	T0–2	N0	M0
Stage I	T1	N0	M0	**Stage IA**	T1a	M0	M0	G1	**Stage II**	T3	N0	M0
Stage IIA	T1	N1	M0		T1a	N0	M0	GX	**Stage IIIA**	T0–2	N1	M0
Stage IIB	T2	N0	M0	**Stage IB**	T1a	N0	M0	G2	**Stage IIIB**	T3	N1	M0
Stage III	T2	N1	M0		T1b	N0	M0	G1–2		T0–3	N2	M0
	T3	N0–1	M0		T1b	N0	M0	GX		T4a	N0	M0
	T4a	N0–1	M0	**Stage IC**	T1	N0	M0	G3	**Stage IVA**	T4a	N1–2	M0
Stage IVA	T1-4a	N2	M0		T2	N0	M0	G1–2		T4a	NX	M0
	T4b	N0–2	M0	**Stage IIA**	T2	N0	M0	G3		T4b	N0–2	M0
	Any T	N3	M0		T2	N0	M0	GX		Any T	N3	M0
Stage IVB	Any T	Any N	M1	**Stage IIB**	T1	N1	M0	Any	**Stage IVB**	Any T	Any N	M1
					T3	N0	M0	Any				
				Stage IIIA	T1	N2	M0	Any				
					T2	N1	M0	Any				
				Stage IIIB	T2	N2	M0	Any				
					T3	N1–2	M0	Any				
					T4a	N0–1	M0	Any				
				Stage IVA	T4a	N2	M0	Any				
					T4b	N0–2	M0	Any				
					Any T	N3	M0	Any				
				Stage IVB	Any T	Any N	M1	Any				

Table 32.3 American Joint Committee on Cancer eighth edition staging for adenocarcinoma and squamous cell carcinoma of the esophagus and esophagogastric junction: groupings for squamous cell carcinoma

Clinical staging (cTNM)				Pathological (pTNM)						Post-neoadjuvant therapy (ypTNM)			
	cT	cN	M		pT	pN	M	G	Location		ypT	ypN	M
Stage 0	Tis	N0	M0	**Stage 0**	Tis	N0	M0	N/A	Any	**Stage I**	T0–2	N0	M0
Stage I	T1	N0–1	M0	**Stage IA**	T1a	N0	M0	G1	Any	**Stage II**	T3	N0	M0
Stage II	T2	N0–1	M0		T1a	N0	M0	GX	Any	**Stage IIIA**	T0–2	N1	M0
	T3	N0	M0	**Stage IB**	T1a	N0	M0	G2–3	Any	**Stage IIIB**	T3	N1	M0
Stage III	T3	N1	M0		T1b	N0	M0	G1-3	Any		T0–3	N2	M0
	T1-3	N2	M0		T1b	N0	M0	GX	Any		T4a	N0	M0
Stage IVA	T4	N0–2	M0		T2	N0	M0	G1	Any	**Stage IVA**	T4a	N1–2	M0
	Any T	N3	M0	**Stage IIA**	T2	N0	M0	G2–3	Any		T4a	NX	M0
Stage IVB	Any T	Any N	M1		T2	N0	M0	GX	Any		T4b	N0–2	M0
					T3	N0	M0	G1-3	Lower		Any T	N3	M0
					T3	N0	M0	G1	Upper/ middle	**Stage IVB**	Any T	Any N	M1
				Stage IIB	T3	N0	M0	G2–3	Upper/ middle				
					T3	N0	M0	GX	Lower/ upper/ middle				
					T3	N0	M0	Any	Location X				
					T1	N1	M0	Any	Any				
				Stage IIIA	T1	N2	M0	Any	Any				
					T2	N1	M0	Any	Any				
				Stage IIIB	T2	N2	M0	Any	Any				
					T3	N1–2	M0	Any	Any				
					T4a	N0–1	M0	Any	Any				
				Stage IVA	T4a	N2	M0	Any	Any				

(continued)

Table 33.3 (continued)

Clinical staging (cTNM)				Pathological (pTNM)						Post-neoadjuvant therapy (ypTNM)			
	cT	cN	M		pT	pN	M	G	Location		ypT	ypN	M
					T4b	N0–2	M0	Any	Any				
					Any T	N3	M0	Any	Any				
				Stage IVB	Any T	Any N	M1	Any	Any				

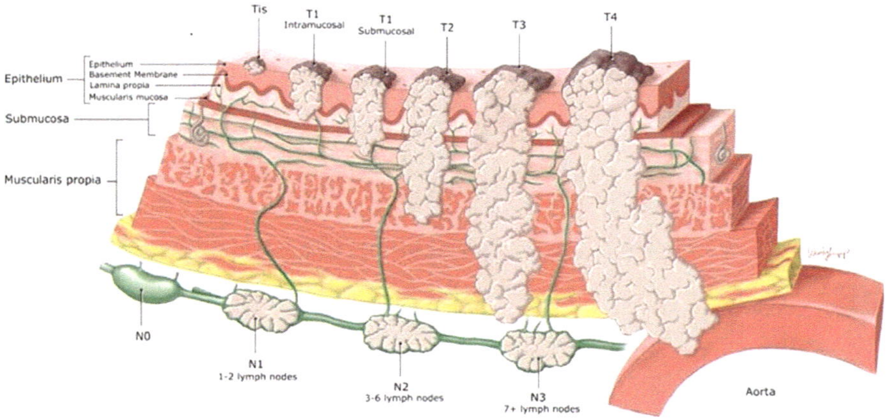

Fig. 32.8 Illustration of TNM staging of esophageal cancer

Treatment

- Choice of treatment must be determined by a multidisciplinary team in a tumor board setting. Input from a gastroenterologist, an esophageal surgeon, a medical oncologist, and a radiation oncologist is advisable.
- As part of the treatment plan, consideration must also be given to smoking cessation, regimens to improve exercise tolerance, and optimization of nutrition.
- Maintenance of nutrition is of utmost importance during therapy
  - Dietary consultation.
  - Supplement with liquid nutrition.
  - Placement of feeding tube – jejunostomy tube is preferred over gastrostomy tube as the stomach will be used for reconstruction.
  - Stent placement should be avoided if there is curative intent as it may complicate/delay therapy, such as worsening esophageal symptoms during radiation; stents play an important role in palliation.
- Barrett's esophagus with high-grade dysplasia is treated as a TisN0M0 cancer (in situ cancer).

- For superficial tumors, endoscopic mucosal resection (EMR) is preferred over endoscopic ablative therapy as it provides pathology confirmation of the T stage of disease.

TisN0M0 and T1aN0M0

- Endoscopic mucosal resection (EMR) or endoscopic submucosal dissection (ESD). If negative radial and deep margins are obtained (i.e., R0 or complete resection), close endoscopic surveillance with possible endoscopic mucosal ablation (cryotherapy or radiofrequency ablation) is recommended for the management of associated Barrett's with dysplasia.
- If negative margins cannot be achieved, or there is extensive long-segment disease, then esophagectomy is indicated.

T1bN0M0

- In general, an esophagectomy is the recommendation, as these patients can have up to 15% occult nodal metastasis.
- EMR/ESD may be considered in superficial T1b adenocarcinomas, and tumors with favorable features (size <3 cm, no lymphovascular invasion, well differentiated), or if the patient is not medically fit for/does not desire surgery. Endoscopic mucosal ablation is recommended for any associated Barrett's with dysplasia.
- Chemoradiation for deep T1b with high-risk features (size ≥3 cm, lymphovascular invasion, poorly differentiated) for patients who are not medically fit for/do not desire surgery.

T2N0M0

- Despite negative clinical nodal staging, up to 30% of patients may have occult nodal disease.
- Neoadjuvant therapy followed by esophagectomy is the most common treatment.
- Alternatively, upfront esophagectomy (without neoadjuvant therapy) is a possibility as long as preoperative staging is deemed to be highly accurate and the tumor has favorable features (size <3 cm, no lymphovascular invasion, well differentiated). Adjuvant therapy is considered if pathology is upstaged.
- Definitive chemoradiation is reserved for patients who are not medically fit for or do not desire esophagectomy.

- Adjuvant immunotherapy is recommended for patients who still have viable residual cancer on their surgical pathologic specimen despite neoadjuvant therapy.

T2N0M0, T3N0M0, T4aN0M0, and TanyN1-3M0

- Neoadjuvant therapy followed by esophagectomy is the most common treatment.
- Definitive chemoradiation is for patients who are not medically fit for or do not desire an esophagectomy.
- Adjuvant immunotherapy is recommended for patients who still have viable residual cancer on their surgical pathologic specimen after neoadjuvant therapy.
- Salvage surgical strategy
  - Observation if clinical complete remission (negative CT, PET/CT, endoscopic biopsies) is found after chemoradiation
  - Reserving surgery if after chemoradiation there is residual/persistent disease or if there is local recurrence after initial clinical complete remission
  - Can be considered for squamous cell carcinoma
  - Being evaluated in clinical trials for adenocarcinoma

T4bNanyM0

- Definitive chemoradiation therapy
  - Paclitaxel/carboplatin or fluorouracil/oxaliplatin
  - 50.5 Gy radiation

TanyNanyM1

- Systemic therapy as well as treatments to palliate symptoms of dysphagia or pain.
- Treatment regimens will depend on tumor molecular markers.
- Surgical resection not indicated.

Neoadjuvant Therapy (Administered Before Surgical Resection)

- Specific regimens of neoadjuvant therapy vary by region in the world and by institution.
- Treatment consists of chemoradiation, less often perioperative chemotherapy (only considered for adenocarcinoma).

- The chemoradiation
  - Regimen is a platinum-based doublet (two chemotherapy agents); commonly used doublets are carboplatin/paclitaxel or fluorouracil/oxaliplatin.
  - Radiation with intensity-modulated radiation therapy (IMRT) with respiratory gating to 50.4Gy, less common 3D-conformal radiation to 40–45 Gy.
- Perioperative chemotherapy (no radiation) for adenocarcinoma – fluorouracil/leucovorin/oxaliplatin/docetaxel (FLOT) or fluoropyrimidine/oxaliplatin
- Restaging with imaging (CT scan or PET/CT) is performed 4–6 weeks following completion of neoadjuvant therapy, and the decision to proceed with surgical resection is confirmed at this point.
- Ideal timing of surgery is 6–10 weeks after neoadjuvant therapy, to allow the patient time to recover from induction therapy, but not beyond as radiation fibrosis will increase the difficulty of surgical resection.

Adjuvant Therapy (Administered After Surgical Resection)

- For patients not receiving neoadjuvant therapy
  - R0 adenocarcinoma: adjuvant chemotherapy or chemoradiation is considered for high-risk T2N0, T3N0, T4aN0, or TanyNany.
  - R1/R2: chemoradiation.
- For patients who have received neoadjuvant therapy
  - R0 adenocarcinoma: adjuvant chemotherapy is considered if there is residual disease after receiving preop chemotherapy.
  - R1/ R2 adenocarcinoma: consider adjuvant chemoradiation if radiation is not given preop.
  - Immunotherapy is used if patients did not have a pathologic complete response after neoadjuvant chemoradiation (still have viable residual cancer in the resection specimen despite receiving neoadjuvant chemoradiation).

Key Reference

- van Hagen P, Hulshof MC, van Lanschot JJ, Steyerberg EW, van Berge Henegouwen MI, Wijnhoven BP, Richel DJ, Nieuwenhuijzen GA, Hospers GA, Bonenkamp JJ, Cuesta MA, Blaisse RJ, Busch OR, ten Kate FJ, Creemers GJ, Punt CJ, Plukker JT, Verheul HM, Spillenaar Bilgen EJ, van Dekken H, van der Sangen MJ, Rozema T, Biermann K, Beukema JC, Piet AH, van Rij CM, Reinders JG, Tilanus HW, van der Gaast A; CROSS Group. Preoperative chemoradiotherapy for esophageal or junctional cancer. N Engl J Med. 2012;366(22):2074–84.

Further Reading

Ajani JA, D'Amico TA, Bentrem DJ, Cooke D, Corvera C, Das P, Enzinger PC, Enzler T, Farjah F, Gerdes H, Gibson M, Grierson P, Hofstetter WL, Ilson DH, Jalal S, Keswani RN, Kim S, Kleinberg LR, Klempner S, Lacy J, Licciardi F, Ly QP, Matkowskyj KA, McNamara M, Miller A, Mukherjee S, Mulcahy MF, Outlaw D, Perry KA, Pimiento J, Poultsides GA, Reznik S, Roses RE, Strong VE, Su S, Wang HL, Wiesner G, Willett CG, Yakoub D, Yoon H, McMillian NR, Pluchino LA. Esophageal and esophagogastric junction cancers, version 2.2023, NCCN clinical practice guidelines in oncology. J Natl Compr Cancer Netw. 2023;21(4):393–422.

Bedenne L, Michel P, Bouché O, Milan C, Mariette C, Conroy T, Pezet D, Roullet B, Seitz JF, Herr JP, Paillot B, Arveux P, Bonnetain F, Binquet C. Chemoradiation followed by surgery compared with chemoradiation alone in squamous cancer of the esophagus: FFCD 9102. J Clin Oncol. 2007;25(10):1160–8.

Eyck BM, van Lanschot JJB, Hulshof MCCM, van der Wilk BJ, Shapiro J, van Hagen P, van Berge Henegouwen MI, Wijnhoven BPL, van Laarhoven HWM, Nieuwenhuijzen GAP, Hospers GAP, Bonenkamp JJ, Cuesta MA, Blaisse RJB, Busch OR, Creemers GM, Punt CJA, Plukker JTM, Verheul HMW, Spillenaar Bilgen EJ, van der Sangen MJC, Rozema T, Ten Kate FJW, Beukema JC, Piet AHM, van Rij CM, Reinders JG, Tilanus HW, Steyerberg EW, van der Gaast A, CROSS Study Group. Ten-year outcome of neoadjuvant chemoradiotherapy plus surgery for esophageal cancer: the randomized controlled CROSS trial. J Clin Oncol. 2021;39(18):1995–2004.

Kelly RJ, Ajani JA, Kuzdzal J, Zander T, Van Cutsem E, Piessen G, Mendez G, Feliciano J, Motoyama S, Lièvre A, Uronis H, Elimova E, Grootscholten C, Geboes K, Zafar S, Snow S, Ko AH, Feeney K, Schenker M, Kocon P, Zhang J, Zhu L, Lei M, Singh P, Kondo K, Cleary JM, Moehler M, CheckMate 577 Investigators. Adjuvant nivolumab in resected Esophageal or gastroesophageal junction cancer. N Engl J Med. 2021;384(13):1191–203.

Rice TW, Ishwaran H, Ferguson MK, Blackstone EH, Goldstraw P. Cancer of the esophagus and esophagogastric junction: an eighth edition staging primer. J Thorac Oncol. 2017;12(1):36–42.

Siegel RL, Miller KD, Wagle NS, Jemal A. Cancer statistics, 2023. CA Cancer J Clin. 2023;73(1):17–48. https://doi.org/10.3322/caac.21763.

Stahl M, Stuschke M, Lehmann N, Meyer HJ, Walz MK, Seeber S, Klump B, Budach W, Teichmann R, Schmitt M, Schmitt G, Franke C, Wilke H. Chemoradiation with and without surgery in patients with locally advanced squamous cell carcinoma of the esophagus. J Clin Oncol. 2005;23(10):2310–7. https://doi.org/10.1200/JCO.2005.00.034. Erratum in: J Clin Oncol. 2006 Jan 20;24(3):531

Chapter 33
Esophagectomy: Approaches and Surgical Techniques

Mohamed El Zaeedi and Travis Geraci

Introduction

The first thoracic esophageal resection was described by Torek in 1915. While esophagectomy has been considered a relatively morbid operation, modern minimally invasive approaches have resulted in improved clinical outcomes. Indications for esophagectomy include esophageal cancer, Barrett's esophagus with extensive high-grade dysplasia, and, rarely, benign esophageal diseases such as recalcitrant esophageal stricture and mega-esophagus from end-stage achalasia. For patients with esophageal cancer, the choice of surgical approach for esophagectomy depends on the anatomic location of the tumor (proximal versus distal esophagus), the available choices for conduit reconstruction, and surgeon preference.

Anatomy

- The esophagus is 18–26 cm muscular tube that travels between the pharynx and the stomach (Fig. 33.1).
- The esophagus has four layers: mucosa, submucosa, muscularis propria, and adventitia (Fig. 33.2). Unlike the remaining part of the gastrointestinal tract, the esophagus has no serosal layer or mesentery.

M. El Zaeedi · T. Geraci (✉)
Division of Thoracic Surgery, Department of Cardiothoracic Surgery, New York University Langone Health, New York, NY, USA
e-mail: mohamed.elzaeedi@nyulangone.org; travis.geraci@nyulangone.org

T. Ng, T. Geraci (eds.), *Thoracic Surgery Clerkship*, Contemporary Surgical Clerkships, https://doi.org/10.1007/978-3-031-44645-0_33

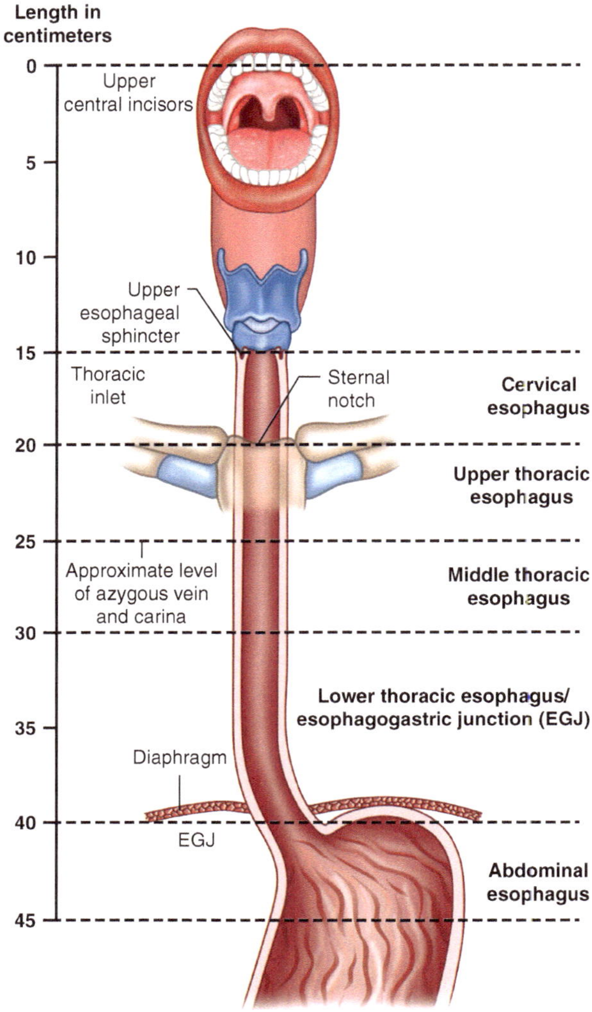

Fig. 33.1 Anatomy of the esophagus

- The esophagus is lined with stratified squamous epithelium which transitions to columnar gastric mucosa at the gastroesophageal junction (Z-line). Patients with severe and/or prolonged gastroesophageal reflux are at risk of developing Barrett's esophagus where squamous cells are replaced by columnar epithelium (metaplasia), a condition that can progress to epithelial cell dysplasia and, subsequently, esophageal adenocarcinoma.
- The arterial supply of the esophagus is dependent on the anatomic location: the cervical portion arises from the inferior thyroid artery, the mid-esophagus or thoracic portion from the branches of the descending thoracic aorta, and the abdominal portion by the left gastric and inferior phrenic arteries.

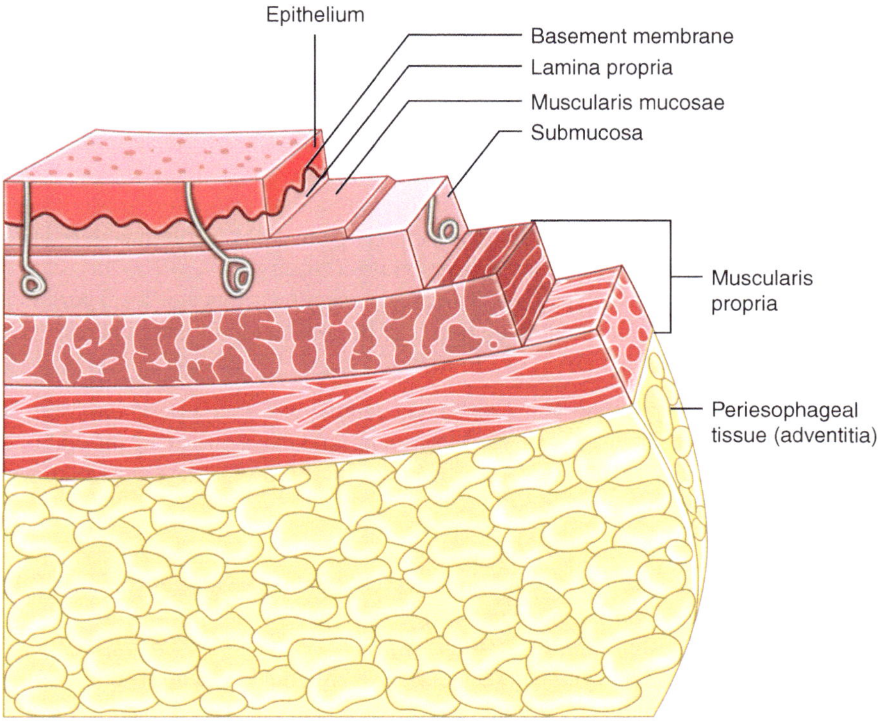

Fig. 33.2 Layers of the esophageal wall

- Lymphatic drainage of the cervical, thoracic, and abdominal portions of the esophagus drains to the cervical, mediastinal, and celiac and gastric lymph nodes respectively. However, due to rich lymphatic submucosal plexus, esophageal cancer can spread to any of the above lymph node stations regardless of the tumor location in the esophagus.

Indications for Esophagectomy

Esophageal Cancer

- Esophageal cancer is the most common indication for esophagectomy.
- The management of esophageal squamous cell carcinoma and adenocarcinoma varies slightly but generally follows guidelines based on the extent of local, regional, or distant disease.
- Barrett's esophagus with high-grade dysplasia (also referred to as carcinoma in situ, Tis) or esophageal cancer limited to the mucosa (T1a) or superficial submucosa (T1b) can be treated with endoscopic mucosal resection. However, esopha-

gectomy is often recommended for T1 cancers with "high risk" features, such as size >3 cm, lymphovascular invasion, or poor tumor differentiation, or incomplete endoscopic resection.
- Esophagectomy is indicated for localized, resectable esophageal cancer (T1-T4a); T4a tumors involve the pericardium, pleura, or diaphragm and are often resectable.
- Patients with tumors that invade beyond the submucosa to the muscularis propria (T2) or beyond, and/or with regional lymph node metastasis, often undergo neoadjuvant chemotherapy or chemoradiation prior to surgery.
- Salvage esophagectomy: patients with local cancer recurrence or local persistent disease after definitive chemoradiation may be considered for surgical resection.
- Contraindications
  - Cervical or cervicothoracic esophageal carcinomas—tumors <5 cm from the cricopharyngeus muscle are rarely surgical candidates due to the morbidity of surgery (often requiring concomitant laryngectomy) and are treated with definitive chemoradiation.
  - Unresectable tumors:

    Tumors involving the heart, great vessels, trachea, or adjacent organs (T4b).
    Supraclavicular lymphadenopathy.
    Distant sites of metastasis (stage IV).
    Multiple sites of lymph node metastasis with multiple lymph nodes (bulky) involved (relative contraindication that must be weighed against all other relevant clinicopathologic information).

End-Stage Achalasia

- Defined radiologically by an esophageal diameter > 6 cm, with absent peristalsis and failure of lower esophageal sphincter relaxation (pressure > 15 mm Hg) on manometry.
- Clinically, patients typically have chronic, intractable symptoms of dysphagia, aspiration, and/or recurrent pneumonia and have failed other interventions such as balloon dilatation, peroral endoscopic myotomy (POEM), or Heller myotomy.

Uncommon Indications for Esophagectomy

- Esophageal stricture: refractory or recurrent stricture causing significant dysphagia despite serial mechanical dilations.
- Esophageal trauma: non-salvageable esophageal tissue, not amenable to repair, stenting, or other less morbid interventions.
- Esophageal perforation: option of last resort for patients with uncontrolled leak not amenable to stenting or surgical repair. Unstable patients who are not candidates for

immediate resection may undergo surgical exclusion, drainage, and diversion (esophagostomy; referred to as a "spit fistula"), then reconsideration for esophagectomy when more stable (see Chap. 32).
- Caustic injury: severe injury resulting in transmural necrosis or perforation (see Chap. 32).

Surgical Principles for Esophagectomy for Cancer

- There are three common approaches to esophagectomy: transhiatal, transthoracic (Ivor Lewis), and three-field (McKeown) esophagectomy. In general, the principal steps of each operative phase are preserved among the three approaches to esophagectomy.
- The location of the tumor in the esophagus, the available choices for conduit reconstruction, and surgeon preference all influence which approach is utilized.
- Postoperative outcomes and long-term cancer survival for esophagectomy are superior when performed in high-volume centers by experienced surgeons.

Surgical Margins

- An R0 resection (no microscopic residual tumor) should be the goal of any surgical resection for esophageal cancer.
- A 5 cm proximal and distal margin to the primary tumor is recommended.
- The status of resection margin has been identified as one of the strongest predictors of recurrence and overall survival.

Extent of Lymph Node Dissection

- It is recommended that 15 lymph nodes be removed for lymph node staging.
- The number of lymph nodes removed (higher is better) is a predictor of survival after esophagectomy.
- Typically, lymph nodes are removed en bloc with the esophageal specimen.

Minimally Invasive Esophagectomy (MIE)

- Minimally invasive laparoscopic, thoracoscopic, and robotic techniques have been utilized for any of the above three techniques of esophagectomy, with strong surgical and oncologic outcomes.
- Minimally invasive techniques have been shown to reduce perioperative morbidity with comparable oncologic results versus an open approach.

- Hybrid approaches which use a combination of minimally invasive and open techniques have also been employed.

Transthoracic Esophagectomy (Ivor Lewis)

- Described by British surgeon Ivor Lewis in 1946.
- Surgery is performed in two stages, two incisions: abdominal then right chest.
  - Abdominal portion with mobilization of the stomach, resection of celiac and gastric lymph nodes, and creation of a gastric conduit
  - Right chest portion with resection of the esophagus, pull-up of the gastric conduit, and an intrathoracic esophagogastric anastomosis
- Indications
  - Tumors of the distal esophagus or gastroesophageal junction
- Advantages
  - Allows for more resection of the proximal stomach as less length of the stomach is required for thoracic anastomosis compared to cervical anastomosis; thus, Ivor Lewis approach may be ideal for gastroesophageal junction tumors.
  - A greater ability to perform an intrathoracic lymph node dissection as compared to transhiatal.
  - No morbidity related to cervical incision (recurrent nerve injury).
  - A lower incidence of anastomotic leak as compared to cervical anastomosis, as there is less tension and better gastric blood supply at the anastomosis.
- Disadvantages
  - A higher incidence of thoracic complications such as postoperative pain, atelectasis, respiratory distress, and pneumonia.
  - Anastomotic leak, if it occurs, is more problematic in the chest; management potentially requires re-operative surgery.
  - Inadequate for tumors of the mid and upper esophagus given an inability to gain adequate proximal esophageal margin in the chest.

  A brief surgical description of an Ivor Lewis esophagectomy

- Abdominal phase
  - Patient positioned supine on the operating table.
  - The liver is retracted to expose the hiatus.
  - The abdomen is evaluated for resectability and for sites of metastasis. The stomach is evaluated for suitability as a conduit.
  - The abdominal esophagus is mobilized from the hiatus, and the lower thoracic esophagus/tumor is dissected up into the mediastinum under vision through the hiatus.

- The stomach is mobilized such that the pylorus can reach the hiatus; this involves dividing the short gastric, left gastric, and left gastroepiploic arteries but preserving the right gastric and right gastroepiploic arteries, with the right gastroepiploic artery being the major source of perfusion for the conduit
- Optional but recommended:

  Kocher maneuver of the duodenum is performed to increase mobility.
  Pyloric emptying procedure is performed, either pyloroplasty or pyloromyotomy.

- The gastric conduit is constructed with serial stapler firing along the greater curvature (Fig. 33.3).

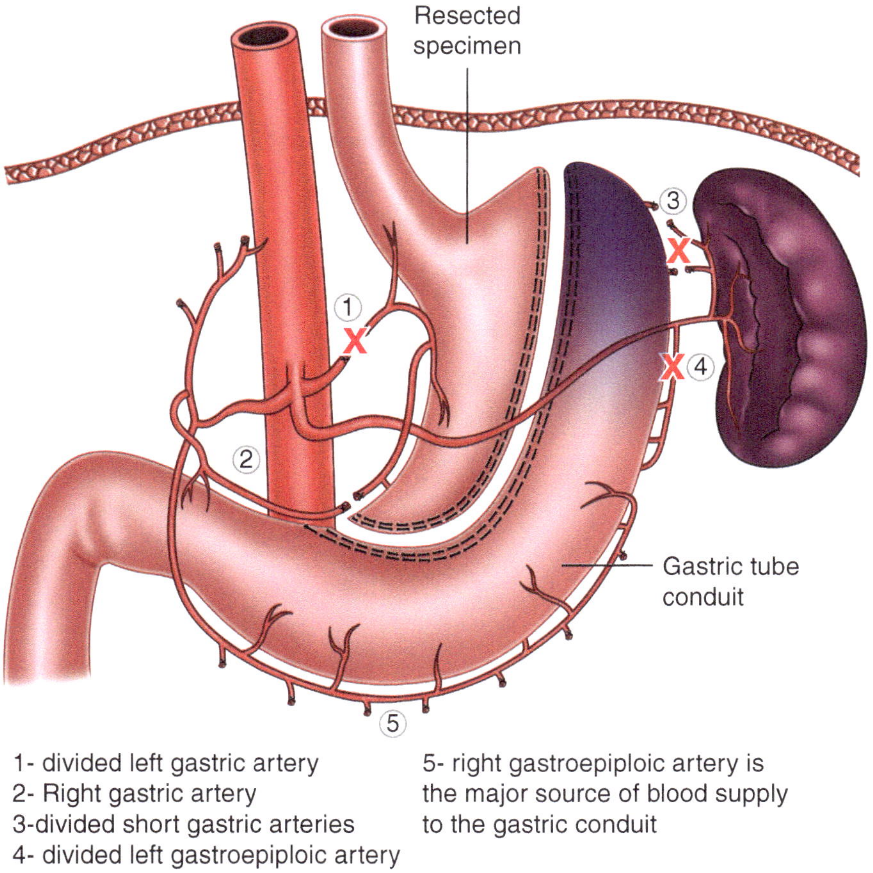

Fig. 33.3 Mobilization of the stomach, gastric conduit tube creation. (1) Divided left gastric artery. (2) Right gastric artery. (3) Divided short gastric arteries. (4) Divided left gastroepiploic artery. (5) The right gastroepiploic artery is the major source of blood supply to the gastric conduit

- Celiac and left gastric lymph nodes are resected en bloc with the specimen.
- The conduit is placed through the hiatus for subsequent retrieval in the right chest.
- Optional: a jejunal feeding tube is placed for postoperative enteral nutrition.

• Thoracic phase

- The patient is positioned in left lateral decubitus with the right chest up.
- A double-lumen endotracheal tube is utilized for single-lung ventilation.
- The esophagus is mobilized and freed from the surrounding mediastinal tissue to above the azygos vein, resecting paraesophageal lymph nodes and thoracic duct (optional) en bloc.
- The azygos vein is divided.
- The distal esophagus and gastric conduit are brought up through the hiatus into the chest.
- The proximal esophagus is divided at or above the level of the azygos vein, and margins are confirmed negative by frozen section.
- Redundancy of the gastric conduit is removed, but without tension, and the specimen is delivered out of the patient.
- Intrathoracic esophagogastric anastomosis is performed, above the level of the azygos vein (Fig. 33.4).

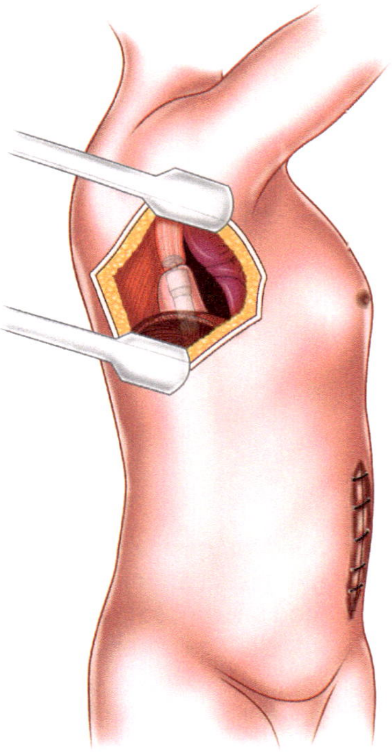

Fig. 33.4 Ivor Lewis esophagectomy, thoracic anastomosis with circular stapler

- A nasogastric tube is placed for decompression.
- Chest drains are placed in the posterior mediastinum.

Transhiatal Esophagectomy

- Surgery is performed in one stage, two incisions: abdominal and left cervical.
  - Simultaneous abdominal and left neck incisions are made.
  - Abdominal portion with mobilization of the stomach, resection of celiac and gastric lymph nodes, and creation of a gastric conduit.
  - Left cervical incision in combination with laparotomy allows for simultaneous blunt dissection of the thoracic esophagus from above and below.
  - Followed by conduit pull-up and esophagogastric anastomosis in the left neck.
- Indications
  - Tumors of the distal esophagus and gastroesophageal junction
  - Less ideal for tumors of the middle and upper thoracic esophagus as tumors in these locations will be dissected bluntly, rather than under direct vision, thus risking injury to adjacent structures or violating oncologic principles.
- Advantages
  - There is no need for a thoracic phase with this approach, resulting in fewer postoperative pulmonary complications such as atelectasis and pneumonia.
  - Easier of management of an esophageal anastomotic leak in the neck as compared to one that occurs in the chest, often requiring opening the neck incision for drainage.
- Disadvantages
  - Blunt/blind dissection of the thoracic esophagus limits the extent of lymphadenectomy and, therefore, potentially impacts long-term oncologic outcomes.
  - Blunt/blind dissection risks of injury to intrathoracic structures and/or bleeding.
  - A higher reported incidence of leaks with neck anastomosis as compared with thoracic anastomosis:

    More tension for cervical as compared to thoracic anastomosis.

    More stomach length is required to reach the neck as compared to the chest; thus, the stomach for anastomosis has more relative ischemia being further away from the vascular pedicle of the right gastroepiploic artery.

The tight space of the thoracic inlet may result in compression of the gastric conduit as it passes through, causing venous congestion.

- Cervical approach risks injury to recurrent nerve, vagus nerve, carotid artery, and jugular vein.
- May not be ideal for esophagogastric junction tumors as resection of the proximal stomach for adequate margin may not allow for enough gastric length to reach the neck for anastomosis.

A brief description of transhiatal esophagectomy:

- Abdominal phase
  - Abdominal phase identical to that described above for Ivor Lewis esophagectomy.
  - In addition, the rest of the non-diseased mid and upper thoracic esophagus is dissected bluntly from below, with the surgeon's hand placed through the hiatus and up the mediastinum.
- Left neck phase
  - Left neck incision can be made simultaneously with the abdominal phase.
  - The neck is extended by placing shoulder rolls and then turned to the right side to expose the left side.
  - An oblique incision is made along the anterior border of the sternoclavicular muscle.
  - Dissection carried deep to the prevertebral fascia. Care must be taken not to injure the recurrent laryngeal nerve at the tracheoesophageal groove.
  - The cervical esophagus is dissected free and encircled with a soft drain for traction.
  - Blunt dissection with the surgeon's hand/fingers down the mediastinum through the cervical incision frees up the remaining part of the upper thoracic esophagus, meeting up with the blunt dissection from below (Fig. 33.5), thus dissecting free the entire esophagus.
  - Cervical esophagus is transected, gastric conduit creation is completed, and the specimen is delivered from the patient.
  - Gastric conduit is pulled up through the hiatus into the left neck, in the original route of the native esophagus, and cervical esophagogastric anastomosis is performed (Fig. 33.6).
  - Soft drain is left in the neck.

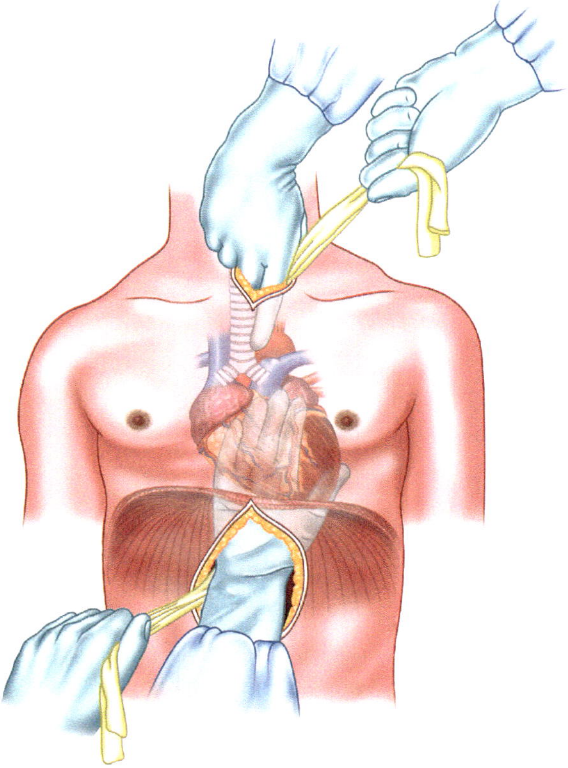

Fig. 33.5 Transhiatal esophagectomy, blunt dissection of the esophagus from laparotomy through the hiatus from below, and cervical incision from above

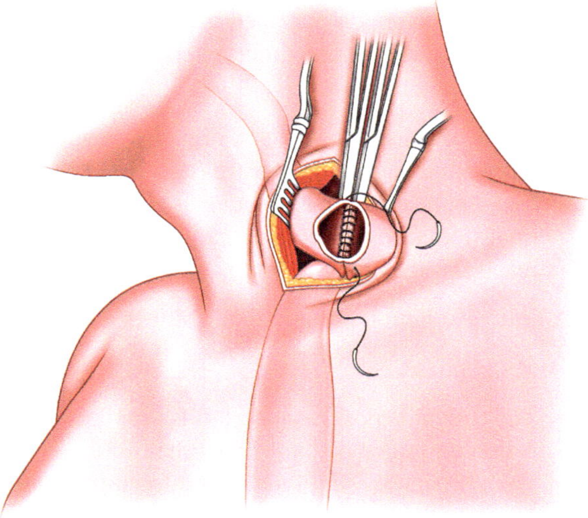

Fig. 33.6 Cervical anastomosis, hand-sewn

Three-Field Esophagectomy (McKeown)

- Surgery is performed in two stages, three incisions: right chest, then abdominal, and left cervical.
  - Begins with the right chest portion to mobilize the esophagus, en bloc with the periesophageal lymph nodes and thoracic duct (optional), from the hiatus to the apex of the chest.
  - Then simultaneous abdominal and cervical portions for gastric mobilization, resection of celiac and gastric lymph nodes, conduit creation, conduit pull-up, and anastomosis in the left neck.
- Indications
  - Tumors of the proximal, middle, or distal thoracic esophagus or gastroesophageal junction.
- Advantages
  - Easier of management of an esophageal leak in the neck as compared to one occurring in the chest, often requiring opening the neck incision for drainage.
  - Ideal for mid and upper thoracic esophageal tumors as it allows for greater esophageal margin distance than Ivor Lewis, and dissection of the tumor is under direct vision rather than blunt/blind dissection of transhiatal.
  - Greater ability to perform an intrathoracic lymph node dissection than transhiatal.
- Disadvantage
  - Incurs the morbidity of all three incisions:

    Thoracotomy—postoperative pain, atelectasis, and pneumonia
    Cervical incision—injury to recurrent nerve, vagus nerve, carotid artery, and jugular vein

  - Cervical anastomosis has a higher leak rate than intrathoracic anastomosis, although easier to manage (reasons listed above as for transhiatal).
  - May not be ideal for esophagogastric junction tumors as resection of the proximal stomach for adequate margin may not allow for enough gastric length to reach the neck for anastomosis.

A brief description of three-field (McKeown) esophagectomy:

- Thoracic phase
  - The patient is positioned in left lateral decubitus with the right chest up.
  - A double-lumen endotracheal tube is utilized for single-lung ventilation.
  - The esophagus is mobilized and freed from the surrounding mediastinal tissue from the hiatus to the apex of the right chest, resecting the paraesophageal lymph nodes and thoracic duct (optional) en bloc.
  - Chest drains are placed in the posterior mediastinum.

- Abdominal and left cervical phase
  - The patient is placed in supine position, and simultaneous laparotomy and left cervical incision are made.
  - The procedure is then completed as described above for transhiatal, except there is no need for blunt dissection of the thoracic esophagus.

Choice of Conduit

- The goal of esophageal replacement after resection is to re-establish continuity of the gastrointestinal tract and allow patients to eat and drink with acceptable transient time through the new conduit.
- Passage of the conduit can be performed in the route of the native esophagus in the posterior mediastinum (most common), substernal (if the mediastinum is obliterated), transpleural, or subcutaneous routes.

Gastric Conduit (Fig. 33.3)

- The primary choice for esophageal replacement in esophagectomy due to adequate length, ease of mobilization, adequate perfusion, and requiring only a single anastomosis.
- The gastric conduit is constructed by tubularization using sequential fires of a surgical stapler along the lesser curvature.
- The conduit is created to approximately 4–5 cm in diameter.
- The right gastroepiploic artery is the main blood supply to the conduit.

Colonic Interposition

- Usually it is the second choice for conduit if the stomach is not suitable.
- Preoperative computed tomography with angiography (CTA) is used to determine the colonic blood supply, and colonoscopy is performed to evaluate for colonic lesions and tissue suitability.
- Requires three anastomoses, a colo-colonic anastomosis to re-establish colonic continuity, along with colo-gastric and colo-esophageal.
- The left colon (Fig. 33.7), in an isoperistaltic manner, is most commonly utilized due to its consistent marginal artery, adequate length of conduit, and good size match with the esophagus. Major blood supply from the ascending branch of the left colic artery.
- Right colon (Fig. 33.8) can also be used, based on the middle colic artery. However, its marginal artery is less consistent and its larger-diameter matches less well with the esophagus as compared to the left colon.

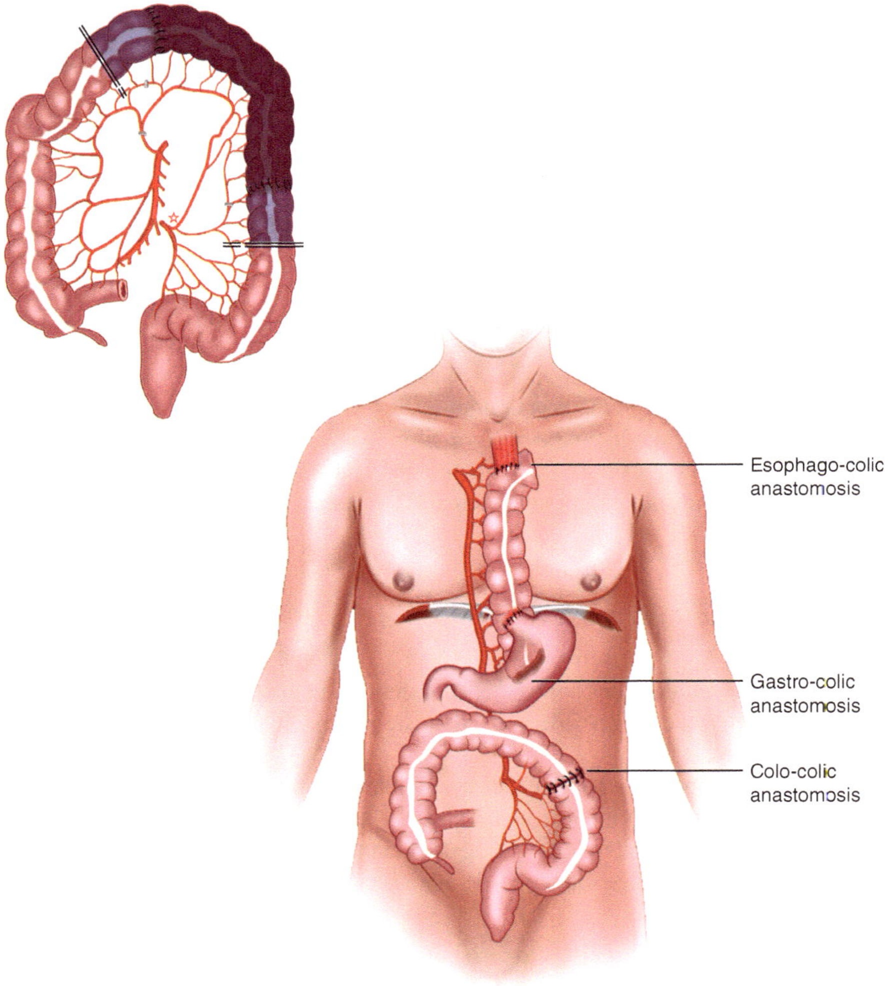

Fig. 33.7 Left colon conduit, isoperistaltic, with arterial supply from the left colic artery (star)

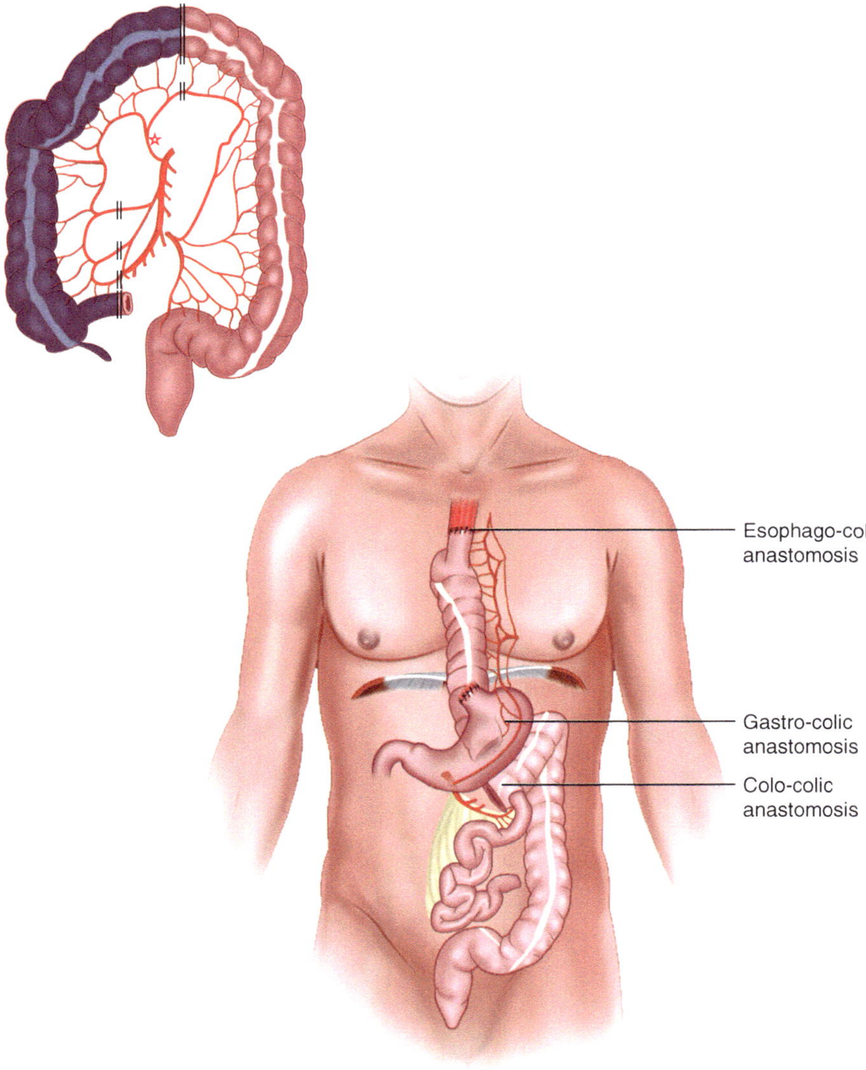

Fig. 33.8 Right colon conduit, isoperistaltic, with arterial supply from the middle colic artery (star)

Jejunal Conduit

- A pedicled jejunal conduit (Fig. 33.9) is utilized in tumors with limited esophageal involvement but extensive gastric involvement mandating total gastrectomy. Length of reach is limited, usually to the level of the inferior pulmonary vein, where a Roux-en-Y esophagojejunostomy is performed.
- For certain cases where resection is performed for cervical esophageal cancer, a free jejunal graft (Fig. 33.10) may be utilized, requiring a vascular anastomoses to cervical vessels (referred to as a "supercharged" jejunum), to re-establish arterial inflow and venous outflow.

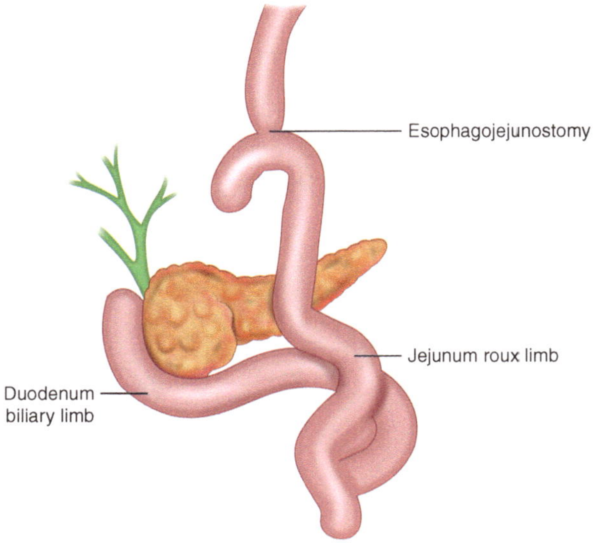

Fig. 33.9 Pedicle jejunal conduit

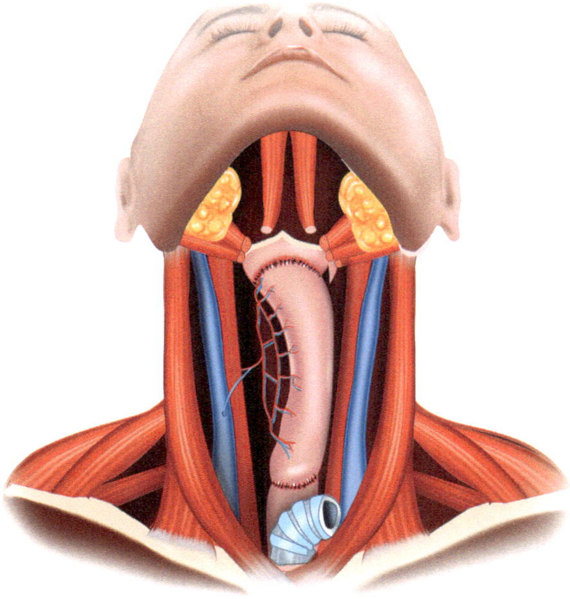

Fig. 33.10 Free jejunal conduit, with microvascular anastomosis to re-establish arterial inflow and venous outflow

Techniques for Anastomosis

Basic Principles

- Tension-free.
- Anastomosis in vascularized tissue, meaning there is good perfusion/no tissue ischemia to the regions of planned anastomosis.
- Anastomosis outside radiation field.
- Aligned, straight, and nonredundant conduit.
- No one technique for anastomosis is shown to be superior to another.

Hand-Sewn (Fig. 33.11)

- Silk sutures are used as stay sutures to align the esophagus and conduit.
- Two layers of sutures are placed: the first, a full-thickness absorbable suture layer, and the second, a row of nonabsorbable Lembert imbricating sutures.

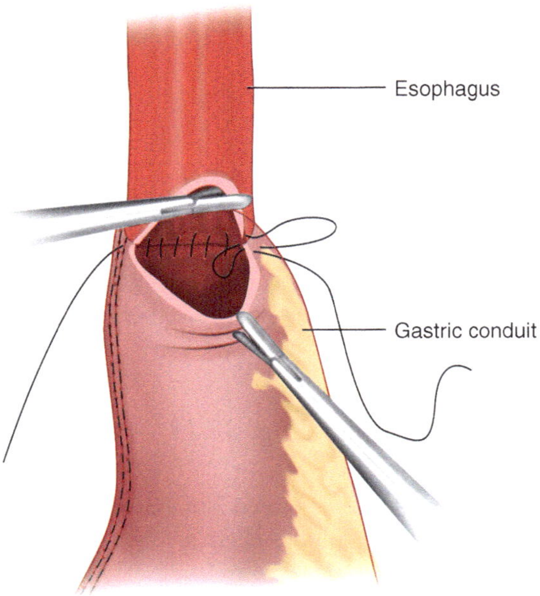

Fig. 33.11 Hand-sewn anastomosis

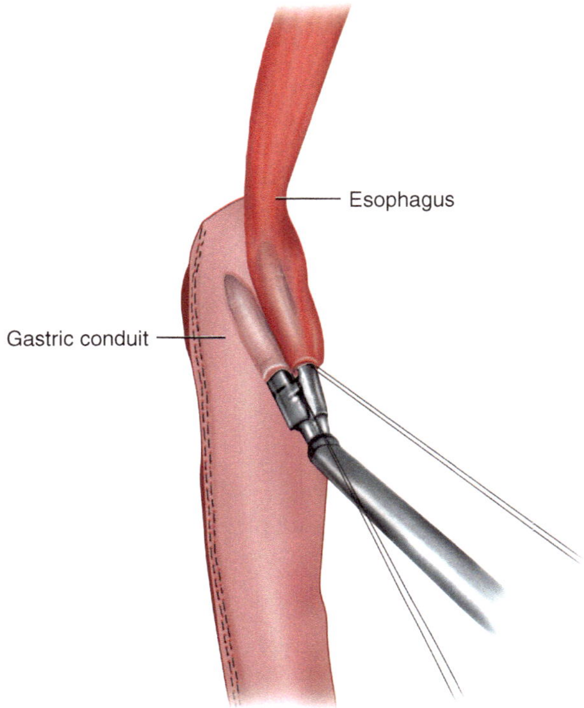

Fig. 33.12 Linear stapled anastomosis

Linear Stapled (Fig. 33.12)

- The gastric conduit is aligned with the native esophagus, and a linear stapler is placed into both structures and fired, creating a posterior anastomosis. The remaining anterior opening is either sewn or stapled closed.

Circular Stapled (Fig. 33.13)

- An anvil stapler is placed into the end of the native esophagus and secured with a purse-string suture; alternatively, the anvil can be placed trans-orally into a staple-ended esophagus.
- The gastric conduit is opened, a circular stapler is advanced and paired with the anvil, and the stapler is fired to create the circular anastomosis.
- The gastrotomy is then closed with a linear stapler.

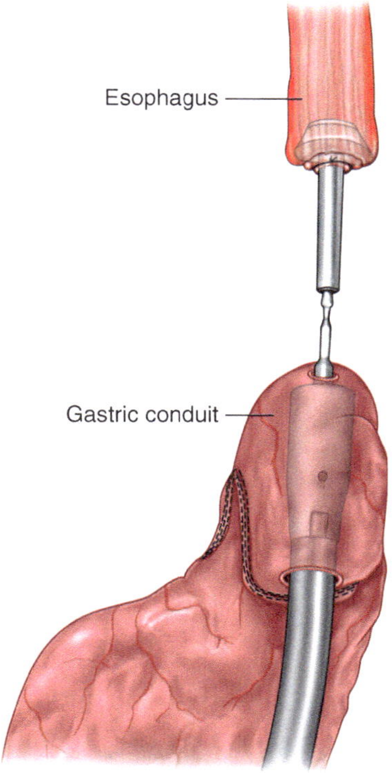

Fig. 33.13 Circular stapled anastomosis

Additional Surgical Considerations

Reinforcement of the Anastomosis

- Greater omentum may be preserved along the greater curvature to cover the anastomosis and/or placed between the esophagus and airway to prevent fistula formation.
- The divided azygos vein can be sutured over the anastomosis.

Enteral Feeding Tube

- While not absolutely required, the placement of a feeding jejunostomy is recommended, allowing access for postoperative enteral nutrition.
- Direct oral feeding has been shown to be safe after esophagectomy, but concern remains regarding the potential to increase the risk of anastomotic leaks and aspiration events.

Pyloric Procedure

- During esophagectomy, vagal nerve innervation of the stomach is often interrupted, potentially leading to delayed gastric emptying and/or functional gastric outlet obstruction.
- A pyloric drainage procedure such as pyloromyotomy or pyloroplasty can be performed during esophagectomy to facilitate gastric emptying.
- There is no consensus regarding whether a pyloric drainage procedure is mandatory or improves outcomes after esophagectomy.
- There are a number of potential interventions to address the pylorus: the data does not support one procedure over another.
  - Pyloromyotomy (Fig. 33.14): performed by incising the serosa and dividing the pyloric muscles longitudinally while maintaining the mucosa.
  - Pyloroplasty (Fig. 33.15): performed by opening the pylorus full thickness (including the mucosa) longitudinally and closing it horizontally.
  - Injection of Botulinum toxin at the pylorus.
  - Endoscopic balloon dilation.

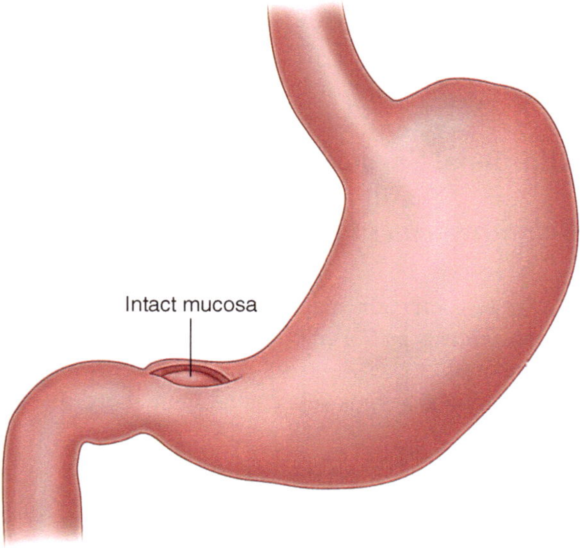

Fig. 33.14 Pyloromyotomy, pylorus muscle divided with mucosa left intact

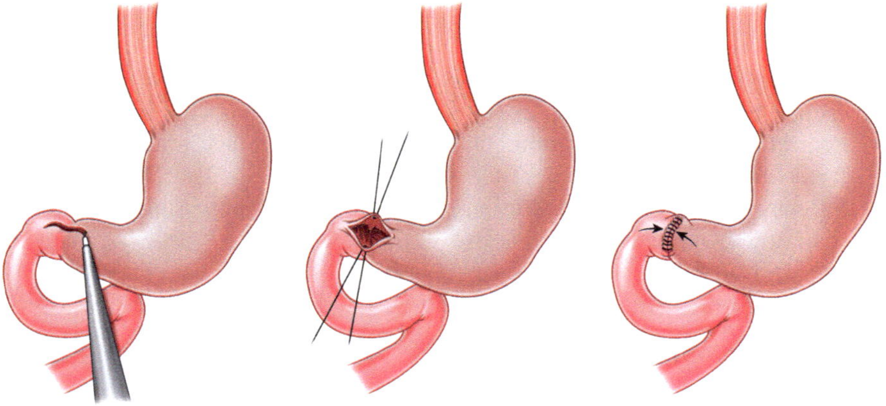

Fig. 33.15 Pyloroplasty, longitudinal full-thickness incision with transverse closure

Complications of Esophagectomy

Anastomotic Leak

- Early leaks occur within 2–3 days of surgery and are most commonly attributed to a technical issue with the anastomosis.
- Late leaks occur 5–7 days or more and may result from conduit ischemia.
- Serial pleural amylase levels can accurately predict an anastomotic leak.
- An esophagram with esophageal contrast is another study that can evaluate for anastomotic leak.
- Patients with an anastomotic leak and sign of sepsis should be evaluated with chest imaging and/or endoscopy to confirm conduit viability and ischemia.
- Minor and contained postoperative leak can be treated initially without surgical intervention. The patient is kept without oral feeding (NPO), given antibiotics, and provided parenteral or enteral nutrition, followed by anastomosis reevaluation with an interval contrast study to document healing.
- An uncontained leak results in sepsis, requiring resuscitation, antibiotics given, and intervention. Intervention may be surgical (repair of leak or anastomotic takedown with esophageal diversion for unsalvageable anastomosis, thoracic washout), endoscopic (stenting, endoscopic vacuum sponge therapy), or a combination of these (endoscopic stenting with thoracoscopic washout). Choosing the appropriate therapy is a complex decision and requires surgical judgment.

Anastomotic Stricture

- A benign anastomotic stricture occurs in approximately a third of patients post-esophagectomy anastomosis.
- Poor blood supply and anastomotic leak are the two strongest independent risk factors for stricture.
- Strictures are initially treated using endoscopy and dilation. Surgical intervention is rarely needed.

Gastric Conduit Necrosis

- Rare, but morbid and potentially mortal complication, due to failure of gastric conduit perfusion.
- Emergent endoscopy is diagnostic, and surgical resection of the necrotic stomach is required, along with esophageal diversion. Reconstruction with another conduit, such as colon, can be considered many months down the line when the patient has fully recovered.

Delayed Gastric Emptying

- With transection of the vagal nerves during esophagectomy, a significant number of patients have some degree of delayed gastric emptying.
- This can also occur due to a narrowed or dysfunctional pylorus, lack of drainage procedure such as pyloromyotomy/pyloroplasty during the esophagectomy, or redundant and kinked gastric conduit in the chest.
- Initially treatment involves endoscopic dilation and botulinum toxin injection of the pylorus.
- If endoscopy fails, surgery with pyloromyotomy or pyloroplasty should be performed.
- Revision of the conduit may be required if symptoms are due to redundancy/kinking.

Esophageal Reflux

- More common when an intrathoracic anastomosis is performed, compared to a cervical anastomosis.
- Patients should be instructed to eat small and more frequent meals and avoid a supine position after meals.
- Acid reflux can be treated with proton pump inhibitors.

Recurrent Laryngeal Nerve Injury

- Approximately 10–20% patients who undergo a cervical anastomosis sustain an injury to the recurrent laryngeal nerve, which manifests as a hoarse, soft voice (dysphonia), aspiration, and/or dysphagia.
- Patients are managed with a period of observation as a minor percentage of patients will resolve spontaneously. For patients with ongoing dysphonia, medialization of the vocal cord can be performed via laryngoscopy.

Chylothorax (Also See Chap. 23)

- Given the close proximity to the esophagus, an injury to the thoracic duct or its branches can occur during esophageal dissection. A chylothorax occurs in approximately 1–5% of the patients.
- Presents with milky color pleural effusion with fluid triglyceride level > 110 mg/dl.
- Patients with a "low output" chyle leak (generally <10 ml/kg/day) can be managed conservatively by initiating NPO, followed by consideration of low-fat or medium-chain triglyceride diet, with close monitoring of pleural drainage volumes for spontaneous closure of the chyle leak.
- When pleural fluid volume remains high output (>10 ml/kg/day), which usually indicates injury to the main thoracic duct rather than its tributaries, an intervention (surgical or interventional radiology) should be considered as persistent loss of chyle can be fatal.
- With interventional radiology, lymphangiography can be performed to identify the cisterna chyli, the thoracic duct, and the site of a chyle leak. This can be followed by accessing the thoracic duct and performing therapeutic coil embolization.
- Surgery therapy involves ligation of a target branch of the thoracic duct or, more commonly, with mass ligation of the main thoracic duct close to its origin.

Key Reference

- Herron R, Abbas G. Techniques of Esophageal Anastomoses for Esophagectomy. Surg Clin North Am. 2021;101(3):511–524.

Further Reading

Ajani JA, D'Amico TA, Bentrem DJ, et al. Esophageal and esophagogastric junction cancers, version 2.2019, NCCN Clinical Practice Guidelines in Oncology. J Natl Compr Cancer Netw. 2019;17(7):855–83.

Berkelmans GHK, Fransen LFC, Dolmans-Zwartjes ACP, et al. Direct Oral feeding following minimally invasive esophagectomy (NUTRIENT II trial): an international, multicenter, open-label randomized controlled trial. Ann Surg. 2020;271(1):41–7.

Biere SS, van Berge Henegouwen MI, Maas KW, Bonavina L, Rosman C, Garcia JR, Gisbertz SS, Klinkenbijl JH, Hollmann MW, de Lange ES, Bonjer HJ, van der Peet DL, Cuesta MA. Minimally invasive versus open oesophagectomy for patients with oesophageal cancer: a multicentre, open-label, randomised controlled trial. Lancet. 2012;379(9829):1887–92.

Birkmeyer JD, Siewers AE, Finlayson EV, et al. Hospital volume and surgical mortality in the United States. N Engl J Med. 2002;346(15):1128–37.

Birkmeyer JD, Stukel TA, Siewers AE, Goodney PP, Wennberg DE, Lucas FL. Surgeon volume and operative mortality in the United States. N Engl J Med. 2003;349(22):2117–27.

Birkmeyer JD, Sun Y, Wong SL, Stukel TA. Hospital volume and late survival after cancer surgery. Ann Surg. 2007;245(5):777–83.

Hulscher JB, van Sandick JW, de Boer AG, Wijnhoven BP, Tijssen JG, Fockens P, Stalmeier PF, ten Kate FJ, van Dekken H, Obertop H, Tilanus HW, van Lanschot JJ. Extended transthoracic resection compared with limited transhiatal resection for adenocarcinoma of the esophagus. N Engl J Med. 2002;347(21):1662–9.

Linden PA, Towe CW, Worrell SG, et al. Drain amylase: a simple and versatile method of detecting esophageal anastomotic leaks. Ann Thorac Surg. 2022;113(6):1794–800.

Mariette C, Markar SR, Dabakuyo-Yonli TS, Meunier B, Pezet D, Collet D, D'Journo XB, Brigand C, Perniceni T, Carrère N, Mabrut JY, Msika S, Peschaud F, Prudhomme M, Bonnetain F, Piessen G, Fédération de Recherche en Chirurgie (FRENCH) and French Eso-Gastric Tumors (FREGAT) Working Group. Hybrid minimally invasive esophagectomy for esophageal cancer. N Engl J Med. 2019;380(2):152–62.

McKeown KC. Total three-stage oesophagectomy for cancer of the oesophagus. Br J Surg. 1976;63(4):259–62.

Omloo JM, Lagarde SM, Hulscher JB, Reitsma JB, Fockens P, van Dekken H, Ten Kate FJ, Obertop H, Tilanus HW, van Lanschot JJ. Extended transthoracic resection compared with limited transhiatal resection for adenocarcinoma of the mid/distal esophagus: five-year survival of a randomized clinical trial. Ann Surg. 2007;246(6):992–1000. discussion 1000-1

Orringer MB. Transhiatal esophagectomy without thoracotomy for carcinoma of the thoracic esophagus. Ann Surg. 1984;200(3):282–8.

van der Sluis PC, van der Horst S, May AM, Schippers C, Brosens LAA, Joore HCA, Kroese CC, Haj Mohammad N, Mook S, Vleggaar FP, Borel Rinkes IHM, Ruurda JP, van Hillegersberg R. Robot-assisted minimally invasive thoracolaparoscopic esophagectomy versus open transthoracic esophagectomy for resectable esophageal cancer: a randomized controlled trial. Ann Surg. 2019;269(4):621–30.

Straatman J, van der Wielen N, Cuesta MA, Daams F, Roig Garcia J, Bonavina L, Rosman C, van Berge Henegouwen MI, Gisbertz SS, van der Peet DL. Minimally invasive versus open esophageal resection: three-year follow-up of the previously reported randomized controlled trial: the TIME trial. Ann Surg. 2017;266(2):232–6.

Torek F. The operative treatment of carcinoma of the oesophagus. Ann Surg. 1915;61(4):385–405.

Varshney VK, Suman S, Garg PK, Soni SC, Khera PS. Management options for post-esophagectomy chylothorax. Surg Today. 2021;51(5):678–85.

Visser E, Markar SR, Ruurda JP, et al. Prognostic value of lymph node yield on overall survival in esophageal cancer patients: a systematic review and meta-analysis. Ann Surg. 2019;269(2):261–8.

Chapter 34
Tracheal Stenosis

Marcus Alvarez and Thomas Ng

Introduction

Tracheal and subglottic stenosis is characterized by anatomic narrowing of the airway below the level of the vocal cords and above the bifurcation into the right and left mainstem bronchi (main carina). The most common nonneoplastic cause of intrinsic tracheal stenosis is due to complications of endotracheal intubation, creating inflammation and stricture. Clinically this can result in central airway obstruction and subsequent respiratory insufficiency requiring intervention.

Anatomy

- Subglottic space
  - Begins below the level of the vocal cords, which are located at the midpoint of the thyroid cartilage, and terminates at the cricoid cartilage.
  - The narrowest portion of the airway is at the cricoid, the only portion completely encircled by cartilage.
  - Receives blood supply from the superior and inferior pharyngeal arteries.

M. Alvarez
Department of Surgery, University of Tennessee Health Science Center, College of Medicine, Memphis, TN, USA
e-mail: malvare2@uthsc.edu

T. Ng (✉)
Division of Thoracic Surgery, University of Tennessee Health Science Center, College of Medicine, Memphis, TN, USA
e-mail: tng4@uthsc.edu

T. Ng, T. Geraci (eds.), *Thoracic Surgery Clerkship*, Contemporary Surgical Clerkships, https://doi.org/10.1007/978-3-031-44645-0_34

  - As the recurrent laryngeal nerve (left and right) ascend, it runs along the posterior aspect of the cricoid and enters the thyroid near the inferior horn of the thyroid cartilage.
- Trachea
  - 10–12 cm length, on average, begins from the cricoid cartilage and ends at the main carina.
  - Supported by approximately 20 cartilage rings that encircle the anterior 75% of the trachea.
  - The posterior aspect, without cartilaginous support, is termed membranous trachea.
  - Receives blood supply from the inferior thyroid artery and segmental end arteries from the aorta, including bronchial arteries.
  - Blood supply enters laterally, left and right sides; thus, its anterior and posterior planes are avascular.
  - The recurrent laryngeal nerves (left and right) run alongside the trachea in the tracheal-esophageal groove.

Presentation

- Epidemiology
  - Post-intubation, by oral endotracheal, cricothyroidotomy, or tracheostomy tubes, is the most common cause of nonneoplastic intrinsic tracheal stenosis:

    The incidence of stenosis is correlated to the duration of tube placement.
    Up to 20% incidence in long-term tracheal intubation.
    Less than 10% of long-term intubations have severe stenosis requiring intervention.
    Injury is due to the balloon cuff, end tip of tube, complications at the stoma (in cases of tracheostomy), or a combination of these.
    Stenosis can be combined with segments of malacia.

  - Other causes:

    Chemical burns and inhalation injuries
    Infectious: tuberculosis, histoplasmosis
    Inflammatory: relapsing polychondritis, Wegener's granulomatosis, sarcoidosis
    Idiopathic (often young female, subglottic in location)
    Any laryngotracheal trauma
    Any laryngotracheal surgery
    Any prior endoscopic tracheal intervention including dilation, stenting, laser therapy, cryoablation

- History
  - Patients present with one or more of the following: cough, dyspnea on exertion, wheezing, stridor, or hoarseness.
  - Prior history of prolonged intubation (>48 hours) or tracheostomy.
  - History of burn/inhalation injury, laryngotracheal trauma, laryngotracheal procedures/surgery.
  - Be aware of patients who have been treated for their "COPD or asthma" and have no or minimal resolution of symptoms with appropriate medical therapy. If this patient has any history of intubation, tracheostomy, airway surgery/procedures, or airway trauma, then the diagnosis of tracheal stenosis must be considered.
- Physical exam
  - Physical exam findings may include upper airway stridor and possibly wheezing.
  - Pay special attention to the head and neck exam, looking for any scars that indicate prior tracheostomy or surgery on the neck.

Imaging and Workup

- Computed tomography (CT) scan of the neck and chest
  - For diagnosis of stenosis.
  - Assess location and extent of stenosis (Fig. 34.1a, b).
  - Rule out any external compression.
- Flexible bronchoscopy
  - Perform awake, as patient may have critical stenosis.

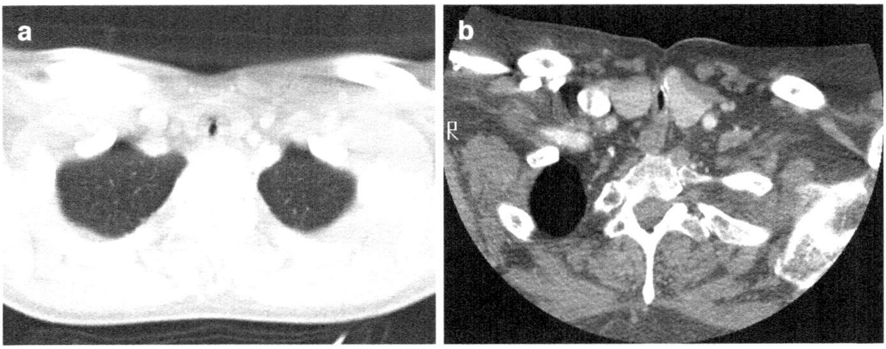

Fig. 34.1 CT scan of post-intubation tracheal stenosis. (**a**) Circumferential stenosis from endotracheal tube cuff; (**b**) A-shaped stenosis at the stoma site of prior tracheostomy

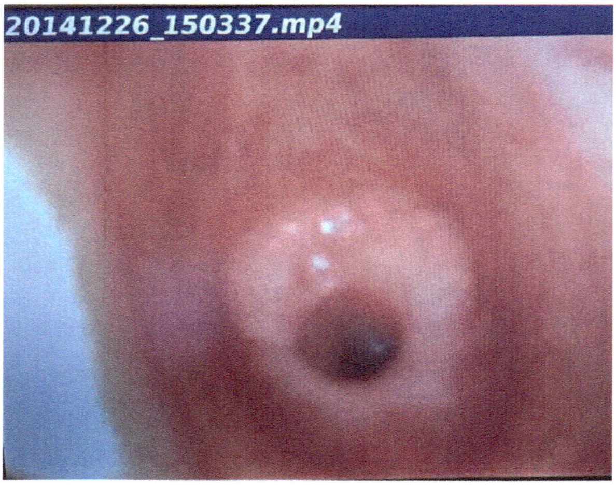

Fig. 34.2 Bronchoscopic view of patient with post-intubation stenosis of the very proximal trachea

- Examine function of the vocal cords.
- Make diagnosis of stenosis (Fig. 34.2); if critical do not pass through.
- If stenosis is not critical, it can pass through to make measurements, note the location and extent of stenosis, assess for concomitant malacia, perform biopsies for pathology and culture, and consider balloon dilation of the stenosis.

- Rigid bronchoscopy
  - For critical stenosis.
  - Initially avoid paralytic agents, to allow for spontaneous respirations, until critical stenosis is bypassed.
  - Dilate critical stenosis, serially with increasing size of rigid scope or with bougie or balloon dilation passed through the rigid scope.
  - Perform biopsies for pathology and culture.
  - Perform measurements of location and extent of stenosis.

Treatment

- Nonsurgical
  - Due to the diffuse extent, generally indicated for infectious/inflammatory and burn etiologies of stenosis.
  - Medical treatment as indicated for infectious and inflammatory etiologies.
  - Endoscopic intervention:

    Relief often not permanent unless underlying cause can be successfully treated

    Dilation: with rigid scope increasing size serially, with serial bougies or balloon dilation

Dilation often not successful in patients with significant post-intubation stenosis due to fibrotic nature and concomitant malacia segment(s)

Laser: limited utility for nonneoplastic stenosis, may risk doing more damage

- Stent:

  Can provide short-term relief but not optimal for long-term use due to complications of occlusion, bleeding, erosion, and migration, requiring frequent re-interventions.

  Options include internal stents (self-expanding: metal covered or uncovered, silicone) or stent with external limb (silicone t-tube).

- Surgical resection
  - Performed most commonly for symptomatic post-intubation stenosis that has failed nonsurgical therapy; resection is the most definitive treatment for this.
  - May be indicated in the rare situation of infectious or inflammatory conditions that have resolved with treatment but with sequelae of focal stenosis.
  - Reconstruction is by primary anastomosis as there is currently no reliable prosthesis; thus, the length of disease is a major determinant of eligibility for resection.
  - With tension-releasing maneuvers (see below), it may be possible to resect approximately half (or 6 cm in an average adult), but factors such as age, posture, BMI, and prior tracheal interventions/radiation may influence this.
  - Tracheal resection:

    Oral endotracheal intubation: dilation of the stenosis may be required prior, can use a small-caliber endotracheal tube if necessary.

    Cervical incision for the upper trachea (Fig. 34.3a), cervical incision and sternotomy for the mid trachea (Fig. 34.3b), and high right thoracotomy for the lower trachea (Fig. 34.3c).

    Lateral dissection is restricted to the diseased segment, avoiding devascularization of the remaining trachea for anastomosis.

    Dissect immediately against the diseased airway to avoid recurrent laryngeal nerves.

    Initial airway transection is below the pathology to allow for across-field ventilation into the distal unobstructed airway (Fig. 34.3a, b, c).

    Retract oral endotracheal tube out of the airway, followed by insertion of the across-filed endotracheal tube.

    Transect airway above the disease, and deliver specimen to pathology (Fig. 34.4).

    Perform one or all of the tension-releasing maneuvers, which includes from least to most complex: neck flexion (routinely performed), pretracheal dissection (routinely performed, may use mediastinoscope to release all the way to carina), laryngeal release (suprathyroid or suprahyoid), and hilar release.

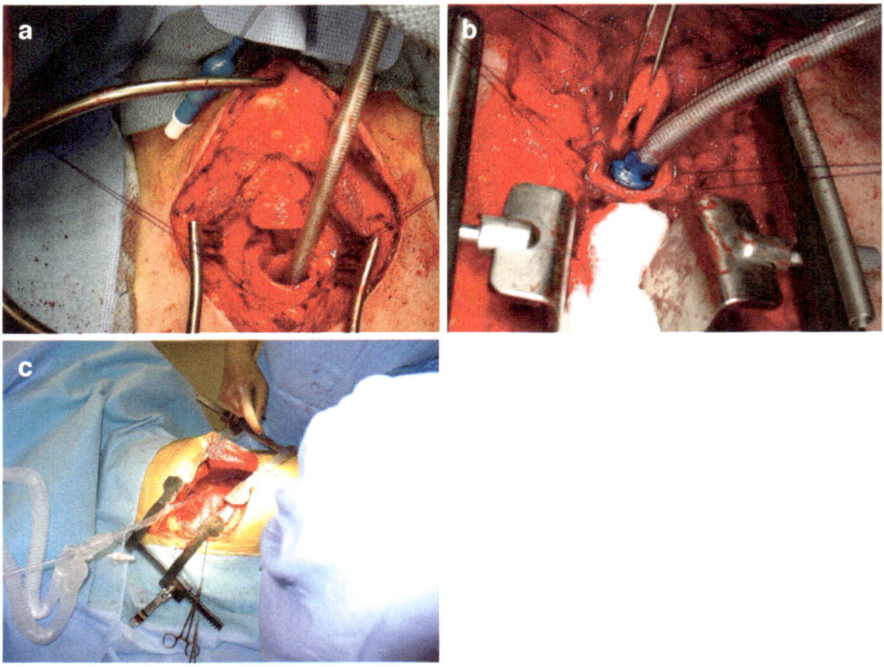

Fig. 34.3 Initial airway transection is below the pathology to allow for across-field ventilation into the distal unobstructed airway. (**a**) Cervical incision for disease in upper trachea; (**b**) cervical incision with sternotomy for disease in the mid trachea; (**c**) high right thoracotomy for disease in the distal trachea

Fig. 34.4 Resected specimen of a complex post-intubation stenosis with malacia from prior tracheostomy

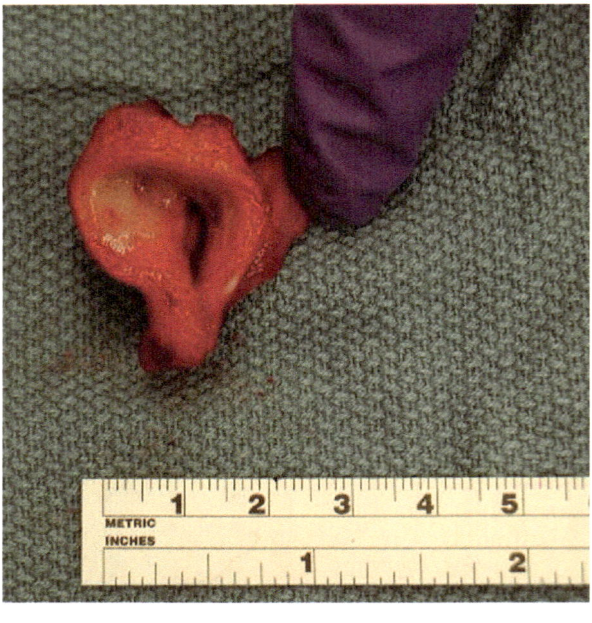

Perform posterior wall anastomosis, then remove across-field ventilation, advance oral endotracheal tube distally, and complete anterior wall anastomosis (Fig. 34.5).

Wound closure followed by chin stitch to prevent neck extension in the postoperative period (Fig. 34.6).

At postoperative day 7, perform bronchoscopy to confirm healing (Fig. 34.7); if so then remove chin stitch.

- Subglottic stenosis (idiopathic or post intubation):

  Oral endotracheal intubation: dilation of the stenosis may be required prior, can use small caliber endotracheal tube if necessary.

  Cervical incision for the upper trachea (most common); if needed add sternotomy for disease extending to the mid trachea.

  Lateral dissection restricted to the diseased segment, avoiding devascularization of the remaining trachea for anastomosis.

  Dissect immediately against the diseased airway to avoid recurrent laryngeal nerves.

  Initial airway transection is below the pathology to allow for across-field ventilation into the distal unobstructed airway.

  Retract oral endotracheal tube out of the airway, followed by insertion of the across-filed endotracheal tube.

  Transection of the airway above the pathology: this may be right up to the cricoid, or resection may include the anterior cricoid cartilage with resection of the diseased mucosa overlying the posterior cricoid cartilage (full resection of posterior cricoid cartilage is to be avoided as this risks injury to both recurrent laryngeal nerves).

  Perform one or all of the tension-releasing maneuvers, which includes from least to most complex: neck flexion (routinely performed), pretracheal dissection (routinely performed, may use mediastinoscope to release

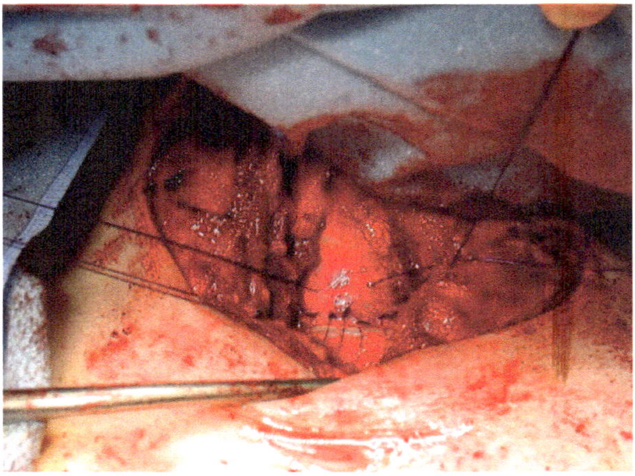

Fig. 34.5 Completion of the trachea anastomosis, in this case using interrupted 4–0 polydioxanone suture (a long-lasting absorbable suture) with all knots on the outside

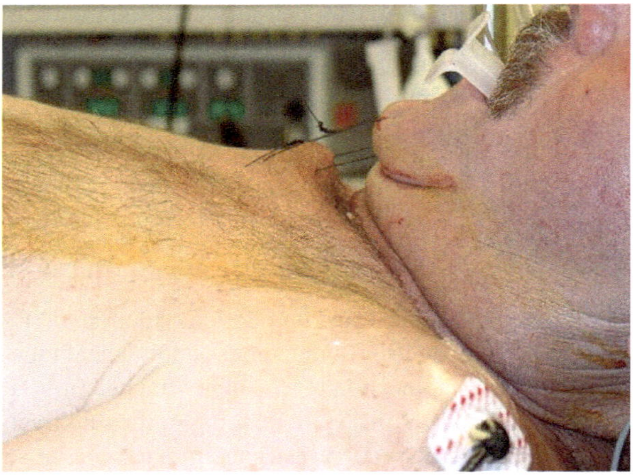

Fig. 34.6 The chin stitch is placed to prevent neck extension in the postoperative period

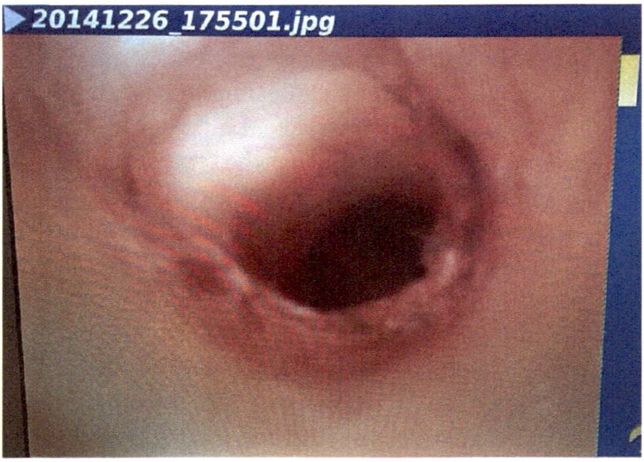

Fig. 34.7 Postoperative bronchoscopy shows a widely patent anastomosis that is healing well

all the way to carina), laryngeal release (suprathyroid or suprahyoid), and hilar release.

Perform posterior wall anastomosis, which may be trachea to cricoid or trachea (with posterior membranous extension flap) to bare posterior cricoid cartilage with the membranous tracheal flap used to resurface the posterior cricoid with mucosa.

Remove across-field ventilation, advance oral endotracheal tube distally, and complete anterior wall anastomosis, which may be trachea to cricoid or trachea to thyroid cartilage.

Wound closure followed by chin stitch to prevent neck extension in the postoperative period.

At postoperative day 7, perform bronchoscopy to confirm healing; if so then remove chin stitch.

Prognosis

- For post-intubation stenosis, success is seen in 93%, as defined by symptom relief that is durable, without requiring long-term tracheal appliance. Success is higher for resections confined to the trachea as compared to resections involving the subglottic region, 96% vs 85%, respectively.
- Operative mortality is less than 1%.

Key Reference

- Wright CD, Li S, Geller AD, Lanuti M, Gaissert HA, Muniappan A, Ott HC, Mathisen DJ. Postintubation Tracheal Stenosis: Management and Results 1993 to 2017. Ann Thorac Surg. 2019;108:1471–7.

Further Reading

Grillo HC, Donahue DM, Mathisen DJ, Wain JC, Wright CD. Postintubation tracheal stenosis: treatment and results. J Thorac Cardiovasc Surg. 1995;109:486–93.

Grillo HC, Mathisen DJ, Wain JC. Laryngotracheal resection and reconstruction for subglottic stenosis. Ann Thorac Surg. 1992;53:54–63.

Ott HC, Mathisen DJ. Tracheal lesions. In: Selke FW, del Nido PJ, Swanson SJ, editors. Sabiston and Spencer surgery of the chest. 9th ed. Elsevier; 2016. Chapter 8. p. 132–49.

Chapter 35
Tracheal Malignancies

Natalie Ostro, Travis Geraci, and Michael Zervos

Introduction

Primary tracheal tumors are rare, representing less than 0.2% of all respiratory malignancies. Tracheal tumors can be primary or secondary. The most common primary malignant tumors are squamous cell carcinoma (SCC) and adenoid cystic carcinoma (ACC). Secondary tumors are either metastatic or a result of direct invasion.

Presentation

The clinical presentation of tracheal tumors is often insidious.

- Patients present with symptoms similar to asthma, with progressive dyspnea and wheezing.
- Stridor is a late finding that occurs when there is near-complete collapse of the airway.
- A large, locally invasive tumor may also present with symptoms of hemoptysis from invasion of an adjacent vessel, dysphagia from compression of the esophagus, or hoarseness from recurrent nerve involvement.

N. Ostro · T. Geraci (✉) · M. Zervos
Division of Thoracic Surgery, Department of Cardiothoracic Surgery, New York University Langone Health, New York, NY, USA
e-mail: natalie.ostro@nyulangone.org; michael.zervos@nyulangone.org; travis.geraci@nyulangone.org

T. Ng, T. Geraci (eds.), *Thoracic Surgery Clerkship*, Contemporary Surgical Clerkships, https://doi.org/10.1007/978-3-031-44645-0_35

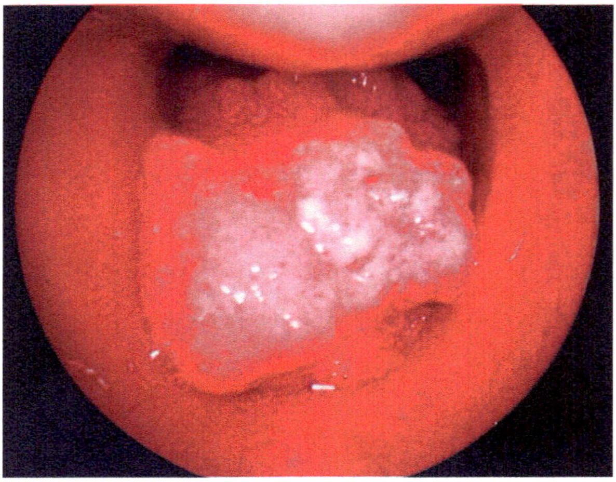

Fig. 35.1 Bronchoscopy view of squamous cell carcinoma of the trachea

Diagnosis

Definitive diagnosis is made using flexible (Fig. 35.1) and/or rigid bronchoscopy for direct visualization of the tumor to obtain biopsy for tissue diagnosis; at the same time, the tumor can be cored out to provide initial relief of a critical airway, the location of the tumor should be noted, and endoscopic measurements of the length of tracheal involvement can be performed.

Cross-Sectional Imaging (Fig. 35.2)

- Can be used to gather information on whether a tumor is likely to be benign or malignant, the extent of invasion, the length of invasion, vascularity, and presence of metastatic disease.
- Benign tumors, such as a hamartoma, have smooth borders and may contain fat.
- Malignant tumors have irregular borders and increased vascularity and may have invaded nearby structures.
- For tumors found to be malignant on histologic analysis, PET/CT and brain MRI are obtained to evaluate whether disease is confined to the airway or has metastatic spread.

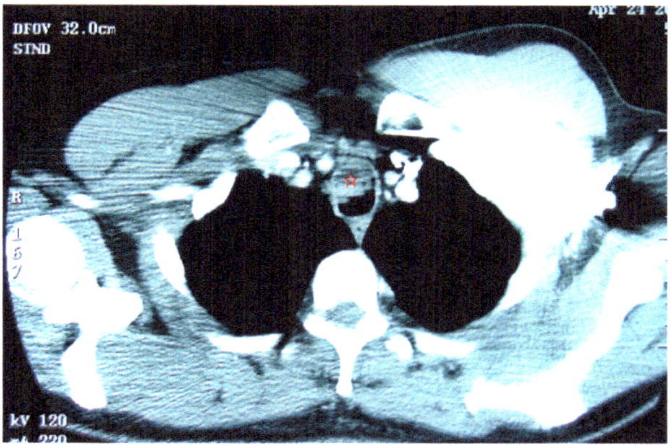

Fig. 35.2 CT scan of patient with resectable upper tracheal squamous cell carcinoma (star)

Primary Malignant Tumors of the Trachea

Squamous Cell Carcinoma (SCC)

- SCC is the most common primary tracheal malignancy.
- It is strongly associated with cigarette smoking.
- It is more common in men (3:1) with a peak incidence in the sixth and seventh decades.
- SCC occurs less commonly in the trachea compared with the larynx or bronchus because of the high laminar flow and improved mucociliary clearance in the trachea.
- SCC is more likely to have lymph node involvement and invade locally as compared with ACC.

Adenoid Cystic Carcinoma (ACC)

- ACC is the second most common tracheal malignancy.
- It makes up over one third of all tracheal tumors.
- It is equally distributed among men and women with a peak incidence in the fifth decade of life. It is not associated with smoking and is a slow-growing tumor which produces symptoms late in the course of disease.
- The extent of tracheal involvement may be more than what is first suspected as these tumors tend to spread submucosally. Resection is the treatment of choice and with radiation an option for any residual disease at the resection margin.

Carcinoid Tumor

- Carcinoid tumors are separated into typical and atypical types.
- Typical carcinoid tumors are less aggressive and have a very good prognosis when completely resected.
- Atypical carcinoid tumors are aggressive, highly malignant tumors. They also generally do not respond to radiation, but may have some response to chemotherapy.

Mucoepidermoid Tumor

- Mucoepidermoid tumors are rare tumors originating from the minor salivary glands of the airway.
- They are typically found in young people less than 40 years old. There are both high-grade and low-grade variants.
- Resection is the treatment of choice, but the tumor is also radiosensitive.

Benign Tumors of the Trachea

Benign tumors of the trachea include pleomorphic adenoma, squamous papilloma, multiple papillomatosis, and globus tumor.

- These are most commonly treated with resection and have an excellent prognosis.
- Pleomorphic adenoma is a mixed-salivary gland tumor which is rarely found in the airway. Multiple papillomatosis is associated with human papillomavirus (HPV) and is treated with laser ablation rather than surgical resection.
- Glomus tumor is usually found in the dermis but can rarely present in the airway.

Secondary Tracheal Neoplasms

Secondary tumors of the trachea originate from other organs and subsequently invade the airway.

- The most common types of these invasive cancers are lung, esophageal, thyroid, and laryngeal cancer.
- Rarely hematogenous spread can occur from other organs including metastatic breast cancer, melanoma, renal cell, ovarian, sarcoma, and lymphoma.
- Treatment in this situation is most commonly palliative with a combination of chemotherapy, radiation, endoscopic treatment (core out, laser, cryotherapy, argon) and/or stent placement to alleviate airway obstruction.

Management of Primary Malignant Tumors of the Trachea

Resectable Tumors

- Surgical resection, when possible, provides the best long-term outcomes and prognosis.
- There is no role for neoadjuvant radiation or chemotherapy prior to surgery because these treatments increase the risk of poor healing at the site of future tracheal anastomosis.
- Tracheal stents should also be avoided if surgical resection is planned because they can damage tracheal tissue and make resection difficult.
- Some institutions routinely use adjuvant radiation, but there is no definitive data to support this practice with complete resection (R0-negative margin).

Tracheal Resection

- Many of the key principles of tracheal resection have already been detailed in Chap. 35.
- The approach for surgery to resect tracheal tumors depends on the location of the tumor. Tumors in the upper or mid-trachea can be resected through a low-collar incision in the neck.
- Hyperextension of the cervical spine, especially in a young person with good neck mobility, allows a significant length of the trachea to be brought into the neck for resection through a collar incision.
- For mid-tracheal tumors, the addition of median sternotomy to the cervical collar incision can provide further exposure if required. Tumors of the distal trachea or carina are best approached through a right thoracotomy.
- The tumor and the required extent of resection are identified with direct visualization using intraoperative bronchoscopy.
- The portion of the trachea to be resected is mobilized circumferentially.
- Great care during dissection must be used to maintain the blood supply to the portion of the trachea that will remain for anastomosis and avoid injury to the esophagus and recurrent laryngeal nerve. Following resection of the diseased portion of the trachea, the remaining ends are brought together in an end-to-end fashion.
- As there is no reliable prosthesis for reconstruction, minimizing tension during primary anastomosis is critical.
- Common tension-releasing maneuvers include paratracheal dissection and neck flexion; more complex maneuvers such as laryngeal release or hilar release can be performed if necessary.
- The anastomosis is completed with a series of interrupted absorbable sutures starting at the posterior midline. A muscle flap or pericardial tissue may be used

to cover the anastomosis or separate it from proximity to a large blood vessel like the innominate artery.
- A "guardian stitch" or Grillo stitch may be placed between the chin and the chest to maintain the patient's neck in flexion in the first week postoperatively to ensure tension is not placed on the anastomosis.

Complications of Tracheal Resection

The most feared complication of resection is failure of the tracheal anastomosis.

- Risk can be minimized by following the rules of creating a good anastomosis, including using healthy tissue that has not been previously irradiated, minimizing tension, and ensuring good blood supply.
- It is generally better to leave a positive margin and treat with adjuvant radiation than risk failure of the anastomosis from too much tension.
- Management of anastomotic failure includes endoscopic therapy (dilation, stenting), reoperation (higher risk for poor outcome than the index resection), or tracheostomy.

More common complications include:

- Development of granulation tissue at the anastomosis causing stenosis, which can be treated by endoscopic procedures.
- Vocal cord dysfunction from recurrent laryngeal nerve injury/involvement, treated with vocal cord medialization.

Unresectable Tumors

Tumors with distant metastatic disease, extensive mediastinal lymphadenopathy, or invasion into adjacent organs or those encompassing a large length of the trachea that would not allow reconstruction are considered unresectable.

- The maximum length of resection is approximately half of the entire length of the trachea, about 4–5 cm or 7–8 cartilaginous rings.
- Treatment includes definitive chemotherapy with or without radiation and endoscopic therapy to alleviate symptoms of tracheal obstruction, which may include tumor core out (Fig. 35.3a, b), laser therapy, cryotherapy, argon beam coagulation, and tracheal stenting.

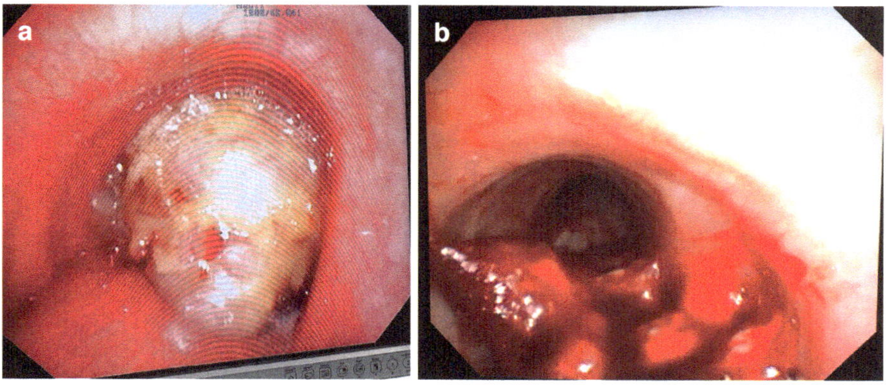

Fig. 35.3 Bronchoscopy view of patient with near-obstructing squamous cell carcinoma of the mid-trachea. (**a**) Before endoscopic therapy; (**b**) after core out to alleviate life-threatening obstruction

Survival Outcomes

Primary tracheal malignancies continue to be a difficult cancer to cure, with a 5-year overall survival of 45%.

Factors that are associated with improved survival include:

- ACC histology
- Younger age
- Ability to achieve an R0 resection

Key Reference

- Gaissert HA, Honings J, Gokhale M. Treatment of tracheal tumors. Semin Thorac Cardiovasc Surg. 2009;21(3):290-5.

Further Reading

Gaissert HA, Grillo HC, Shadmehr MB, Wright CD, Gokhale M, Wain JC, Mathisen DJ. Long-term survival after resection of primary adenoid cystic and squamous cell carcinoma of the trachea and carina. Ann Thorac Surg. 2004;78(6):1889–96. discussion 1896-7

Gaissert HA, Grillo HC, Shadmehr MB, Wright CD, Gokhale M, Wain JC, et al. Uncommon primary tracheal tumors. Ann Thorac Surg. 2006;82(1):268–72. discussion 72-3

Geraci TC, Prokopakis EP, Bizekis C, Zervos MD. Benign and malignant disorders of the trachea. In: Lalwani AK, editor. Current Diagnosis & treatment otolaryngology—head and neck surgery, 4e. New York, NY: McGraw-Hill Education; 2020.

Raz DJ, Weiser TS, Mathisen DJ. Tracheal diseases. In: Yuh DD, Vricella LA, Yang SC, Doty JR, editors. Johns Hopkins textbook of cardiothoracic surgery. New York, NY: McGraw-Hill Education; 2014.

Chapter 36
Tracheostomy and Tracheoinnominate Fistula

Jennifer Nishimura

Introduction

Tracheostomy procedure creates an opening from the skin of the neck through the anterior wall of the trachea where a tracheostomy tube (or other airway tube) can be inserted for airway access. The most common indication for this procedure is respiratory failure requiring prolonged ventilation. It can be performed via an open or percutaneous technique. A rare, but life-threatening, complication of tracheostomy is a tracheoinnominate fistula. It is associated with a high mortality and is a surgical emergency.

Anatomy

Trachea

- Located anterior in the neck and descends posteriorly into the mediastinum.
- Approximately 10–13 cm in length (two rings per centimeter length).
- Begins at the inferior border of the cricoid cartilage and ends at the carina.
- The anterolateral wall is cartilaginous (18–22 incomplete C-shaped rings), and the posterior wall is membranous with the trachealis muscle, a smooth muscle, at its posterior aspect.
- Lumen is circular at birth and takes an ovoid shape in adulthood.

J. Nishimura (✉)
Division of Cardiothoracic Surgery, Department of Surgery, University of New Mexico, Albuquerque, NM, USA
e-mail: jnishimura@salud.unm.edu

T. Ng, T. Geraci (eds.), *Thoracic Surgery Clerkship*, Contemporary Surgical Clerkships, https://doi.org/10.1007/978-3-031-44645-0_36

- Mucosa is lined by ciliated pseudostratified columnar epithelium with goblet cells and mucous glands.
- Main functions include air flow to and from the larynx and bronchi, mucociliary clearance, and warming and humidifying air.

Anatomical Relationships with the Trachea

- Proximal esophagus: left posterior membranous trachea
- Vertebral body: posterior membranous trachea
- Thyroid lobes: anterolateral cervical trachea
- Thyroid isthmus: anterior cervical trachea at the second or third tracheal ring
- Recurrent laryngeal nerve: tracheoesophageal groove
- Innominate artery: anterior trachea
- Left common carotid artery: left anterior/anterolateral trachea

Vascular Anatomy of the Trachea

- Arterial blood supply enters the trachea laterally and has a segmental arrangement of flow.
  - Cervical trachea: tracheoesophageal branches of inferior thyroid artery
  - Thoracic trachea: branches of bronchial arteries
- Venous drainage: inferior thyroid venous plexus which drains into the brachiocephalic vein.

Innominate Artery (Brachiocephalic Artery)

- The first great vessel branch of the aortic arch (Fig. 36.1)
- Crosses the anterior trachea in oblique fashion from left to right at approximately the ninth tracheal ring
  - High-riding innominate artery refers to an innominate artery that crosses the anterior trachea at a higher level (sixth ring or above).
- Bifurcates into two arteries
  - Right common carotid artery
  - Right subclavian artery

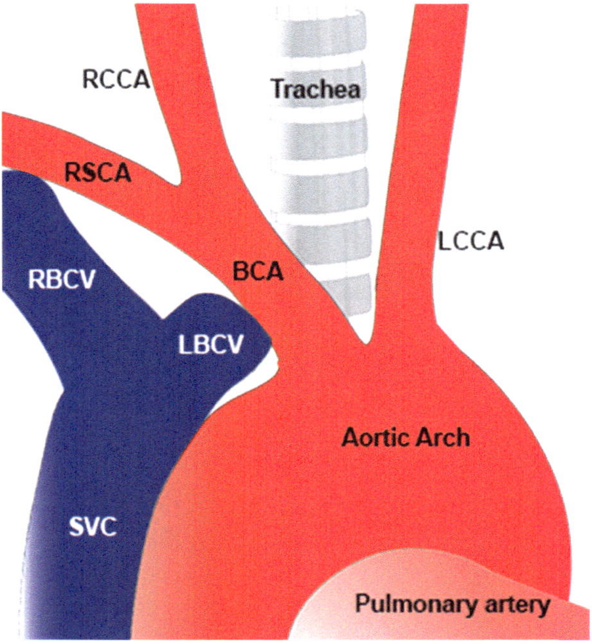

Fig. 36.1 Anatomy of the trachea and innominate artery. Please note there are variations of the anatomy described above. Abbreviations: *SVC* superior vena cava; *RBCV* right brachiocephalic vein; *LBCV* left brachiocephalic vein (truncated to show underlying innominate artery); *BCA* brachiocephalic artery (innominate artery); *RSCA* right subclavian artery; *RCCA* right common carotid artery; *LCCA* left common carotid artery

Tracheostomy Tubes

Cuffless (Uncuffed) and Cuffed Tracheostomy Tubes

- Cuffless tubes (Fig. 36.2a)
  - Allow air to move around the tube facilitating phonation (augmented with the use of a speaking tracheostomy valve) and respiration through the vocal cords while maintaining the airway
  - Typically used in alert patients off the ventilator
  - Removes the risk of tracheal injury from over inflated cuff
  - As intermediate step towards tracheostomy decannulation
- Cuffed tubes (Fig. 36.2b, c)
  - Most commonly used during initial placement of tracheostomy.
  - Used when positive pressure ventilation is required.
  - When the cuff is inflated, a seal is created preventing a significant air leak around the tube resulting in a closed circuit.
  - Theoretically prevents aspiration when the cuff is inflated.
  - Important: avoid overinflating the cuff (which may lead to injury to the trachea – stenosis, malacia).

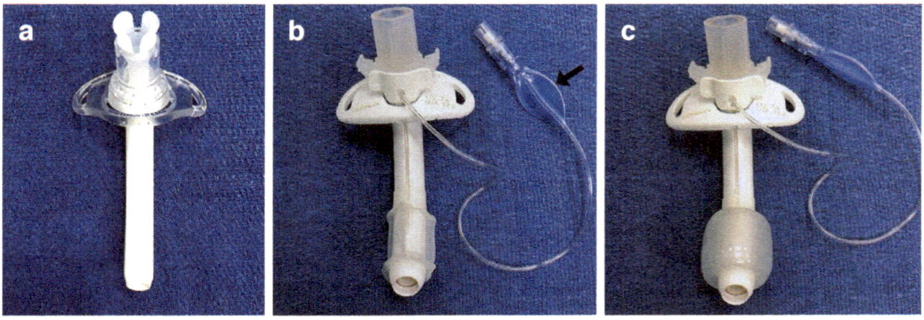

Fig. 36.2 Cuffless and cuffed tracheostomy tubes with inner cannula. The neck plate (flange) extends from the sides of each tracheostomy tube. (**a**) Cuffless tracheostomy; (**b**) cuffed tracheostomy with deflated cuff; (**c**) cuffed tracheostomy with inflated cuff. The pilot balloon is noted by the arrow

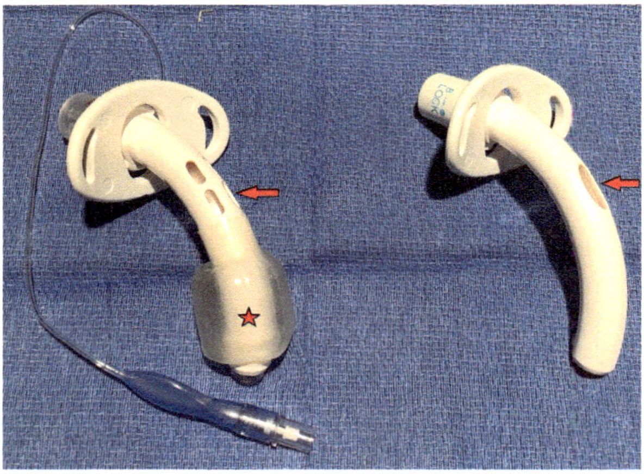

Fig. 36.3 Fenestrated tracheostomy tubes (arrows), cuffed (star) and uncuffed

Non-fenestrated and Fenestrated Tracheostomy Tubes

- Non-fenestrated tubes are more commonly used, whether when on or off mechanical ventilation.
- Fenestrated tubes have single or multiple hole(s) in the tube that permit airflow through the fenestration(s) to the vocal cords (Fig. 36.3):
  - Allows phonation and breathing through the upper airway when tracheostomy is capped.
  - May be utilized as an intermediate step towards tracheostomy decannulation.
  - Note: fenestrated tubes may have increased risk of tracheal wall trauma and granulation tissue formation.

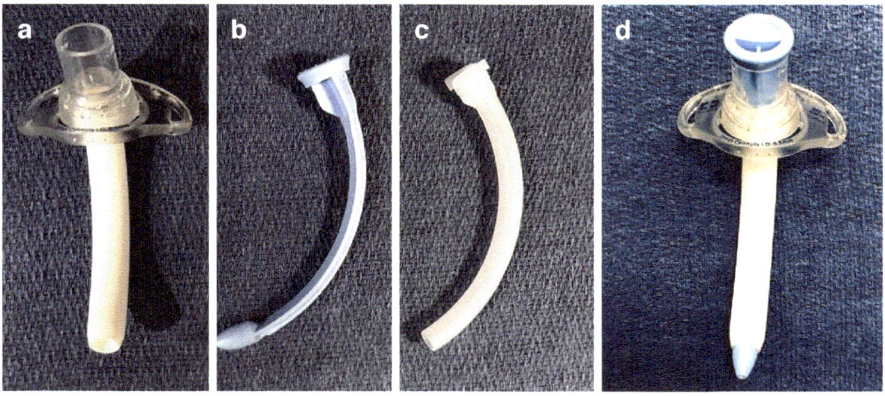

Fig. 36.4 Uncuffed, non-fenestrated tracheostomy tube. (**a**) Outer cannula with flange; (**b**) obturator; (**c**) inner cannula; (**d**) outer cannula with obturator in place

Components of Tracheostomy Tube

- Outer cannula with flange (Fig. 36.4a)
  - Constructed with polyvinyl chloride (PVC), silicone, and metal (uncommon)
  - Stents the tracheostomy open
  - Has flanges that extend from its sides with openings to allow attachment of a collar or ties to secure around the neck
- Obturator (Fig. 36.4b, d)
  - Placed into the outer cannula to facilitate tracheostomy tube insertion
- Inner cannula (Fig. 36.4c)
  - Inserted into the outer cannula.
  - Removed to clean or replaced (disposable inner cannula) for airway hygiene or if a blockage is present.
  - Note: inner cannula reduces the inner diameter of the tracheostomy tube lumen which increases resistance and work of breathing.

Tracheostomy Placement

- The following covers tracheostomy procedure in the adult patient.
- Tracheostomy can be performed using open or percutaneous dilational technique.
- Temporary or permanent.

Indications for Tracheostomy

- Respiratory failure requiring prolonged mechanical ventilation (most common indication)
- Airway protection
  - Traumatic brain injury
  - Spinal cord injury
  - Stroke
  - Other neurological diseases
- Upper airway obstruction
  - Tumors
  - Major head and neck trauma
  - Angioedema
  - Burn injury
  - Bilateral vocal cord paralysis
  - Definitive management for obstructive sleep apnea and obesity hypoventilation syndrome
  - Adjunct to major head and neck surgery

Timing of Tracheostomy for Respiratory Failure

- Depends on its indication and varies by practice.
- Optimal timing remains controversial.
- Definition of early versus late tracheostomy differs with some studies reporting 5–10 days as a cutoff.

Benefits of Tracheostomy over Oral Endotracheal Intubation

- Improves patient comfort.
- Less need for sedation.
- Facilitates weaning off the ventilator.
- Improves speech and swallow.
- Decreases dead space and work of breathing.
- Note: oral endotracheal tubes pass through the pharynx and vocal cords versus tracheostomy tubes which is located below the larynx/vocal cords.

Contraindications to Tracheostomy

- Neck infection at surgical site (absolute).
- Uncorrectable coagulopathy.
- Inability to tolerate periods of apnea or loss of positive pressure ventilation.
- Severe hypoxemia with high PEEP or FiO2 requirement.

Contraindications Specific to Percutaneous Tracheostomy

- Cervical spine instability (absolute).
- Uncorrectable coagulopathy (absolute).
- Difficult anatomy (relative) – consider open tracheostomy.
- Short or obese neck:
  - Difficulty identifying external landmarks
  - Tracheal deviation
  - Limited ability to extend neck

History and Physical Examination

- Specific history to determine indication for procedure, presence of contraindications, risks specific to the patient, and other information that may determine best approach (open versus percutaneous).
- Focused examination
  - Identify anatomical landmarks: thyroid cartilage, cricoid cartilage, and suprasternal notch.
  - Inspect for signs of infection at the planned surgical site.
  - Palpate the neck for a high-riding innominate artery (open tracheostomy preferred).
- Pertinent medications (anticoagulation, antiplatelet, immunosuppression).
- Labs (hemoglobin/hematocrit, platelets, coagulation studies).
- Review imaging for surgical planning and aberrant anatomy.
- Ventilator settings (FiO2 and PEEP).

Preparation for Procedure and Patient Positioning

- Tracheostomy is an aerosolizing procedure requiring appropriate personal protective equipment.
- Position supine with shoulder roll to facilitate neck extension if not contraindicated.
- Ensure all equipment is available and functioning before starting the procedure.
- The endotracheal tube should be easily accessible the entire time including after the patient is prepped and draped.

Key Points for Tracheostomy

- Always maintain control of the airway.
- Avoid placement of tracheostomy tube higher than the second and lower than the fourth tracheal ring if possible.
  - Insertion site is commonly described between the second and third tracheal rings.
  - High tracheostomy placement increases risk of subglottic stenosis.
  - Low tracheostomy placement increases risk of tracheoinnominate fistula (TIF).

Open Tracheostomy Technique

- Typically performed in the operating room under general anesthesia.
- Can be performed "awake" when there is upper airway obstruction and no other means to secure the airway.

Variations of Tracheotomy

- Bjork flap (inferior-based tracheal flap)
- Horizontal incision
- Vertical incision
- Horizontal "H" incision
- Cruciate incision

General Steps of Open Tracheostomy

- Make skin incision at the planned insertion site (below cricoid cartilage).
- Dissect down to the anterior wall of the trachea.
  - Through subcutaneous tissue, platysma, and midline raphe of strap muscles.
  - Strap muscles are retracted laterally.
  - The anterior jugular veins, inferior thyroid vein, and thyroid isthmus may be encountered during dissection and can be sources of early postoperative bleeding.
  - Isthmus may need to be retracted or divided.
- Reduce FiO2 to decrease risk of an airway fire and deflate the endotracheal tube cuff before tracheal incision.
- Make tracheotomy (see variations above), ideally at the second tracheal ring.
- Endotracheal tube is slightly retracted, to just above the tracheotomy but still maintained inside the airway below the vocal cords.
- Through the tracheotomy, place tracheostomy tube with obturator into the trachea under direct visualization.
- Remove obturator, place inner cannula, and inflate the tracheostomy cuff.
- Connect the ventilator circuit to tracheostomy tube, and confirm placement by return of end-tidal carbon dioxide (ETCO2), auscultation of lung fields, and/or bronchoscopy.
- Secure tracheostomy tube with sutures to the flange and/or tracheostomy collar around the neck.
- Remove endotracheal tube after proper position of the new airway is confirmed.

Percutaneous Tracheostomy Technique

- Performed at bedside (ICU) or in the operating room
- Uses (modified) Seldinger technique
- Performed under bronchoscopic visualization

General Steps of Percutaneous Tracheostomy

- Make skin incision directly overlying the trachea at the planned insertion site, ideal over the second tracheal ring.
- Bluntly dissect down to the anterior tracheal wall.

- Insert bronchoscope through oral endotracheal tube (ETT) for direct visualization of the trachea and all the steps described below.
- Slowly retract ETT until subglottic landmarks are identified. Maintain the endotracheal tube below the vocal cords.
- Insert introducer needle (with or without sheath) through the anterior tracheal wall into the tracheal lumen. If a sheath is used, remove the needle leaving the sheath in place. Needle or sheath should be midline, reposition if seen off to the side of the trachea.
- Feed guidewire through needle/sheath, and advance towards the carina.
- Remove needle/sheath over wire.
- Dilate the tract over guidewire (note: there are different types of dilators; and guiding catheters may be used over the wire).
- Remove the dilator over guidewire, maintaining position of the wire.
- Insert tracheostomy tube over the guidewire.
- Remove wire (and guiding catheter if used).
- Inflate cuff of tracheostomy tube.
- Connect tracheostomy tube to the ventilator circuit.
- Confirm position with return of ETCO2, bronchoscopy, and/or breath sounds.
- Secure tracheostomy tube with sutures to the flange and/or tracheostomy collar around the neck.
- Remove endotracheal tube after proper position of the new airway is confirmed.

Complications and Risks of Tracheostomy

- Intraoperative complications: bleeding, damage to surrounding structures (esophagus, trachea, blood vessels, nerves including the recurrent laryngeal nerve), pneumothorax, tracheal ring fracture, creation of false passage, loss of airway, hypoxemia, hypercarbia, and death.
- Early complications: bleeding, infection (cellulitis and tracheitis), tube obstruction (mucus plug), unintentional decannulation, pneumothorax/pneumomediastinum, subcutaneous emphysema, false passage creation, and TIF.
- Late complications: infection (pneumonia), tube obstruction (mucus plug), unintentional decannulation, TIF, tracheoesophageal fistula, subglottic stenosis, tracheal stenosis, dysphagia, tracheomalacia, granulation tissue formation, and persistent tracheocutaneous fistula.

Postoperative Management

- Fresh tracheostomy precautions
  - Tracheostomy tubes (same size and smaller), obturator, and equipment for tracheotomy and oral endotracheal intubation should be readily available at bedside.

- Routine tracheostomy maintenance
  - Monitor cuff pressure.
  - Gently perform tracheal suctioning.
  - Keep stoma clean and dry.
  - Change or clean inner cannula.
  - Change tracheostomy tube after tract matures (typically around postoperative day 7).

Weaning and Decannulation

- Decannulation is considered if the following criteria are met:
  - Mechanical ventilation is no longer needed.
  - Able to protect airway.
  - No upper airway obstruction.
  - Minimal secretions.
  - Effective cough.
  - Indications for tracheostomy placement resolved.
- Weaning strategies
  - Exchange cuffed tube for cuffless (with or without fenestration) when patient no longer requires positive pressure ventilation and is at low aspiration risk.
  - Downsize tracheostomy tube.
  - Capping trial.

Tracheoinnominate Fistula

Clinical Presentation

- Incidence: overall incidence after tracheostomy reported to be less than 1%.
- Typically critically or chronically ill with multiple comorbidities.

Pathogenesis

- The innominate artery crosses the anterior trachea at approximately the ninth tracheal ring. This anatomical relationship provides a setting to develop a tracheoinnominate fistula (TIF) after tracheostomy.

- Pressure from the cuff or other part of the tracheostomy tube leads to erosion into the innominate artery resulting in a TIF.

Risk Factors

- High-riding innominate artery
- Low positioned tracheostomy
- Poorly fitting tracheostomy tube with excessive movement
- Overinflated cuff
- Prolonged intubation
- Other patient factors: prior radiation therapy, chronic steroid use, inflammation, and infection

Presentation

- Tracheal bleeding through tracheostomy tube, peristomal bleeding, or hemoptysis.
- Bleeding can be minor to massive.
- Some present with minor bleeding that spontaneously stops and precedes massive hemorrhage (sentinel or herald bleed).
- Any post-tracheostomy bleeding starting at 48 hours postop should be presumed TIF until ruled out.

Diagnosis

- Any episodic bleeding or active bleeding should be evaluated in a controlled environment with flexible bronchoscopy and/or ventilating rigid bronchoscopy to evaluate for TIF. The tracheostomy should be retracted/removed to allow for complete visualization of the entire of the anterior tracheal wall.
- Angiography and computed tomography angiography have limited sensitivity – may show contrast extravasation from the innominate artery into the trachea.
- Differential: post-procedure bleeding from inadequate hemostasis or coagulopathy (<24 h post procedure), tracheitis, bleeding from stomal or tracheal granulation tissue, necrotizing pneumonia, and pulmonary artery injury.
- Massive hemorrhage from the trachea post-tracheostomy is pathognomonic for TIF.

Initial Management of Tracheoinnominate Fistula

Initial Main Objectives During Massive Bleeding

- Secure airway.
- Tamponade bleeding.
- Large-bore intravenous access.
- Get appropriate help.
- Get to the operating room for definitive control of bleeding.
- Volume resuscitation and distal airway clearance of blood.

Temporizing Maneuvers to Control Massive Bleeding

- Tracheostomy tube or endotracheal tube cuff is overinflated to tamponade bleeding.
- If bleeding persists, airway is secured via cuffed oral endotracheal intubation, tracheostomy tube is removed, and digital compression to the innominate artery is applied against the posterior aspect of the sternum by one of the techniques below:
  - Pretracheal space through the tracheostomy wound is developed inferiorly along the anterior trachea and behind the innominate artery, and digital compression to the innominate artery is applied against the posterior aspect of manubrium (Utley).
  - Alternatively, a finger is inserted directly through the stoma and into the trachea alongside the oral endotracheal tube, and digital compression is applied against the posterior aspect of manubrium – preferred as this avoids dissection of the artery which may increase the size of the arterial defect.
- Percutaneous stent-graft or other endovascular technique to control acute hemorrhage as a bridging procedure has been described in the literature.

Definitive Treatment of Tracheoinnominate Fistula

Resect and Ligate Innominate Artery

- Median sternotomy (provides optimal exposure).
- Expose innominate artery.
- Obtain proximal and distal control of innominate artery.
- Resect involved segment of artery and oversew/ligate the proximal and distal ends.
- Note: primary repair is not recommended given the higher risk of rebleeding.

Manage Tracheal Defect

- Debride to healthy tissue then repair or cover defect with viable tissue.
- Place a vascularized flap (strap muscle, sternocleidomastoid muscle, thymus) to buttress the repair and separate the divided artery ends from airway.

Other Approaches Described

- Innominate artery reconstruction with interposition graft or extra-anatomical bypass.
  - Generally not considered first-line, given its association with a higher risk of recurrent bleeding and postoperative death
  - Considered in the presence of known severe left carotid artery stenosis/occlusion, right internal mammary artery coronary bypass graft, or evidence of cerebral or limb ischemia after ligation of the innominate artery, in which case extra-anatomic bypass may be preferred due to infection risk of an interposition graft placed in a contaminated field
- Endovascular intervention is described in the literature for definitive treatment in patients with prohibitive risk for open surgery but is currently not considered standard of care; endovascular grafts are at a high risk for infection from the contaminated field.

Postoperative Complications

- Recurrent bleeding
- Sternal wound complications and mediastinitis
- Stroke or right upper extremity hypoperfusion
  - Rare but may occur if there is poor cerebral collateralization and/or severe left carotid artery stenosis or occlusion
- Death

Prognosis

- Overall prognosis is poor and is related to the difficulty in gaining control of the massive hemorrhage and the pre-existing illness.
- Neurologic complications from ligation of the innominate artery are rare.
- High mortality rate despite successful and timely surgical management; therefore, prevention is key.

Key Reference

- Furlow PW, Mathisen DJ. Surgical anatomy of the trachea. Ann Cardiothorac Surg 2018;7(2):255–260.

Further Reading

Ailawadi G. Technique for managing tracheo-innominate artery fistula. Oper Tech Thorac Cardiovasc Surg. 2009;14:66–72.

Allan JS, Wright CD. Tracheoinnominate fistula: diagnosis and management. Chest Surg Clin N Am. 2003;13(2):331–41.

Cheung NH, Napolitano LM. Tracheostomy: epidemiology, indications, timing, technique, and outcomes. Respir Care. 2014;59(6):895–915. discussion 916-9

Furlow PW, Mathisen DJ. Surgical anatomy of the trachea. Ann Cardiothorac Surg. 2018;7(2):255–60.

Furukawa K, Kamohara K, Itoh M, Morokuma H, Morita S. Operative technique for tracheo-innominate artery fistula repair. J Vasc Surg. 2014;59(4):1163–7. https://doi.org/10.1016/j.jvs.2013.09.013. Epub 2013 Nov 14

Hashimoto DA, Axtell AL, Auchincloss HG. Percutaneous tracheostomy. N Engl J Med. 2020;383(20):e112. https://doi.org/10.1056/NEJMvcm2014884. Epub 2020 Oct 2

Minnich DJ, Mathisen DJ. Anatomy of the trachea, carina, and bronchi. Thorac Surg Clin. 2007;17(4):571–85.

O'Malley TJ, Jordan AM, Prochno KW, Saxena A, Maynes EJ, Ferrell B, Guy TS, Entwistle JW, Massey HT, Morris RJ, Abai B, Tchantchaleishvili V. Evaluation of endovascular intervention for Tracheo-innominate artery fistula: a systematic review. Vasc Endovasc Surg. 2021;55(4):317–24. https://doi.org/10.1177/1538574420980625. Epub 2021 Feb 2

Utley JR, Singer MM, Roe BB, Fraser DG, Dedo HH. Definitive management of innominate artery hemorrhage complicating tracheostomy. JAMA. 1972;220(4):577–9.

Chapter 37
Chest Wall Tumors

Hamza Durrani and Adam Bograd

Introduction

- Chest wall tumors are a heterogeneous and rare group of tumors that, combined, account for approximately 5% of all thoracic tumors.
- They can be benign or malignant (~55%) (Table 37.1).
- The average age at presentation for patients with benign tumors is 26 years versus 40 years for malignant tumors.
- The male-to-female ratio for most tumors is 2:1 except for desmoid tumors where the ratio is reversed.
- Chest wall tumors are considered primary if they arise from any chest wall tissue, including nerves, blood vessels, muscle, bones, cartilage, connective tissue, or fatty tissue.
- Secondary tumors are those that arise by direct extension either from a lung/pleural tumor or from a metastatic lesion; along with lung cancer, more common neoplasms to metastasize include melanomas, breast cancer, and renal cell cancer.

H. Durrani · A. Bograd (✉)
Division of Thoracic Surgery, Swedish Medical Center, Seattle, WA, USA
e-mail: Adam.Bograd@swedish.org

T. Ng, T. Geraci (eds.), *Thoracic Surgery Clerkship*, Contemporary Surgical Clerkships, https://doi.org/10.1007/978-3-031-44645-0_37

Table 37.1 Most common benign and malignant chest wall tumors

Benign tumors	**Percentage (%)**
Fibrous dysplasia	40
Chondromas	15–20
Langerhans cell histiocytosis	10–20
Aneurysmal bone cyst	
Desmoid	
Malignant tumors	**Percentage (%)**
Chondrosarcomas	50
Solitary plasmacytomas	10–30
Ewing's sarcomas	8–22
Osteosarcomas	10–15
Lymphomas	10
Malignant fibrous histiocytoma	
Rhabdomyosarcoma	

Presentation

- Enlarging masses of varying growth velocity.
- Benign chest wall tumors tend to grow slower than malignant lesions.
- Most benign tumors are asymptomatic, but progress to becoming painful.
- May experience pain due to bone invasion and pathologic fractures or secondary to displacement or invasion of surrounding structures.
- Many are found incidentally on imaging obtained for other reasons.
- Patients may present with fever, weight loss, shortness of breath, neuropathy, night sweats, or even malaise; these systemic symptoms are typically less common.

Workup

- History and physical examination
  - It is important to know about any comorbidities and the patient's nutritional status, as well as history of prior malignancies, radiation, and thoracic operations, as all these factors must be considered when planning reconstructive options and subsequent healing.
- Imaging generally includes the following:
  - Chest radiograph (CXR).
  - CT scan: evaluate the primary chest wall tumor, assess for metastatic disease especially to the lung.

  - MRI: especially if the tumor is near vital structures such as the brachial plexus, spine, major vasculature, and heart.
  - PET scan may be required for staging purposes.
- Tissue diagnosis
  - Core needle biopsy can be attempted in all lesions but can consider performing excisional biopsy with 1–2 cm margins for lesions <5 cm.
  - For larger lesions, consider core needle biopsy or incisional biopsy if core is not diagnostic.
  - Care must be taken to ensure the biopsy does not compromise future definitive resection, as the biopsy tract will need to be resected en bloc with the tumor.
- Pulmonary function tests (PFTs) should be obtained as part of the workup of a chest wall mass, as most patients undergoing chest wall resection will have some degree of postoperative respiratory dysfunction.

Benign Tumors

Benign chest wall tumors may arise from any tissue of the chest wall. In general, even if imaging suggests a tumor is benign, it may still be necessary to establish a histologic diagnosis.

Chondroma (Fig. 37.1)

- Account for 15–20% of all benign chest wall tumors.
- These include enchondromas (benign bone tumor arising from the medulla) and osteochondromas (benign bone and cartilage tumor), with osteochondromas being more common in the first two decades of life.

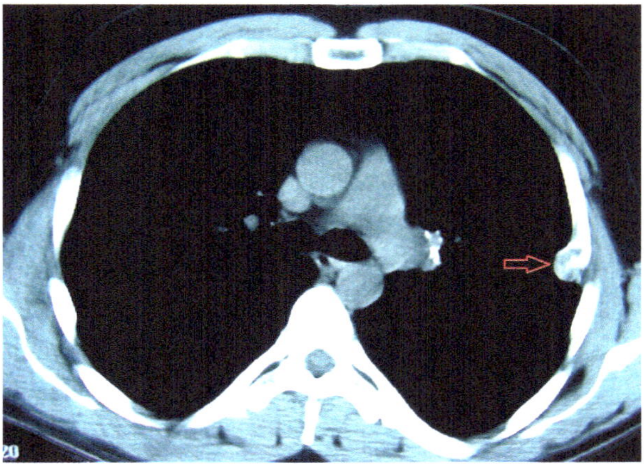

Fig. 37.1 CT scan of osteochondroma, showing a stalked bony protuberance arising from a rib (arrow)

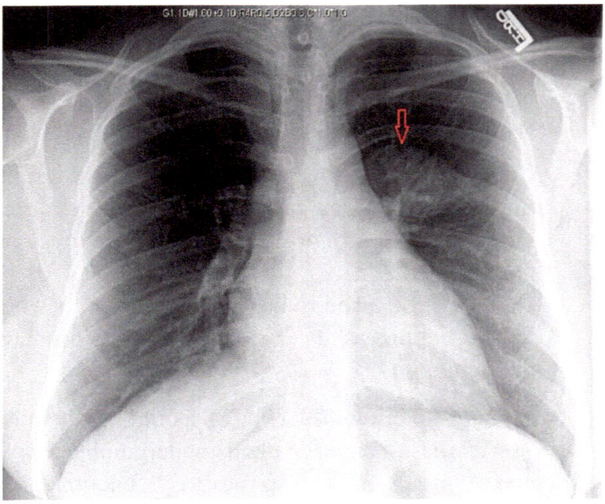

Fig. 37.2 Chest X-ray of fibrous dysplasia, showing an expansile lesion at the posterior aspect of a rib (arrow)

- Typically occur at the costochondral junction, painless, and can present as masses associated with rib fractures.
- Because their presentation, imaging, and biopsy are difficult to distinguish from that of low-grade malignant chondrosarcomas, and because of the possible risk of malignant degeneration, surgical resection is recommended.

Fibrous Dysplasia of the Bone (Fig. 37.2)

- Most common benign lesions in children and young adults.
- Thought to be a result of maturation defects and can be associated with trauma.
- Present as a painless, asymptomatic mass, most frequently in the lateral or posterior chest wall.
- On chest radiograph, it can appear as a fusiform, expanded ground-glass mass with cortical thickening of the posterior portion.
- If multiple lesions then consider the diagnosis of Albright's syndrome (skin pigmentation, precocious puberty, and other endocrinopathies).
- Treatment is resection if there is a question regarding diagnosis and for providing symptom relief, otherwise observation.
- If resection cannot be performed, bisphosphonates may be utilized.

Desmoid Tumor (Fig. 37.3)

- Develop from muscular aponeuroses; they contain sheets of fibroblasts with abundant collagen but lack a capsule.
- Although classified as benign and slow-growing, these tumors are locally aggressive, extending along tissue planes, and encase structures such as brachial plexus and vasculature.
- They recur frequently but do not metastasize (for this reason they are considered by some to be low-grade fibrosarcomas).
- More commonly in females (2:1 female-to-male predominance), in the third or fourth decades of life, at sites of prior scarring, and in people with familial adenomatous polyposis (FAP) syndrome.
- Present as a slow-growing, painful mass, fixed to deep, underlying tissues but not the skin, can be by neurovascular deficits.
- Management
  - Observation can be considered in asymptomatic lesions that are not growing.
  - Wide resection (2–4 cm margins) as these tumors spread along facial planes; re-resections for local recurrences are not uncommon with rates of recurrence ranging from 5 to 50%.
  - Radiation is considered for incomplete resections, unresectable tumors, or poor surgical candidates.
  - Systemic therapy (chemotherapy, radiation anti-inflammatory, hormonal and targeted therapy) for unresectable tumors or for poor surgical candidates.

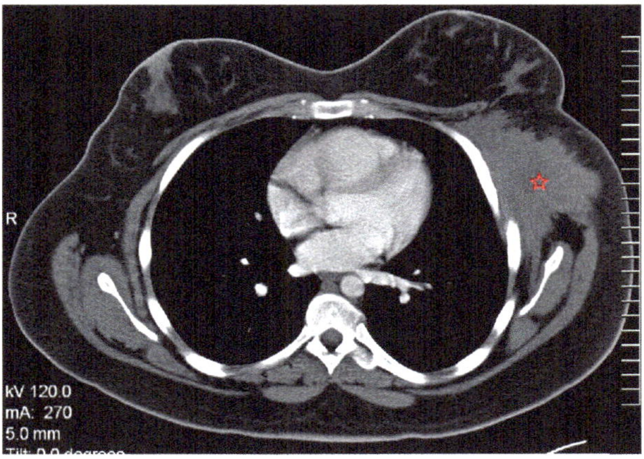

Fig. 37.3 CT scan of desmoid tumor, showing an infiltrative, locally invasive chest wall mass (star)

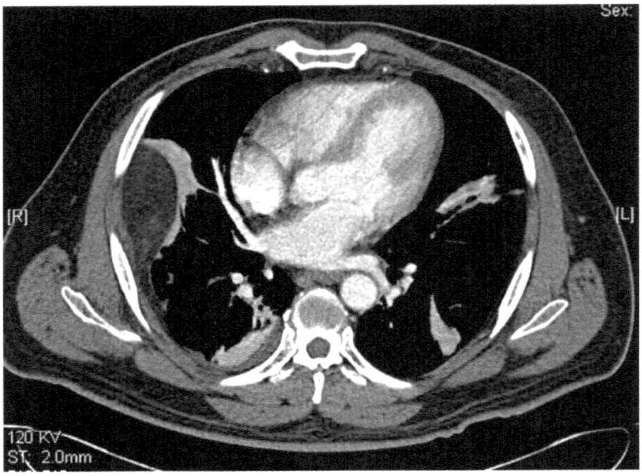

Fig. 37.4 CT scan of lipoma, showing a fat density subpleural mass

Eosinophilic Granulomas (Langerhans Cell Histiocytosis)

- Unknown etiology, controversy as to whether they are true tumors, but more an inflammatory cell infiltration.
- More commonly seen in men.
- May be solitary or multifocal.
- Can present with pain and fever; destructive lesion of ribs and sternum, thus can be confused with Ewing's sarcoma or osteomyelitis.
- Treatment is excisional biopsy for solitary lesions or radiation for multiple lesions.

Other Notable Benign Chest Wall Tumors

- Fibromas
- Lipomas (Fig. 37.4): subcutaneous, intramuscular, or extrapleural
- Neurogenic tumors: schwannomas, neurofibromas; arising from intercostal nerves and spinal nerve roots
- Lymphangiomas
- Aneurysmal bone cyst

Primary Malignant Tumors

Chondrosarcoma (Fig. 37.5a, b)

- Most common primary malignant chest wall tumor, accounting for 50%.
- Most originate from the costochondral junction (~80%), with the remainder arising from the sternum.
- May be seen in patients with a prior history of trauma.
- May progress from benign cartilage tumors.
- Most commonly presents in the third and fourth decades of life.
- Typical presentation is of a solitary, slowly enlarging, hard, fixed mass associated with pain.
- CT scan shows a well-defined lobulated mass with foci of dense chondroid matrix calcification; however, calcification can also be absent.
- 10% of patients will have synchronous lung metastases/evidence of metastases on imaging.
- Treatment is resection with wide margins of at least 4 cm; for high-grade lesions, consider resection of portions of normal rib above and below and the entire bone from which the tumor arises (such as sternum).
- Recurrence rates are around 10% in patients with negative margins and 75% in patients with positive resection margins.
- These tumors do not respond well to radiation or chemotherapy.

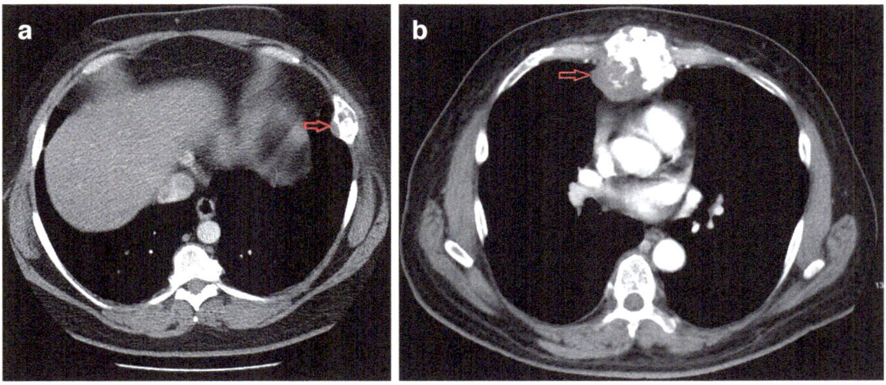

Fig. 37.5 CT scan of chondrosarcoma, showing a lobulated mass with dense chondroid matrix calcification (arrow). (**a**) Of rib; (**b**) of sternum

Solitary Plasmacytomas (Solitary Plasma Cell Tumor Myeloma)

- Accounts for 10–30% of chest wall malignancies.
- Occur in the elderly with a mean age of 60 years.
- Present with pain without obvious mass.
- Classic osteolytic appearance on chest radiograph.
- Originate from the ribs and sternum and generally progress to multiple myeloma with greater frequency than extraosseous plasmacytomas.
- As part of the workup, extra-thoracic lesions should be ruled out.
- Treatment of solitary plasmacytomas is radiation, surgical resection is rarely considered for refractory cases, and systemic chemotherapy is used for progression of disease.

Ewing's Sarcoma

- Originate from neural crest cells and are the most common malignant lesion of the ribs in children; they also account for 8–22% of malignant chest wall tumors in adults.
- Male predominance.
- Aggressive and can invade or displace adjacent structures.
- Present with a single or multiple masses, with one or more ribs being involved, present with metastasis to the lungs or bones.
- Painful and are commonly associated with fever and malaise.
- Workup often reveals leukocytosis and elevated ESR.
- The classic "onion peel" appearance on CXR is due to multiple layers of periosteal new bone formation.
- Treatment
  - Initially, with chemotherapy, followed by consideration for wide resection
  - Radiation considered in the adjuvant setting in patients with positive margins

Osteosarcoma

- 10–15% of chest wall malignant tumors.
- Affects both the young and the elderly.
- Can arise from preexisting bone lesions and previous radiation sites
- Occur most frequently in the ribs, scapulae, or clavicles.
- Present as painful, rapidly enlarging mass.
- Metastasis is common (to lung, bone, and liver).
- Elevated alkaline phosphatase levels.

- Classic CXR finding of "sunburst" pattern due to new periosteal bone formation.
- CT scan shows a large heterogeneous mass with necrosis, hemorrhage, or ossification.
- Treatment can be by resection followed by chemotherapy or neoadjuvant chemotherapy followed by wide surgical resection.
- Prognosis is predicted by the response to chemotherapy.
- Radiation is usually not effective.

Soft Tissue Sarcoma

- The most common soft tissue sarcomas are malignant fibrous histiocytoma (Fig. 37.6) and rhabdomyosarcoma.
- Other common tumors include liposarcomas, fibrosarcomas, leiomyosarcomas, angiosarcomas, malignant schwannomas, and neurofibrosarcomas.
- Certain genetic syndromes (von Recklinghausen's disease for neurofibrosarcoma) as well as a history of radiation therapy may predispose patients to the development of soft tissue sarcomas.
- Angiosarcomas are most commonly seen in elderly patients with a previous history of radiation (Fig. 37.7).
- MRI is useful in identifying infiltration and relation to adjacent vital structures.
- Treatment is generally with wide local resection.
- Both local recurrences and radiation-induced sarcomas are treated like an initial occurrence.
- The high recurrence rates following resection are due to the tendency to spread along fascial planes and between muscle fibers.
- Radiation is considered for patients with residual disease, inadequate margins, tumors >5 cm, and high-grade and highly invasive tumors.
- Chemotherapy is generally not effective (with exception for rhabdomyosarcoma).
- For soft tissue sarcoma, histologic grade is associated with prognosis.

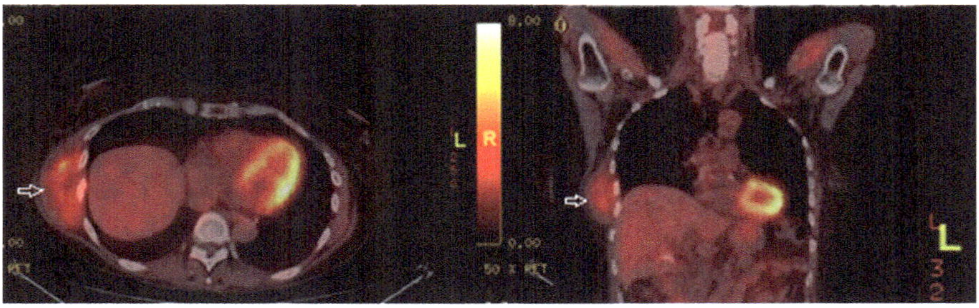

Fig. 37.6 PET/CT scan showing an avid chest wall mass of malignant fibrous histiocytoma (arrow)

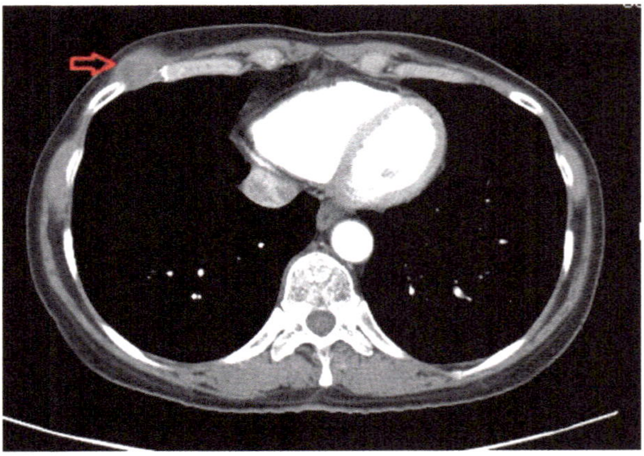

Fig. 37.7 CT scan of pleomorphic chest wall sarcoma (arrow) arising from prior radiation therapy for breast cancer

Lymphoma

- The most common chest wall lymphoma is diffuse large B-cell lymphoma.
- Treatment is generally with radiation and chemotherapy.

Surgical Treatment

- Multidisciplinary/multispecialty approach to management is essential.
- Surgical resection
  - As mentioned previously, most lesions are treated with resection, yet specific treatment nuances still exist.
  - Outcomes of resection of chest wall tumors are related to the extent of resection and the natural history of the underlying tumor.
  - 4 cm margins are preferred for high-grade or highly infiltrative tumors.
  - 1–2 cm margins are usually adequate for more benign processes/lower-grade malignancies.
  - One study analyzing survival in patients with primary malignant chest wall tumors found that 56% of patients remained recurrence-free at 5 years with 4 cm or greater resection margin versus 29% for those with 2 cm margins.
  - For tumors that invade a rib, resection of adjacent ribs may be indicated.
  - Invasion into adjacent structures such as overlying skin or underlying lung needs to be evaluated, and these structures should be resected with the mass en bloc.
- Reconstruction
  - Reconstruction of rigid chest wall

    Restoring skeletal stability helps support respiratory mechanics and minimize paradoxical motion during respiration, as well as protect underlying structures.

In general anterior/lateral defects >2 adjacent ribs or > 5 cm require rigid reconstruction.

Posterior defects >10 cm (as there is scapula coverage) or any size defect that allows the inferior tip of the scapula to fall into and become entrapped will require rigid reconstruction.

Materials used in rigid chest wall reconstruction include polytetrafluoroethylene/Gore-Tex (sewn "tight as a drum," Fig. 37.8), polypropylene/Marlex methyl methacrylate sandwich.

Avoid synthetic materials in the presence of active infection, devitalized tissue, necrosis, or contamination; defer rigid reconstruction to a later date.

- Skin/soft tissue reconstruction

  Muscle flap or myocutaneous flaps, with rotational/pedicle preferred over free flap:

  - Latissimus dorsi (Fig. 37.9a, b)
  - Rectus abdominis (Fig. 37.10a, b, c)
  - Pectoralis major
  - Serratus anterior
  - Trapezius

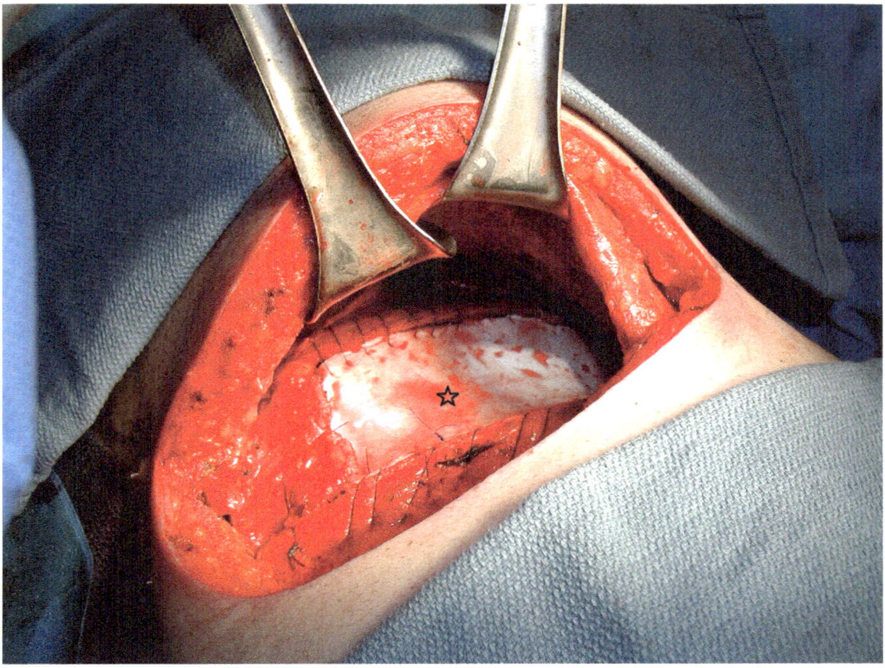

Fig. 37.8 Rigid chest wall reconstruction using polytetrafluoroethylene/Gore-Tex (star), sewn "tight as a drum"

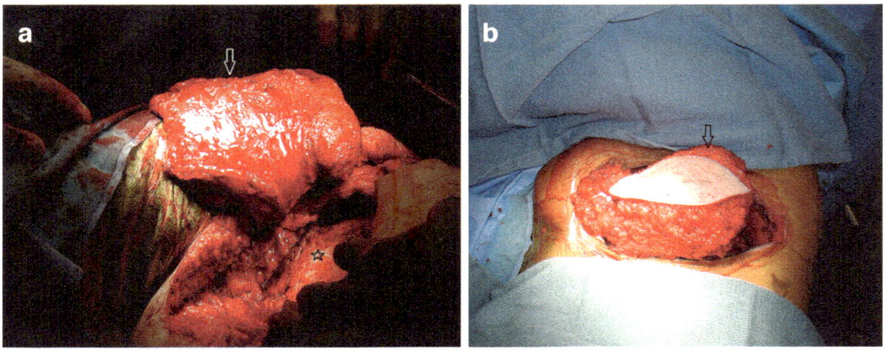

Fig. 37.9 Latissimus dorsi myocutaneous rotational flap (arrow) for soft tissue reconstruction, covering over the polytetrafluoroethylene/Gore-Tex (star) that was used for rigid chest wall reconstruction. (**a**) Flap harvest; (**b**) flap insetting

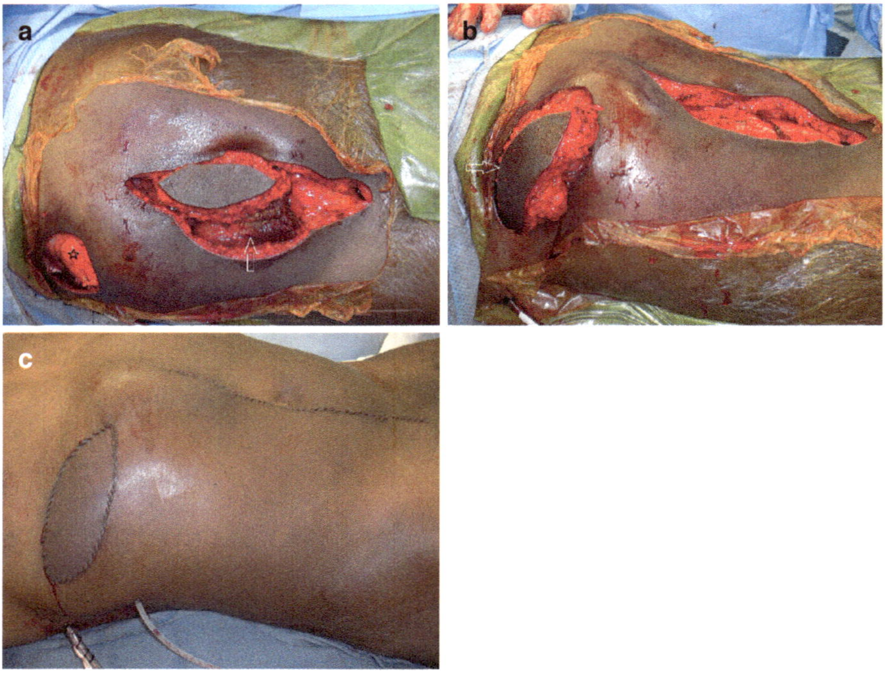

Fig. 37.10 Rectus abdominis myocutaneous rotational flap (arrow) for soft tissue reconstruction, covering over the polytetrafluoroethylene/Gore-Tex (star) that was used for rigid chest wall reconstruction. (**a**) Flap harvest; (**b**) flap insetting; (**c**) completion of flap insetting and wound closure

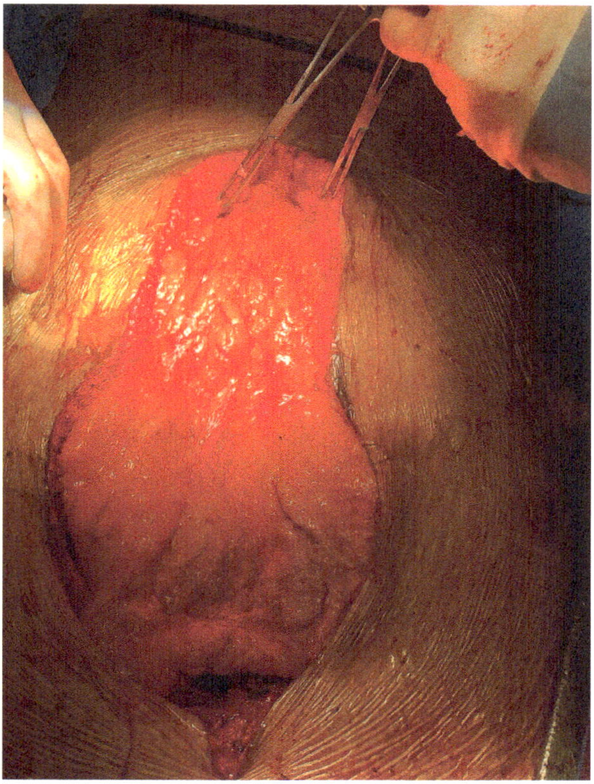

Fig. 37.11 Omental flap used for reconstruction of sternal defect after resection of sternal chondrosarcoma

Muscle flap coverage of prosthetic rigid chest wall reconstruction, beyond the skin and subcutaneous tissue, is vital in preventing infection of the prosthesis.

Omentum can be used for partial thickness reconstruction or as backup when a muscle flap is either not available or has failed previously (Fig. 37.11).

Bioprosthetic mesh such as acellular dermal matrix allows tissue ingrowth and becomes incorporated and revascularized with time; their role in chest wall reconstruction has not been clearly established.

The choice of flap is based on the location and size of defect, the condition of adjacent muscles, and the overall condition of the patient, as well as prior or possible future radiation.

Key Reference

- David EA, Marshall MB. Review of Chest Wall Tumors: A Diagnostic, Therapeutic, and Reconstructive Challenge. Seminars in Plastic Surgery [Internet]. 2011 Feb 1 [cited 2021 Mar 29];25(1):16–24.

Further Reading

Boyd A. Tumors of the chest wall. In: Hood RM, Antman K, Boyd A, et al., editors. Surgical diseases of pleura and Chest Wall. Philadelphia: WB Saunders; 1986.

Burt M, Fulton M, Wessner-Dunlap S, Karpeh M, Huvos AG, Bains MS, et al. Primary bony and cartilaginous sarcomas of chest wall: results of therapy. Ann Thorac Surg. 1992;54(2):226–32.

Clemens MW. UpToDate, Post TW, editors. Surgical management of chest wall tumors. Waltham, MA: UpToDate. (Accessed on June 11, 2022.)

Fong Y-C, Pairolero PC, Sim FH, Cha SS, Blanchard CL, Scully SP. Chondrosarcoma of the Chest Wall. Clin Orthop Relat Res. 2004;427:184–9.

Gordon MS, Hajdu SI, Bains MS, Burt ME. Soft tissue sarcomas of the chest wall. J Thorac Cardiovasc Surg. 1991;101(5):843–54.

Graeber GM, Snyder RJ, Fleming AW, Head HD, Lough FC, Parker JS, et al. Initial and long-term results in the management of primary chest wall neoplasms. Ann Thorac Surg. 1982;34(6):664–73.

Incarbone MDM, Pastorino MDU. Surgical treatment of chest wall tumors. World J Surg. 2001;25(2):218–30.

Ingley KM, Burtenshaw SM, Theobalds NC, White LM, Blackstein ME, Gladdy RA, et al. Clinical benefit of methotrexate plus vinorelbine chemotherapy for desmoid fibromatosis (DF) and correlation of treatment response with MRI. Cancer Med. 2019;8(11):5047–57.

Javaid MK, Boyce A, Appelman-Dijkstra N, Ong J, Defabianis P, Offiah A, et al. Best practice management guidelines for fibrous dysplasia/McCune-Albright syndrome: a consensus statement from the FD/MAS international consortium. Orphanet J Rare Dis. 2019;14:1.

King RM, Pairolero PC, Trastek VF, Piehler JM, Payne WS, Bernatz PE. Primary chest wall tumors: factors affecting survival. Ann Thorac Surg. 1986;41(6):597–601.

McAfee MK, Pairolero PC, Bergstralh EJ, Piehler JM, Unni KK, McLeod RA, et al. Chondrosarcoma of the chest wall: factors affecting survival. Ann Thorac Surg. 1985;40(6):535–41.

McKinnon JG, Neifeld JP, Kay S, et al. Management of desmoid tumors. Surg Gynecol Obstet. 1989;169(2):104–6.

Park BJ, Flores RM. Chest wall tumors. In: Shields TW, LoCicero J, Reed CE, Feins RH, editors. General thoracic surgery. Philadelphia: Lippincott Williams & Wilkins; 2009.

Pass HI. Primary and metastatic chest wall tumors. In: Roth JA, Ruckdeschel JC, Weisenburger TH, editors. Thoracic oncology. Philadelphia: WB Saunders; 1989.

Posner MC. The desmoid tumor. Arch Surg. 1989;124(2):191.

le Roux BT, Shama DM. Resection of tumors of the chest wall. Curr Probl Surg. 1983;20(6):345–86.

Sabanathan S. Surgical treatment of primary malignant chest wall tumours. Eur J Cardiothorac Surg. 1997;11(6):1011–6.

Sabanathan S, Salama FD, Morgan WE, Harvey JA. Primary chest wall tumors. Ann Thorac Surg. 1985;39(1):4–15.

Schwarz RE, Burt M. Radiation-associated malignant tumors of the chest wall. Ann Surg Oncol. 1996;3(4):387–92.

Shamberger RC, Grier HE, Weinstein HJ, Perez-Atayde AR, Tarbell NJ. Chest wall tumors in infancy and childhood. Cancer. 1989;63(4):774–85.

Sherman NE, Romsdahl M, Evans H, Zagars G, Oswald MJ. Desmoid Tumors: a 20-year radiotherapy experience. Int J Radiat Oncol Biol Phys. 1990;19(1):37–40.

Somers J, Faber LP. Chondroma and chondrosarcoma. Semin Thorac Cardiovasc Surg. 1999;11(3):270–7.

Stock CT Jr, Uy KF, Graeber GM. Neoplasms of the chest wall. In: Darling GE, Baumgartner WA, Jacobs JP, editors. Pearson's general thoracic surgery. STS cardiothoracic surgery E-book. Chicago: Society of Thoracic Surgeons; 2020. ebook.sts.org. Accessed June 11, 2022.

Tateishi U, Gladish GW, Kusumoto M, Hasegawa T, Yokoyama R, Tsuchiya R, et al. Chest wall tumors: radiologic findings and pathologic correlation. Radiographics. 2003;23(6):1477–90.
Tomo H, Ito Y, Aono M, Takaoka K. Chest wall deformity associated with osteochondroma of the scapula: a case report and review of the literature. J Shoulder Elb Surg. 2005;14(1):103–6.
Widhe B, Bauer HCF. Surgical treatment is decisive for outcome in chondrosarcoma of the chest wall: a population-based Scandinavian sarcoma group study of 106 patients. J Thorac Cardiovasc Surg. 2009;137(3):610–4.
Winkler K, Beron G, Kotz R, Salzer-Kuntschik M, Beck J, Beck W, et al. Neoadjuvant chemotherapy for osteogenic sarcoma: results of a cooperative German/Austrian study. J Clin Oncol. 1984;2(6):617–24.

Chapter 38
Chest Wall Deformities

Christina Bi and Travis Geraci

Chest Wall Deformities

Chest wall deformities are congenital abnormalities in the development of the musculoskeletal and/or cartilaginous structures of the chest wall, most commonly the anterior portion, including the sternum.

- **Pectus excavatum**, also referred to as "funnel chest," is a deformity of the anterior chest wall, characterized by central depression of the sternum.
- **Pectus carinatum** is an abnormal elevation of the sternum above the normal curvature of the anterior chest.
- **Poland syndrome** is a deformity involving the partial or complete absence of the pectoralis major and minor muscles. May have hypoplastic or absent breast tissue.
- **Sternal cleft** results from a failure of fusion of the sternum during embryogenesis, resulting in an abnormal opening in the central, anterior chest.

Pectus Excavatum

Pectus excavatum is a posterior depression of the sternum relative to the normal curvature of the anterior chest wall.

C. Bi
Grossman School of Medicine, New York University Langone Health, New York, NY, USA
e-mail: christina.bi@nyulangone.org

T. Geraci (✉)
Division of Thoracic Surgery, Department of Cardiothoracic Surgery, New York University Langone Health, New York, NY, USA
e-mail: travis.geraci@nyulangone.org

T. Ng, T. Geraci (eds.), *Thoracic Surgery Clerkship*, Contemporary Surgical Clerkships, https://doi.org/10.1007/978-3-031-44645-0_38

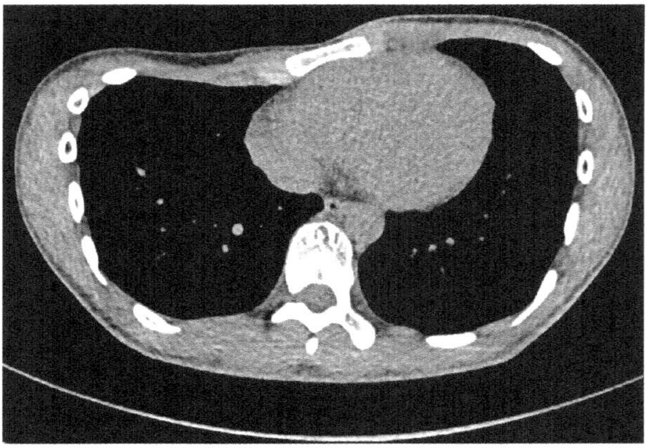

Fig. 38.1 Axial CT image demonstrating Pectus excavatum with greater right-ward defect and rotation with mild left-ward displacement of the heart

- Severity of sternal depression varies and is often asymmetric with a greater deflection or rotation of the right chest with consequent leftward deviation of the heart (Fig. 38.1).
- The associated costal cartilages have a posterior curvature.
- Most commonly involves the middle to lower sternum, preserving the manubrium and first and second ribs.
- Most common congenital chest wall deformity (1 in 400–1000 births).
- There is no decisive embryological pathoetiology of pectus excavatum, but the predominant theories center on abnormalities of the structural tissues and/or abnormal mechanical stress during fetal growth.
  - Excessive and/or abnormal growth of the costal cartilages.
  - Abnormal connective tissues.
  - One theory implicates abnormal in utero diaphragmatic development and abnormal embryonic positioning.

Presentation and Workup

- There is a large range of clinical presentations, in terms of both the visual severity of the deformity and attributed symptoms, most of which are related to the decreased anteroposterior diameter of the chest.
- Computed tomography scan of the chest is used to characterize the anatomy of the defect and determine the severity and relationship of the internal organs of the chest.
- Symptomatic patients report dyspnea, exercise intolerance, chest pain, or palpitations. Untreated patients may become gradually more symptomatic with age due to an increase in skeletal rigidity.

- The cosmetic abnormality of the deformity may cause psychological stress and/or anxiety. Of note, there is only a weak correlation between the severity of the defect and concern regarding its appearance.
- More common in males.
- May have a family history of the deformity.
- Associated with other musculoskeletal abnormalities (such as scoliosis), congenital heart defects, and connective tissue disorders.

Cardiopulmonary Morbidity

- There is controversy as to whether pectus excavatum causes cardiopulmonary impairment.
- As a result of a reduced and abnormal structure of the chest, patients have a decrease in vital capacity and respiratory reserve.
- The depressed sternum may compress the anterior wall of the right ventricle, decreasing stroke volume and cardiac output. The compression may also occur at the level of the tricuspid valve or result in a displacement of the heart to the left.
- There is an elevated incidence of mitral valve prolapse in pectus excavatum patients (10–15%). It is unknown whether mitral valve prolapse is related to tissue abnormalities rather than mechanical cardiac compression alone.
- Pectus excavatum patients also have an increased incidence of conditions causing arrhythmias, including first-degree heart block, right bundle branch block, and Wolff-Parkinson-White syndrome.

Physical Exam

- General appearance: the most common phenotype is tall stature with a narrow chest, sloped ribs, and rounded shoulders. The abdomen may be relatively protuberant.
- Patients often have a clearly apparent sternal depression on physical exam.
- Rare associated thoracic abnormalities: scoliosis, kyphosis.
- Cardiac exam: resting tachycardia and/or functional systolic murmurs (20%).
- Pulmonary exam: tachypnea.
- Measurements of the depth or deformity compared to chest width, or lateral height at the midclavicular lines, can be performed, but there are no standards or guidelines for these values.

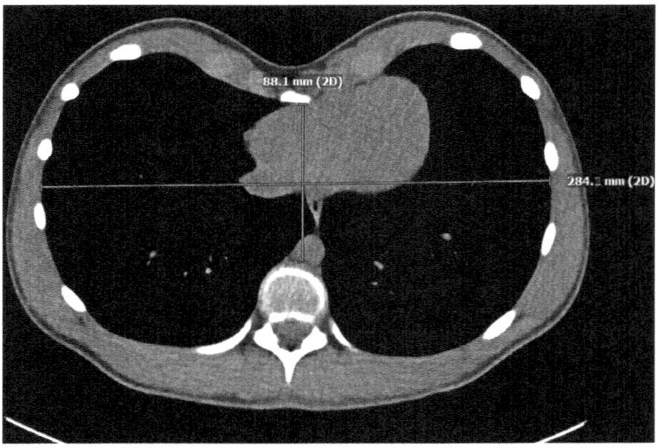

Fig. 38.2 Axial CT image of the chest, demonstrating pectus excavatum. The calculated Haller index is 3.2 based on the transverse diameter and apicoposterior measurements (calculations shown)

Pectus/Haller Index

- Haller index
  - Most common method for determining the severity or grade of the pectus deformity. Of note, the index is not a strict guideline for intervention, but a tool to help quantify the severity of deformity.
  - Ratio of the maximal transverse diameter to the anterior/posterior measurement at the point of deepest depression (Fig. 38.2, Haller index of 3.2).
  - A normal Haller index is 2.5 or less; therefore, a ratio greater than 2.5 is generally considered diagnostic of pectus excavatum. However, the anatomy of the thorax and its dimensions vary depending on age and sex, which must be considered.
  - Classically, a Haller index of 3.25 is considered a severe defect and has been used to recommend surgical correction.
- The Pectus Correction Index
  - An alternative method that accounts for the maximum anterior prominence of the chest.
  - Calculated as the fraction of the difference between corrected anterior/posterior distance and the actual anterior/posterior distance at the deepest depression to the corrected anterior/posterior distance x100%.
  - Correction index of 28% or greater correlates with classic Haller index of 3.25 or greater.

Treatment and Outcomes

Pectus excavatum is of variable severity and therefore does not have a uniform management.

- Exercise and posture programs are recommended for mild-to-moderate defects with the aim of optimizing cardiopulmonary function and improving posture to increase chest wall expansion.
- Candidates for surgical treatment include patients with cosmetic concerns/psychological distress, a high degree of deformity (Haller index >3.25), symptoms including exercise intolerance, abnormal cardiopulmonary function testing, and recurrence after failed repair.
- It is preferable to perform a surgical repair during adolescence, when the thoracic skeleton is malleable, tissues continue to mature, and recovery is faster.
- Surgical repair improves cosmesis of the chest wall but has an undetermined benefit regarding cardiopulmonary function.
  - A meta-analysis of surgical outcomes reported symptomatic improvement, but a decrease in pulmonary function over time, theorized as a loss of chest wall compliance.
  - Cardiac function improves postsurgical repair with shifting of the displaced heart towards the midline.
  - Exercise intolerance does not appear to improve after surgical correction.

Surgical Repair

- The surgical approach is dependent on cardiopulmonary morbidity, cosmetic concerns, and surgical experience/expertise.
- The Ravitch procedure and the Nuss procedure are the two most common surgical repairs for pectus excavatum; however, a number of alternative interventions have been described.
  - The majority of centers performing pectus repair perform the Nuss procedure.
  - There are limited comparisons between the Ravitch and Nuss procedures, but meta-analysis data suggest limited differences in clinical outcomes, albeit a higher rate of reintervention in patients undergoing the Nuss procedure due to bar displacement.

Ravitch Procedure (Also Referred to as Open Repair)

- Surgical technique
  - A midline incision over the sternum is made and the pectoralis major muscles reflected. Parasternal subperichondrial resection of the costal cartilages is performed along the deformed portion (typically cartilages 3–7). A transverse, anterior sternal wedge osteotomy is performed, and the sternum is elevated.

- In addition, select surgeons will place a metal bar or strut beneath the sternum to maintain its shape and structure, which is removed 6 months to a year after surgery.

- A modification to the traditional Ravitch procedure, involves a limited cartilage resection with reduced tissue removal of the parasternal and costal cartilages.
- Complications of the Ravitch procedure: reoperation, pneumothorax, hemothorax, and phrenic nerve injury.

Nuss Procedure (Also Referred to as Minimally Invasive Repair)

- Surgical technique
  - Bilateral incisions are made at the midaxillary line of the chest at the deepest depression of the sternum. Thoracoscopically, a curved metal pectus (Nuss) bar is placed behind the sternum at the deepest point of the depression, with the convexity positioned posteriorly. The bar is then rotated 180 degrees such that the convexity is positioned anteriorly, forcing the sternum anteriorly.
  - Select patients require placement of an additional Nuss bar (Fig. 38.3), distributing tension over a wider anatomy, thus allowing correction of a longer portion of the sternum, and limiting "bowing" of the chest over a single sternal bar.
  - The bar is removed after 3 years as the chest wall remodels. Duration is dependent on growth and patient tolerance.

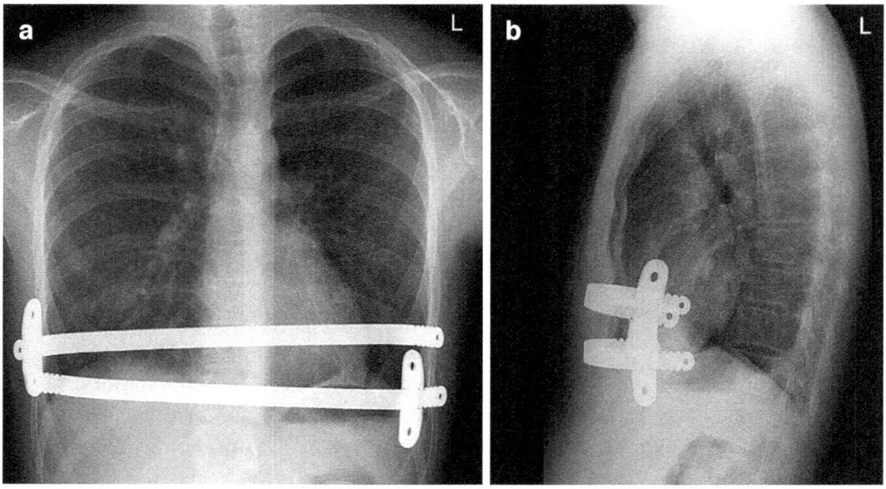

Fig. 38.3 Chest radiograph of a double Nuss bar in place. (**a**) Anteroposterior; (**b**) lateral

- This technique requires no cartilage or sternal resection.
- Assess for metal allergy prior to placing the bar as allergic reactions have been reported.
- Complications of the Nuss procedure: cardiac perforation (rare, but often fatal), pericardial effusion, pneumothorax, hemothorax, reoperation, and bar displacement.
  - Postoperative pain: the Nuss procedure is associated with postoperative pain that complicates the immediate postoperative course and may become chronic, limiting the duration before bar removal. Efforts to reduce pain include epidural and intravenous methods of analgesia as well as intercostal nerve cryoablation.

Alternative Interventions

- **Silicone implants**: customized silicone prosthesis offers a purely cosmetic improvement of the deformity.
  - Implants are placed in a minimally invasive fashion and are safe, effective, and long-lasting.
  - Option for asymptomatic patients with only mild sternal depressions.
  - May need to be removed after two to three decades due to calcifications.
- **Autologous tissue**: autologous cartilage grafts harvested from resection of costal cartilages. Grafts are cut into small chips, wrapped in bioabsorbable hemostyptic and antimicrobial fabric, and placed into a subcutaneous pocket in the sternal depression, where it can be easily contoured.
  - In contrast to silicone implants, autologous implants can be lifelong.
- **Vacuum bell procedure**: application of tension/suction to the sternal depression of the anterior chest using suction cup or vacuum bell.
- **Magnetic mini-mover procedure**: a magnet is implanted into the sternum, with another magnet on an external brace. Daily use of the brace over a prolonged period is designed to move the sternum outwardly into a more normal position.

Pectus Carinatum

Pectus carinatum is an anterior protrusion of the sternum relative to the normal curvature of the anterior chest wall (Fig. 38.4).

- Typically involves the middle and lower sternum and associated costal cartilages. Rarely can involve the entire sternum and manubrium.

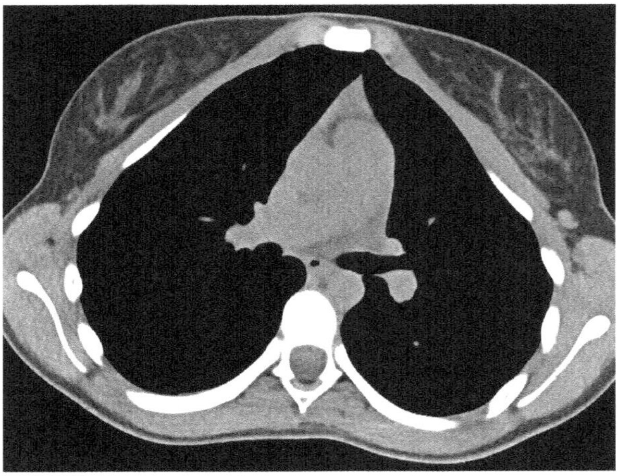

Fig. 38.4 Axial CT image of a pectus carinatum deformity

- Occurs much less frequently than pectus excavatum, constituting 10% of all chest wall deformities.
- More common in males than females (4:1) with approximately 30% reporting a family history.
- Symptoms are uncommon, but may become apparent or more severe with growth in adolescence, such as dyspnea, exercise intolerance, and psychological distress from the cosmetic abnormality.

Treatment

- Surgical correction is the primary form of treatment for patients with pectus carinatum.
- For patients with a mild-moderate deformity, bracing is offered as a nonoperative intervention.
- The surgical technique involves a modified Ravitch repair with resection of the associated costal cartilages and downward displacement of the sternum.

Poland Syndrome

Poland syndrome is a congenital chest wall deformity involving the partial or complete absence of the pectoralis major and minor muscles.

- Associated with finger abnormalities such as syndactyly (fused fingers) or brachydactyly (hypoplasia) and abnormalities of the ribs and/or breast tissue (hypoplasia or complete absence of breast).

- Rare deformity (approximately 1 in 30,000 births), more common in females.
- Pathoetiology is not well understood.

Sternal Clefts

Sternal Clefts are rare congenital fusion defects involving the sternum that result in an abnormal opening in the central, anterior chest. Sternal clefts are often associated with other thoracic anatomic abnormalities.

- **Sternal cleft**: failure of fusion of the manubrium and upper sternum, resulting in a V-shaped opening or absence in the bony structure of the chest. The remaining skin, soft tissues, and solid organs are normal.
- **Ectopia cordis**: a sternal cleft involving the inferior sternum. Associated with abnormalities of the diaphragm and/or pericardium and cardiac anomalies.
- **Thoracic ectopia cordis**: sternal cleft defect with an extra-thoracic displacement of the heart.
- **Pentalogy of Cantrell**: inferior sternal cleft, anterior diaphragmatic defect, absence of pericardium, omphalocele, and cardiac abnormalities.

Thoracic Outlet Syndrome

Thoracic outlet syndrome (TOS) involves compression of the neurovascular structure(s) of the upper extremity, resulting in a varied presentation depending on the affected anatomy.

- There are three types of TOS based on which structure is compressed in the thoracic outlet: neurogenic TOS (brachial plexus), venous TOS (subclavian vein), and arterial TOS (subclavian artery).
- The most common mechanism involves compression against the first rib, but may also involve muscles of the thoracic outlet, including the anterior scalene.
- A cervical rib may be present in a minority of patients (2–5%).

Neurogenic TOS

Progressive and debilitating condition of upper extremity pain and paresthesias caused by dynamic compression of the brachial plexus at the thoracic outlet.

- Most common type of TOS, approximately 90% of all cases
- Presents with pain, paresthesias, and dysfunction of the affected upper extremity, commonly in an ulnar nerve distribution

- Risk factors: repetitive motion of the upper extremity, such as musicians, assembly-line workers, and athletes
- Diagnosis
  - Generally, there is a lack of well-defined diagnostic criteria or tests. Neurogenic TOS is a clinical diagnosis, elicited by exam findings in the setting of an appropriate history/symptoms.
  - Provocative tests include the Adson test, costoclavicular test, the Roos test, and the Wright test.
  - Rule-out tests/conditions

    Neurogenic pectoralis minor syndrome involves the compression of the brachial plexus in the retropectoral space but may present similarly to neurogenic TOS.
    Cervical spine magnetic resonance imaging (MRI) to evaluate for spinal radiculopathy.
    Electromyography to evaluate for ulnar nerve entrapment and carpal tunnel syndrome.
    Vascular ultrasounds are obtained if there are elements of arterial or venous TOS.
    Superior sulcus lung cancer presenting with Pancoast syndrome (severe arm and shoulder pain, Horner's syndrome, and atrophy of the small muscles of the hand) must be ruled out, as symptoms may overlap those of TOS.

- Management
  - Physical therapy with ergonomic modifications and pain management is the first-line treatment for neurogenic TOS.

    The objective is to release the pressure/tension between the clavicle and first rib.
    A number of patients, however, will not be able to tolerate therapy due to symptom exacerbation.

  - Botulinum toxin injection into the anterior scalene muscle may reduce symptoms.
  - First-rib resection with scalenectomy or scalenotomy.

    Indicated for severely symptomatic patients or patients that fail to improve or recur after physical therapy.
    Complete resection of the posterior first rib to the level of the transverse process is necessary to achieve optimal results.
    Common approaches include supraclavicular, transaxillary, thoracoscopic, and robotic (Fig. 38.5).
    A long stump of residual posterior rib is associated with recurrence of neurogenic TOS.

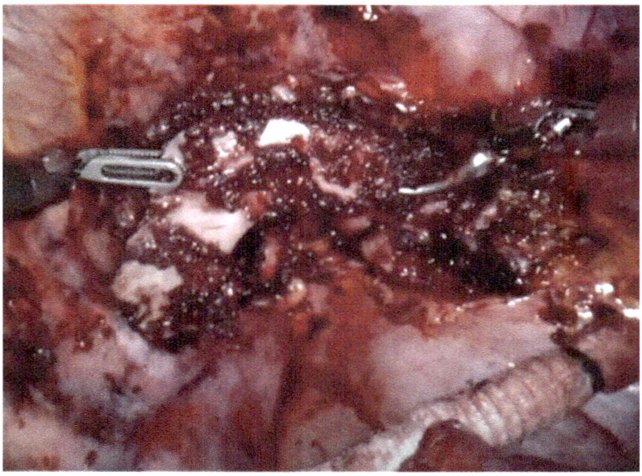

Fig. 38.5 Intraoperative view of a robotic first-rib resection. The robotic instruments are holding a portion of the first rib, which has been removed. Note that the subclavian artery and vein (and brachial plexus), which course beneath the rib, must be preserved without injury

Venous TOS

Tissue swelling and pain from compression of the subclavian vein in the costoclavicular space between the clavicle and first rib.

- Most patients have a congenital abnormality in which the costoclavicular ligament inserts further lateral than normal, predisposing to compression with hypertrophy of the scalene muscles from repetitive motion.
- Thrombosis is commonly caused by trauma and/or excessive repetitive use of the affected extremity.
- Paget-Schroetter syndrome: venous TOS with acute axillo-subclavian vein thrombosis (referred to as "effort thrombosis") after repetitive use of the upper extremity.
  - Most common after repetitive downward motion at the shoulder, such as in baseball pitchers.
- Patients present with a diffusely swollen, discolored, painful upper extremity.
- Diagnosis is established by clinical presentation/history and radiographic imaging, including vascular ultrasound and CT angiography, and venography (may be difficult to obtain in a severely swollen extremity).
- Treatment
  - Catheter-directed thrombolysis or thrombectomy

    May be used as an initial intervention; however, its overall utility is debated as at least half of patients will have continued symptoms and/or recurrence. Best suited for resolving an acute venous thrombosis.
  - First-rib resection with resection of the costoclavicular ligament medially and the anterior scalene muscle laterally

Anticoagulation is required in the postoperative period for patients presenting with thrombosis.

– Venous reconstruction if necessary

Arterial TOS

Upper extremity pain, pulselessness, claudication, paralysis, or digit ischemia from thromboembolism attributed to compression of the subclavian artery at the scalene triangle of the thoracic outlet.

- Least common form of TOS (less than 1%), but most severe symptoms.
- Dynamic obstruction of the subclavian artery between the anterior scalene and a bony structure, most commonly a cervical rib or protuberant transverse process at the C7 level, may be accompanied by post-stenosis aneurysm.
- Diagnosis is established by clinical presentation/history and radiographic imaging, including vascular ultrasound and CT angiography.
- Treatment
  - First (and cervical if present) rib resection.
  - Thrombosis of the subclavian artery or patients with distal thromboembolism should undergo first-rib resection with thrombectomy/embolectomy and arterial reconstruction or bypass.

Key Reference

- Kelly RE Jr. Pectus excavatum: historical background, clinical picture, preoperative evaluation and criteria for operation. Semin Pediatr Surg. 2008;17(3):181–93.

Further Reading

Burt BM, Palivela N, Goodman MB. Transthoracic robotic first rib resection: technique crystallized. Ann Thorac Surg. 2020;110(1):e71–3.

Costantino CL, Schumacher LY. Surgical technique: minimally invasive first-rib resection. Thorac Surg Clin. 2021;31(1):81–7.

Huddleston CB. Pectus excavatum. Semin Thorac Cardiovasc Surg. 16(3):225–32.

Johnson JN, Hartman TK, Pianosi PT, Driscoll DJ. Cardiorespiratory function after operation for pectus excavatum. J Pediatr. 2008;153(3):359–64.

Kelly RE Jr, Shamberger RC, Mellins RB, et al. Prospective multicenter study of surgical correction of pectus excavatum: design, perioperative complications, pain, and baseline pulmonary function facilitated by internet-based data collection. J Am Coll Surg. 2007;205(2):205–16.

Kolvekar SK, Panagiotopoulos N. Pectus excavatum. In: Kolvekar S, Pilegaard H, editors. Chest wall deformities and corrective procedures. Cham: Springer; 2015. https://ebookcentral.proquest.com/lib/nyulibrary-ebooks/detail.action?docID=4189326. Accessed May 20, 2022.

Kuhn JE, Lebus VGF, Bible JE. Thoracic outlet syndrome. J Am Acad Orthop Surg. 2015;23(4):222–32.

Malek MH, Berger DE, Marelich WD, Coburn JW, Beck TW, Housh TJ. Pulmonary function following surgical repair of pectus excavatum: a meta-analysis. Eur J Cardiothorac Surg. 2006;30(4):637–43.

Nuss D, Obermeyer RJ, Kelly RE. Nuss bar procedure: past, present and future. Ann Cardiothorac Surg. 2016;5(5):422–33.

Panda N, Donahue DM. Evaluation of patients with neurogenic thoracic outlet syndrome. Thorac Surg Clin. 2021;31(1):55–9.

Saxena AK. Overview of repair of pectus excavatum type of deformities. In: Saexna AK, editor. Chest Wall deformities. Berlin: Springer; 2017. https://ebookcentral.proquest.com/lib/nyulibrary-ebooks/detail.action?docID=4873433. Accessed April 15, 2022.

Sujka JA, St Peter SD. Quantification of pectus excavatum: anatomic indices. Semin Pediatr Surg. 2018;27(3):122–6.

Chapter 39
Thymic Disorders and Malignancies

Camille C. Yongue, Travis Geraci, and Robert Cerfolio

The Thymus Gland

- The thymus gland is a lymphatic organ with an important role in the development and maturation of the immune system during childhood.
- Over time, the thymus gland involutes and is replaced by adipose tissue; however, the thymus gland often does not disappear completely.
- The thymus gland is in the anterior-superior mediastinum, situated anterior to the pericardium, across the innominate vein, at the base of the ascending aorta.
  - The anterior-superior mediastinum is the compartment anterior to the pericardium, beneath the sternum.
  - The superior mediastinum extends from the thoracic inlet to a theoretical plane from the sternal angle to the junction of T4 and T5.
- The thymus contains all three embryonic germ cell layers and is variable in its relative size and shape (Fig. 39.1).

C. C. Yongue · T. Geraci (✉) · R. Cerfolio
Division of Thoracic Surgery, Department of Cardiothoracic Surgery, New York University Langone Health, New York, NY, USA
e-mail: camille.yongue@nyulangone.org; robert.cerfolio@nyulangone.org; travis.geraci@nyulangone.org

T. Ng, T. Geraci (eds.), *Thoracic Surgery Clerkship*, Contemporary Surgical Clerkships, https://doi.org/10.1007/978-3-031-44645-0_39

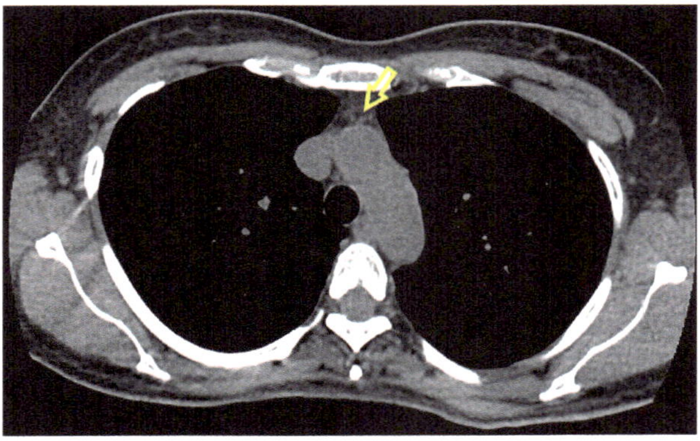

Fig. 39.1 Axial computer tomography scan (CT) image demonstrating a normal thymus gland (arrow) in the anterior mediastinum

Thymic Pathology

- Diseases of the thymus gland manifest in the prevascular mediastinal space, also referred to as the anterior and superior compartments.
- Thymic epithelial tumors include thymoma (the most frequent mediastinal lesion in adults) and thymic carcinoma.
- The majority of thymic lesions are asymptomatic, although they may compress or invade adjacent structures leading to symptoms, such as pain, dyspnea, cough, or swelling of the face and upper extremities.
- A broad differential diagnosis must be maintained during the workup of a mediastinal mass, including thymic lesions, which have a number of pathologies that overlap in presentation and appearance on imaging.

Thymic Hyperplasia

- There are two distinct types of thymic hyperplasia: true cellular hyperplasia and lymphoid (follicular) hyperplasia.
  - Hyperplasia may be a response to physiologic stress, such as surgery, chemotherapy, radiation, burns, or steroid use.
  - Lymphoid hyperplasia is associated with autoimmune diseases, such as myasthenia gravis.
- Thymic hyperplasia appears as a symmetric, diffuse enlargement of the thymus gland on CT imaging (Fig. 39.2).
  - It is often challenging to differentiate hyperplasia from a normal thymus gland and/or thymoma.
  - Magnetic resonance imaging (MRI) may help determine hyperplasia from other pathologies, revealing normal, homogenous, infiltrating fat rather than tumor.

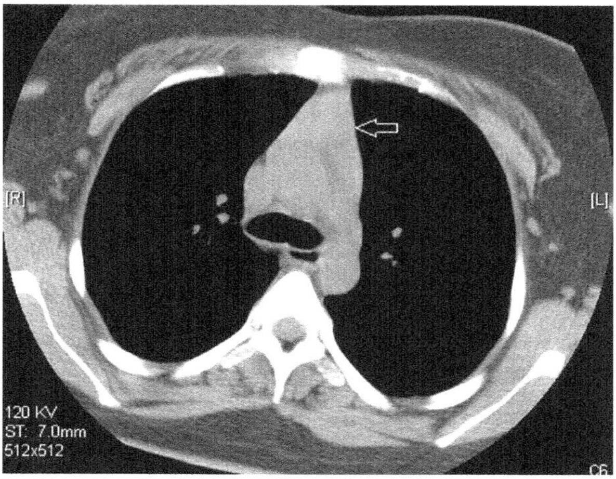

Fig. 39.2 CT scan of thymic hyperplasia in a patient with Graves' disease, the hyperplastic thymus retains its relative concave triangular shape

- Patients with thymic hyperplasia do not require surgical resection.
  - Selective patients may undergo surgery if there is a diagnostic uncertainty.
  - On occasion patients with suspected thymoma may undergo surgical resection and ultimately are found on surgical pathology to have thymic hyperplasia, not thymoma.

Thymic Neoplasms

- **Thymic cysts**
  - Thymic cysts are benign growths that are typically filled with simple serous fluid.
  - On CT they appear as a well-circumscribed uniform-fluid-density lesion (Fig. 39.3).
  - If the lesion is not well defined by CT, MRI may be helpful to define the cystic nature of the lesion with a bright signal on a T2-weighted image.
  - Pure cysts may be observed; however, lesions with septations or soft tissue components, those with growth or compressive symptoms, warrant resection to exclude other diagnoses such as cystic thymoma (Fig. 39.4) or teratoma.
- **Thymolipoma**
  - Thymolipomas are benign hamartomatous tumors of the thymus gland that consist of mature adipose tissue surrounding islands of thymic tissue.
  - Thymolipomas account for less than 10% of all thymic pathologies and can occur in patients of any age.
  - Most thymolipomas are asymptomatic and discovered incidentally, though they tend to be large at the time of diagnosis.

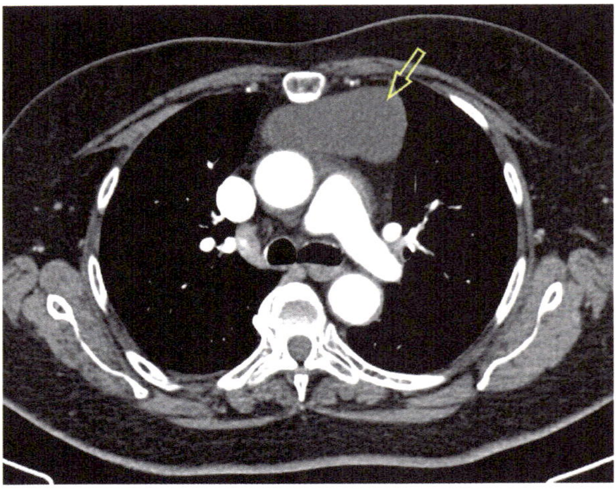

Fig. 39.3 Axial CT image demonstrating an 8 cm fluid density in the anterior mediastinum (arrow), representative of a benign thymic cyst

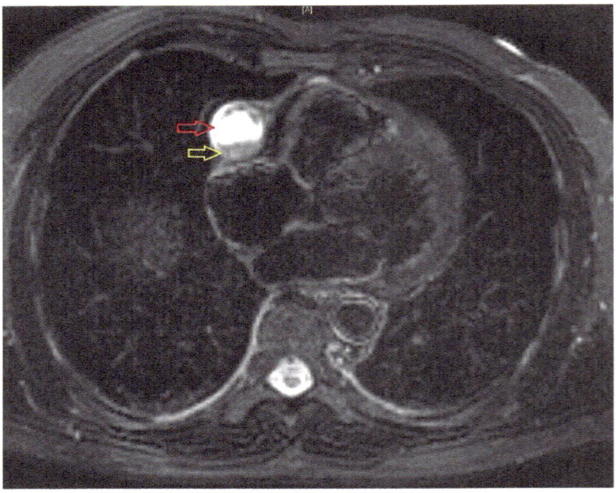

Fig. 39.4 MRI showing a lesion which is not purely cystic, with cystic (bright on T2-weighed image, red arrow) and solid (yellow arrow) components. This was a cystic thymoma

- Unlike thymomas, thymolipomas are only weakly associated with myasthenia gravis and have a stronger association with aplastic anemia, Graves' disease, and Hodgkin lymphoma.
- Large tumors compressing mediastinal structures may require surgical resection.
- Surgical resection may improve associated autoimmune disease.
- There are no reports of metastasis, recurrence, or long-term mortality.

- **Thymoma**
  - Thymomas are rare (1.5 cases/million), though they are the most common tumor of the anterior mediastinum, comprising 50% of all anterior mediastinal tumors and 20–25% of mediastinal masses overall.

- Thymomas develop from thymic epithelial cells, without known environmental or genetic risk factors.
- Thymomas are classified by clinical criteria according to the American Joint Committee on Cancer (AJCC) staging (Tables 39.1 and 39.2) or the Masaoka staging system (Table 39.3) and histologic criteria by the World Health Organization classification (Table 39.4).
- All thymomas have malignant potential, may cause morbidity by invading adjacent structures in the mediastinum, and have potential for locoregional recurrence after resection.
- Presentation and diagnosis

  Thymomas most frequently occur in middle age (ages 40–60) and have an equal sex distribution.

Table 39.1 The American Joint Committee on Cancer 8th edition TNM staging

Primary tumor (T)	
Tx	Primary tumor cannot be assessed
T0	No evidence of primary tumor
T1a	Tumor encapsulated or into mediastinal fat
T1b	Tumor with invasion into mediastinal pleura
T2	Tumor invasion of the pericardium
T3	Tumor invasion of the lung, innominate vein, superior vena cava, phrenic nerve, chest wall, extrapericardial pulmonary artery/vein
T4	Tumor invasion of the aorta, arch great vessels, intrapericardial pulmonary artery, myocardium, trachea, esophagus
Regional lymph nodes (N)	
Nx	Regional nodes cannot be assessed
N0	No regional node metastasis
N1	Metastasis to anterior (perithymic) nodes
N2	Metastasis to deep intrathoracic or cervical nodes
Distal metastasis (M)	
M0	No pleural, pericardial, or distal metastasis
M1a	Pleural or pericardial tumor nodule(s)
M1b	Distant organ metastasis

Table 39.2 The American Joint Committee on Cancer 8th edition groupings

Stage I	T1a,b, N0, M0
Stage II	T2, N0, M0
Stage IIIA	T3, N0
Stage IIIB	T4, N0
Stage IVA	Any T, N1, M0 or any T, N0-N1, M1a
Stage IVB	Any T, N2, any M or any T, any N, M1b

Table 39.3 Masaoka thymoma staging

Stage I	Encapsulated tumor, without tumor invasion into the capsule
Stage II	Tumor invasion into fatty/thymic tissue surrounding the tumor or microscopic invasion into the capsule
Stage III	Tumor invasion into organs surrounding the thymus
Stage IVA	Tumor implants in the pleura or pericardium
Stage IVB	Spread to lymph nodes or via bloodstream to distant organs

Table 39.4 The World Health Organization thymoma classification

Subtype	Criteria
Type A	Occurrence of bland, spindle-shaped epithelial cells (at least focally); paucity or absence of immature (TdT+) T cells throughout the tumor
Atypical type A variant	Criteria of type A thymoma; in addition: comedo-type tumor necrosis; increased mitotic count (>4/2 mm^2); nuclear crowding
Type AB	Occurrence of bland, spindle-shaped epithelial cells (at least focally); abundance of immature (TdT+) T cells focally or throughout tumor
Type B1	Thymus-like architecture and cytology: abundance of immature T cells, areas of medullary differentiation (medullary islands), paucity of polygonal or dendritic epithelia cells without clustering (i.e., < 3 contiguous epithelial cells)
Type B2	Increased numbers of single or clustered polygonal or dendritic epithelial cells intermingled with abundant immature T cells
Type B3	Sheets of polygonal slightly to moderately atypical epithelial cells; absent or rare intercellular bridges; paucity or absence of intermingled TdT+ T cells
Micronodular thymoma with lymphoid stroma	Nodules of bland spindle or oval epithelial cells surrounded by an epithelial cell-free lymphoid stroma
Metaplastic thymoma	Biphasic tumor composed of solid areas of epithelial cells in a background of bland-looking spindle cells; absence of immature T cells

Nearly half of all patients are asymptomatic on presentation with a minority presenting with chest pain, dysphagia, hoarseness, dyspnea, and swelling of the face or upper extremities caused by compression/invasion of mediastinal structures (Fig. 39.5).

May present with autoimmune paraneoplastic syndromes, most commonly myasthenia gravis, which occurs in close to half of all patients with thymoma. Less common syndromes include red blood cell aplasia, hypogammaglobulinemia, and inappropriate antidiuretic hormone secretion.

CT chest imaging is the most common modality to characterize a thymoma in the anterior mediastinum (Fig. 39.6). Typical findings include a homogenous, well-circumscribed, potentially lobulated mass in the anterior-superior mediastinum. Areas of calcification may be present.

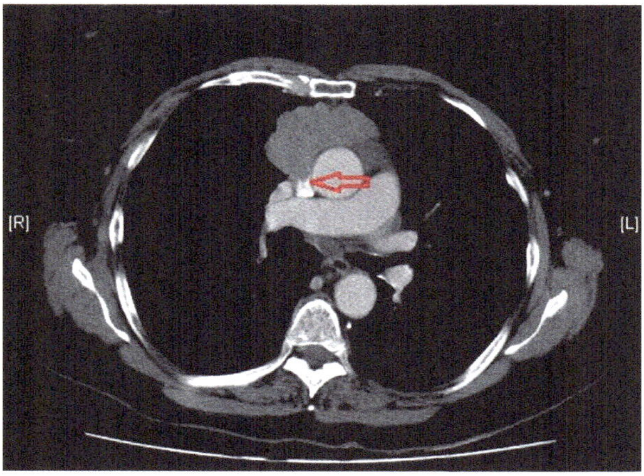

Fig. 39.5 Thymoma invading the superior vena cava (arrow)

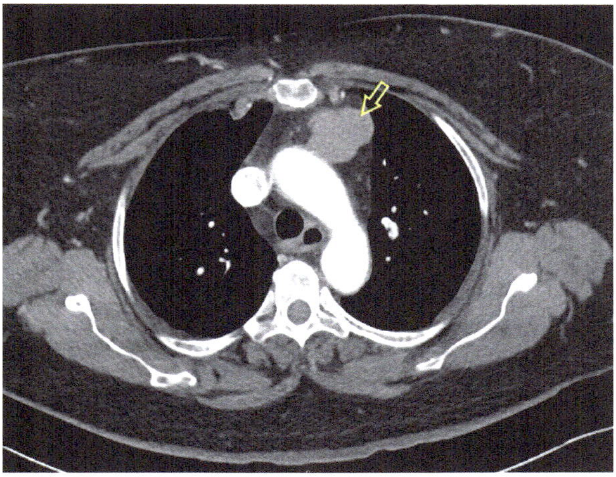

Fig. 39.6 Axial CT imaging demonstrating a 3.5 cm lobulated, well-circumscribed lesion in the left aspect of the anterior mediastinum (arrow), representative of a thymoma

Biopsy is not necessary if the diagnosis of resectable thymoma is strongly suspected, as there is a risk of needle tract or pleural seeding.

Biopsy is warranted in patients with advanced disease or where alternative pathologies are on the differential, such as thymic carcinoma, lymphoma, or germ cell tumor.

– Treatment

Treatment of thymoma involves en bloc surgical resection of the entire thymus gland (total thymectomy), the target mass, pericardial fat, and any resectable structures to which it is adherent (see Operative Technique below).

Complete resection of all microscopic tumor (R0 resection) is the most important predictor of outcome.

After R0 resection, although controversial, tumors with capsular/mediastinal fat invasion on postoperative pathology are considered for postoperative radiation.

After R0 resection, radiation is recommended for tumors invading beyond mediastinal fat (i.e., invasion into adjacent structures).

Postoperative radiation therapy is recommended for microscopic (R1) or gross residual disease (R2) after resection.

For locally advanced thymomas, where resectability is in question, biopsy is indicated to confirm diagnosis, followed by induction chemotherapy and re-evaluation for potential resection.

- Outcomes

  Prognosis and long-term survival in patients with thymoma are based on stage, tumor behavior, and the ability to achieve a complete resection.

  Overall 10-year survival for patients with stage I and II thymomas are approximately 90% and 70%, respectively. Patients with stage III–IV thymoma have a significantly worse survival.

- **Thymic carcinoma**
  - Thymic carcinomas are histologically distinct (typically a squamous cell carcinoma) from thymoma and are rarer and more aggressive neoplasm associated with a poor prognosis.
  - Thymic carcinoma is staged according to the Masaoka classification and/or the AJCC TMN system (Tables 39.1, 39.2, and 39.3).
  - Presentation and diagnosis

    Thymic carcinoma occurs in a wide age range of patients, including adolescents.

    May present symptoms due to tumor invasion of adjacent structures, with local lymph node metastasis or distant metastasis (lung, bone, liver).

    CT scan is most commonly used to characterize the tumor (Fig. 39.7).

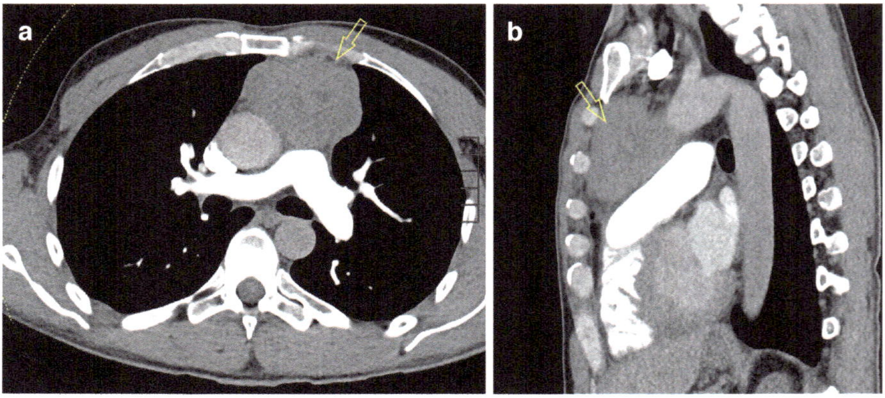

Fig. 39.7 CT images of a 6 cm anterior mediastinal mass (arrows), with core biopsy revealing thymic carcinoma. (**a**) Axial; (**b**) sagittal

Similar to thymoma, biopsy is not necessary if the diagnosis of resectable tumor is strongly suspected.
Biopsy is warranted in patients with more advanced disease, which is more likely to occur in thymic carcinomas than thymomas.

- Treatment

  Treatment is similar to thymoma; for resectable disease, this involves en bloc surgical resection of the entire thymus gland (total thymectomy), the target mass, pericardial fat, and any resectable structures to which it is adherent (see Operative Technique below).
  Complete resection with no residual microscopic tumor (R0 resection) is the most important predictor of outcome.
  After R0 resection, consider postoperative radiation for tumors with capsular/mediastinal fat invasion on postoperative pathology.
  After R0 resection, radiation is recommended for tumors invading beyond mediastinal fat (i.e., invasion into adjacent structures).
  Postoperative radiation therapy with or without chemotherapy is recommended for microscopic (R1) or gross residual disease (R2) after resection.
  For locally advanced thymic carcinomas, where resectability is in question, biopsy is indicated to confirm diagnosis, followed by induction chemotherapy and re-evaluation for potential resection.
  For unresectable disease: referred for concurrent chemoradiation.

- Outcomes

  Overall 5-year survival for Masaoka stage I, II, III, IVA, and IVB is 100%, 81%, 51%, 24%, and 17%, respectively.
  Similar to thymoma, prognosis and long-term survival are based on stage, tumor behavior, and the ability to achieve a complete resection.
  Recurrence and/or disease progression is common, occurring in approximately 50% of potentially resectable/ resected patients, with a median time to recurrence of about 1 year.

- **Thymic carcinoid**
  - Thymic carcinoid tumors, also referred to as thymic neuroendocrine tumors, are rare thymic neoplasms accounting for 2–5% of all thymic tumors, typically arising in the anterior mediastinum.
  - Approximately 25% of thymic carcinoid tumors occur in patients with multiple endocrine neoplasia type 1 (MEN1), and 3–8% of all MEN1 patients develop a thymic carcinoid tumor, particularly in the later stages of the disease.
  - Thymic carcinoid tumors are classified as low (typical carcinoid), intermediate (atypical carcinoid), and high grade (large-cell neuroendocrine and small-cell neuroendocrine carcinoma) according to the World Health Organization system based on histological appearance.
  - Presentation and diagnosis

Often invade adjacent structures leading to symptoms such as hoarseness, cough, dyspnea, chest pain, and facial or upper extremity swelling.

Cushing's syndrome due to ectopic ACTH production.

Between 20 and 40% of patients will present with metastatic disease, commonly in the lung, liver, and bone, and with local lymph node metastasis.

Evaluation and staging are completed most commonly by CT scan, often with contrast to detail areas of hemorrhage and necrosis and to define relationship to vascular structures in the mediastinum.

Somatostatin receptor-based imaging, such as dotatate PET scan (Fig. 39.8), is particularly helpful in identifying thymic carcinoid tumors as somatostatin receptors are overexpressed in neuroendocrine tumors and scans using radiolabeled somatostatin analogues can identify primary masses and metastases.

As disease is commonly advanced on presentation, needle biopsy for tissue diagnosis is often indicated.

- Treatment

For resectable tumor, en bloc surgical resection of the entire thymus gland, the tumor, pericardial fat, and any resectable structures to which it is adherent for R0 resection is the goal.

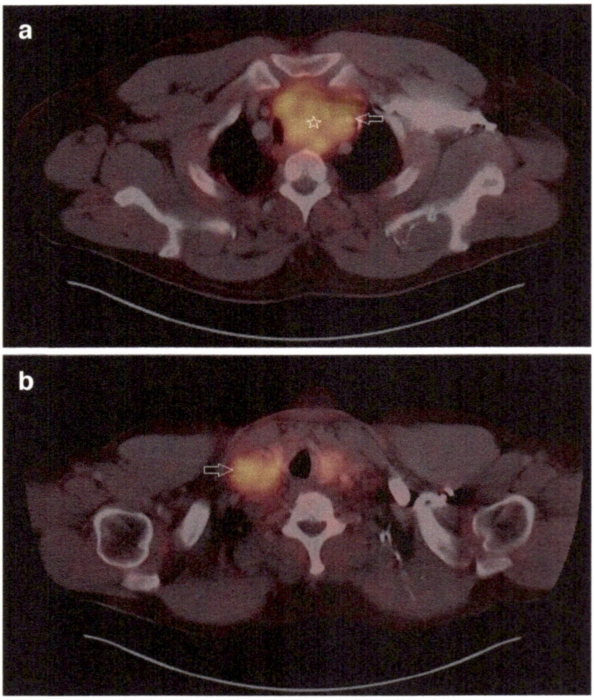

Fig. 39.8 Dotatate PET CT scan of thymic carcinoid, atypical. (**a**) Locally invasive mass (star) encasing left carotid artery (arrow); (**b**) with right cervical/supraclavicular adenopathy (arrow)

Due to the extent of disease and the high risk of recurrence even with R0 resection, postoperative therapy is recommended, although the optimal adjuvant regimen is not clearly known due to the rarity of this disease.
Adjuvant radiotherapy is indicated for residual disease after resection in cases of well-differentiated thymic carcinoid, while poorly differentiated disease should be treated with adjuvant concomitant chemoradiotherapy.
For locally advanced thymic carcinoids (which is often the case), where resectability is in question, biopsy is indicated to confirm diagnosis, followed by induction chemotherapy and re-evaluation for potential resection.
For unresectable disease: referred for concurrent chemoradiation.
For patients whose tumors have evidence of somatostatin receptor expression, long-acting somatostatin analogs, such as octreotide, may help slow tumor growth, though their use is controversial and there is limited data available.

- Outcomes

  Thymic carcinoid tumors have an aggressive biology, respond poorly to chemotherapy and radiation, and thus have a relatively poor prognosis.
  Low-grade thymic carcinoids have 5-year and 10-year survival rates of 50% and 9%, respectively, with high-grade disease having even worse outcomes.

Myasthenia Gravis

- Myasthenia gravis is an autoimmune disease of the neuromuscular junction caused by antibodies targeted at the postsynaptic nicotinic acetylcholine receptors. These autoantibodies lead to destruction and internalization of the receptors and impairment of neurotransmission.
- Patients with myasthenia gravis may have thymic hyperplasia (85%) or thymoma (10–15%).
- Myasthenia gravis is relatively rare, can occur at any age, and has a female predominance.
- Presentation and diagnosis
  - The classic manifestation in patients with myasthenia gravis is diplopia and transient muscle fatigue that worsens with repeated activity (as acetylcholine stores are depleted) and improves with rest.
  - A "myasthenic crisis" is defined as respiratory insufficiency severe enough to require mechanical ventilation.
  - Diagnosis is made by clinical evaluation, blood tests for autoantibodies against the acetylcholine receptor, muscle-specific kinase antibody, and less often electromyography and Tensilon test.

- Treatment
  - Pharmacologic therapy with acetylcholinesterase inhibitors (such as pyridostigmine) and/or immunosuppression.
  - Intravenous immunoglobulin and plasmapheresis are used as acute therapy during myasthenic crises.
  - Total thymectomy in the setting of myasthenia gravis is indicated for patients with thymoma and in patients without thymoma with generalized symptoms.
  - Surgical approach may be by sternotomy or minimally invasive robotic or thoracoscopic approaches (see Operative Techniques below). Transcervical approach for patients without thymoma is also an option.
  - In conjunction with neurology, utilization of preoperative intravenous immunoglobulin and plasmapheresis may be indicated, to optimize patients for surgery.
- Outcomes
  - At 10 years, successful thymectomy results in an 85% improvement rate, a 40–60% remission rate in patients without thymoma, and an 18% remission rate in patients with thymoma.

Operative Technique: En Bloc Total Thymectomy

- Classically, thymic tumors are removed via median sternotomy. However, if oncologic principles are observed, the majority can be safely and effectively resected via minimally invasive approaches, either by robotic or thoracoscopic. Long-term data for minimally invasive surgery, however, are lacking.
- Extent of resection is from phrenic nerve to phrenic nerve and from the diaphragm to the base of the neck/thoracic inlet, resecting the tumor en bloc with total thymectomy, pericardial fat, and any resectable structures it is adherent to (Fig. 39.9). This extent (or borders) of resection is the same for patients with myasthenia gravis without thymoma, with the exception that resection of adjacent structures is not necessary.
- With regard to the thymus, the gland is mobilized from the left innominate vein, where thymic veins drain into (Fig. 39.10). The thymic veins are divided as they are encountered. The right and left thymic horns are reduced from the base of the neck/thoracic inlet; these horns can reach as high as the thyroid (Fig. 39.9).
- For minimally invasive surgery, the approach can be from the left or right side, often dictated by the anatomy of the lesion. Entering the contralateral pleural space aids in dissection and assures removal of all anterior mediastinal tissue from phrenic nerve to contralateral phrenic nerve.
- Adherence/invasion to adjacent structures

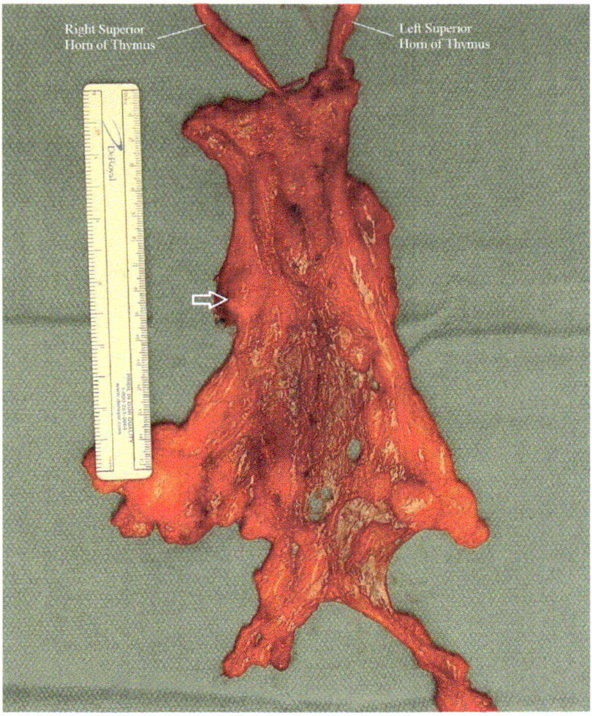

Fig. 39.9 Resected specimen of a small thymoma (arrow). Extent of resection includes the entire thymus and pericardial fat en bloc with the tumor

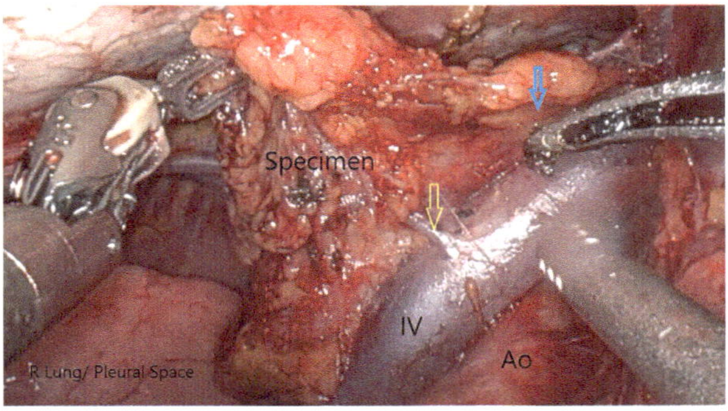

Fig. 39.10 Intraoperative view of a robotic en bloc total thymectomy approached from the left chest. The specimen includes the thymus gland including the left thymic horn (blue arrow), target mass, and pericardial fat. IV, left innominate vein with thymic vein (yellow arrow); Ao, aorta

– Pericardium

Can be resected en bloc.

Lateral defects are reconstructed, especially the right side, due to risk of cardiac herniation.

Reconstruction of anterior defect is optional, but preferred, to avoid cardiac adherence to sternum.

Materials used for reconstruction include bovine pericardium or polytetrafluoroethylene (PTFE).

- Phrenic nerve

  En bloc of one nerve is acceptable in good operative candidates.
  Resection of two nerves is to be avoided as it results in significant loss of pulmonary function and quality of life.
  In situations where both phrenic nerves are invaded, resect the one that is most extensively involved, then skeletonize and mark with clips the other nerve to provide a target for postoperative radiation.

- Left innominate vein

  Can be resected en bloc, by partial resection or resection of the entire circumference of the vein
  If partial resection, then can be primarily repaired or patch repaired with autologous vein patch
  If circumferential resection, can be left as is without reconstruction or reconstructed using autologous vein, bovine pericardium, or PTFE interposition

- Lung

  Often can be resected en bloc by wedge; however, en bloc segmentectomy, lobectomy, bilobectomy, or pneumonectomy may be necessary depending on the extent of tumor invasion and the ability of the patient to tolerate such resection based on preoperative pulmonary function.

- Superior vena cava

  Can be resected en bloc to achieve R0 resection.
  Cardiopulmonary bypass is usually not necessary if the superior vena cava is first bypassed with a graft from one of the innominate veins (or both) to the right atrium. This is then followed by resection of the vena cava.
  Bypass grafts utilized include spiral vein, bovine pericardium, or PTFE (Fig. 39.11).

Key Reference

- Varma V, Alabousi A, Burute N, Haider E. Thymic masses and mimics in adults: review of common and uncommon pathologies. Clin Imaging. 2021;77:98–110.

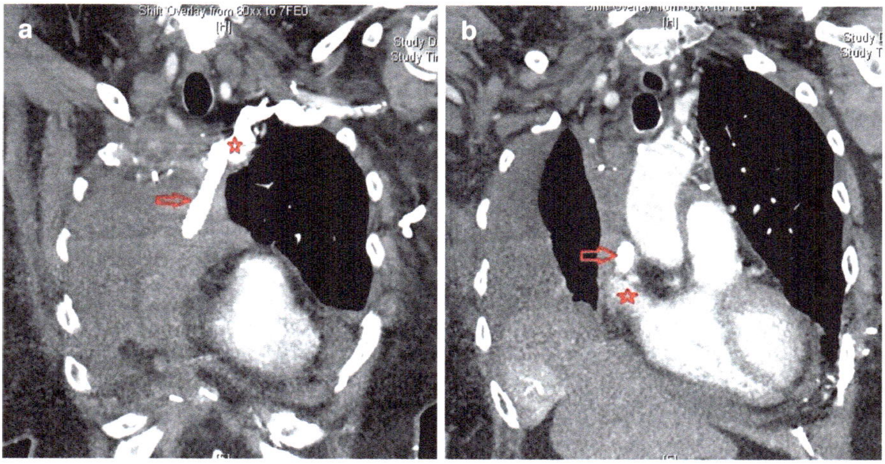

Fig. 39.11 Postoperative CT coronal images after resection of thymoma en bloc with superior vena cava followed by ringed polytetrafluoroethylene reconstruction. (**a**) Proximal aspect of graft (arrow) anastomosed to the left innominate vein (star); (**b**) distal aspect of graft (arrow) anastomosed to the right atrium (star)

Further Reading

Blumberg D, Port JL, Weksler B, et al. Thymoma: a multivariate analysis of factors predicting survival. Ann Thorac Surg. 1995;60(4):908–13. discussion 914

Engels EA. Epidemiology of thymoma and associated malignancies. J Thorac Oncol. 2010;5:S260.

Gamanagatti S, Sharma R, Hatimota P, et al. Giant Thymolipoma. Am J Roentgenol. 2005;185(1):283–4.

Geraci TC, Ferrari-Light D, Pozzi N, Cerfolio RJ. Midterm results for robotic thymectomy for malignant disease. Ann Thorac Surg. 2021;111(5):1675–81.

Keesey JC. Clinical evaluation and management of myasthenia gravis. Muscle Nerve. 2004;4:484–505.

Lausi PO, Refai M, Filosso PL, Ruffini E, Oliaro A, Guerrera F, Brunelli A. Thymic neuroendocrine tumors. Thorac Surg Clin. 2014;24(3):327–32.

Litvak AM, Woo K, Hayes S, et al. Clinical characteristics and outcomes for patients with thymic carcinoma: evaluation of Masaoka staging. J Thorac Oncol. 2014;9:1810–5.

National Comprehensive Cancer Network. Thymomas and Thymic Carcinomas (Version 1.2023). http://www.nccn.org/professionals/physician_gls/pdf/thymic.pdf. Accessed February 13, 2023.

Öberg K, Hellman P, Ferolla P, Papotti M, ESMO Guidelines Working Group. Neuroendocrine bronchial and thymic tumors: ESMO Clinical Practice Guidelines for diagnosis, treatment and follow-up. Ann Oncol. 2012;23(Suppl 7):vii120-3.

Plantmason L, Lui N, Theodore P, Plantmason L. Mediastinal disease. In: Yuh DD, Vricella LA, Yang SC, Doty JR, Yuh DD, Vricella LA, Yang SC, Doty JR, Yuh DD, et al., editors. Johns Hopkins textbook of cardiothoracic surgery, second edition. New York, NY: McGraw-Hill; 2014.

Romi F. Thymoma in myasthenia gravis: from diagnosis to treatment. Autoimmune Dis. 2011;2011:474512.
Rosado-De-Christenson ML, Pugatch RD, Moran CA, et al. Thymolipoma: analysis of 27 cases. Radiology. 1994;193(1):121–6.
Strobel P, Marx A, Chan JKC, et al. Thymic neuroendocrine tumours: typical and atypical carcinoid. In: Travis WD, Brambilla E, Buirke AP, Marx A, Nicholson AG, editors. WHO classification of tumours of the lung, pleura, thymus, and heart. 4th ed. Lyon: International Agency for Research on Cancer; 2015.
Wolfe GI, Kaminski HJ, Aban IB, Minisman G, Kuo HC, Marx A, Ströbel P, Mazia C, Oger J, Cea JG, Heckmann JM, Evoli A, Nix W, Ciafaloni E, Antonini G, Witoonpanich R, King JO, Beydoun SR, Chalk CH, Barboi AC, Amato AA, Shaibani AI, Katirji B, Lecky BR, Buckley C, Vincent A, Dias-Tosta E, Yoshikawa H, Waddington-Cruz M, Pulley MT, Rivner MH, Kostera-Pruszczyk A, Pascuzzi RM, Jackson CE, Garcia Ramos GS, Verschuuren JJ, Massey JM, Kissel JT, Werneck LC, Benatar M, Barohn RJ, Tandan R, Mozaffar T, Conwit R, Odenkirchen J, Sonett JR, Jaretzki A 3rd, Newsom-Davis J, Cutter GR, MGTX Study Group. Randomized trial of thymectomy in myasthenia gravis. N Engl J Med. 2016;375(6):511–22.
Yang CJ, Hurd J, Shah SA, Liou D, Wang H, Backhus LM, Lui NS, D'Amico TA, Shrager JB, Berry MF. A national analysis of open versus minimally invasive thymectomy for stage I to III thymoma. J Thorac Cardiovasc Surg. 2020;160(2):555–67.

Chapter 40
Mediastinal Tumors

Ashley N. Miller and Thomas Ng

Introduction

The mediastinum is the region of the thorax between the two pleural cavities. The mediastinum contains vital organs such as the heart, great vessels, trachea, and esophagus. Mediastinal tumors can originate from any mediastinal structures or tissues that pass through the mediastinum during development. They can be of benign or malignant pathology. This chapter will discuss tumors of the mediastinum apart from those that derive from the thymus gland (discussed in Chap. 40).

Anatomy

- The borders of the mediastinum include the thoracic inlet superiorly, the diaphragm inferiorly, the lungs/pleura laterally, the sternum anteriorly, and the paravertebral sulcus posteriorly (Fig. 40.1).
- The mediastinum is divided into three compartments, which helps to determine the origin of a tumor based on location.
- Anterior mediastinum

A. N. Miller
Department of Surgery, University of Tennessee Health Science Center, College of Medicine, Memphis, TN, USA
e-mail: amill203@uthsc.edu

T. Ng (✉)
Division of Thoracic Surgery, University of Tennessee Health Science Center, College of Medicine, Memphis, TN, USA
e-mail: tng4@uthsc.edu

T. Ng, T. Geraci (eds.), *Thoracic Surgery Clerkship*, Contemporary Surgical Clerkships, https://doi.org/10.1007/978-3-031-44645-0_40

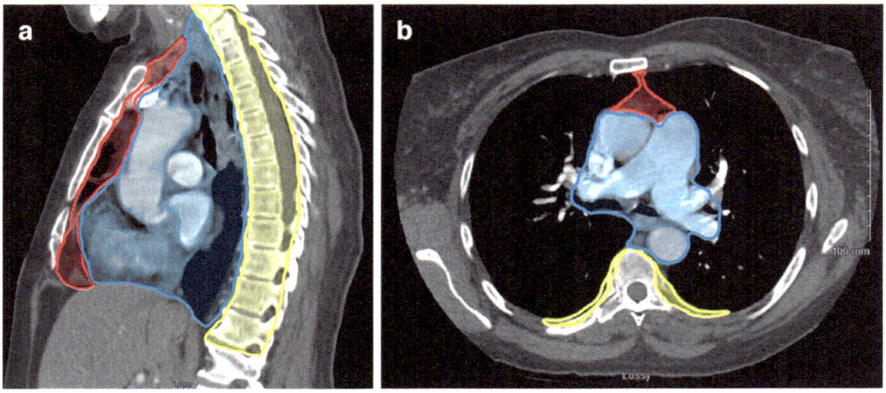

Fig. 40.1 Mediastinal compartments. Red is anterior, blue is middle, and yellow is posterior. (**a**) CT sagittal view; (**b**) CT axial view

- Space from the posterior border of the sternum to the anterior border of the pericardium and great vessels (Fig. 40.1, shaded red).
- The anterior mediastinum contains the thymus, lymphatic tissue, and connective tissue and is the location of germ cell migration embryologic development.

- Middle mediastinum (also termed visceral mediastinum)
  - Space from the anterior pericardium to the anterior border of the thoracic spine (Fig. 40.1, shaded blue).
  - The middle mediastinum contains the pericardium, heart, great vessels, pulmonary hila, trachea, esophagus, lymphatic tissue, connective tissue, vagus nerves, phrenic nerves, and thoracic duct.
- Posterior mediastinum
  - Space from the anterior border of the thoracic spine to the posterior border of the costovertebral sulci (Fig. 40.1, shaded yellow).
  - The posterior mediastinum contains the intercostal neurovascular bundles (nerve, artery, and vein), sympathetic chain ganglia, spinal ganglia, lymphatic tissue, and connective tissue.

Differential Diagnosis of Mediastinal Tumors (Table 40.1)

- Anterior mediastinal tumors
  - The "4 T's": thymoma, thyroid (ectopic or substernal extension), teratoma, or terrible lymphoma; however, this mnemonic is not all inclusive and serves as a guide to expand the differential diagnosis.

Table 40.1 Differential diagnosis of mediastinal masses for each compartment

Anterior compartment	Middle compartment	Posterior compartment
Thymus	Lymphadenopathy	Neurogenic tumors
• Thymoma	• Lymphoma	• Neurofibroma
• Thymic cyst	• Sarcoid	• Neurilemmoma
• Thymic hyperplasia	• Metastatic cancer	• Neurosarcoma
• Thymic carcinoma	Bronchogenic cyst	• Ganglioneuroma
Germ cell tumor	Pericardial cyst	• Ganglioneuroblastoma
• Teratoma/dermoid cyst	Esophageal cyst	• Neuroblastoma
• Seminoma	Esophageal tumors	• Chemodectoma
• Non-seminoma	Tracheal tumors	• Pheochromocytoma
– Yolk sac tumor	Neurogenic tumors	Meningocele
– Embryonal carcinoma	Cardiac tumors	Thoracic spine lesions
– Choriocarcinoma	Vascular masses	Lymphoma
Intrathoracic thyroid		
• Substernal thyroid		
• Ectopic thyroid tissue		
Lymphoma		
Parathyroid adenoma/carcinoma		
Hemangioma		
Lipoma		
Liposarcoma		
Fibroma		
Fibrosarcoma		
Foramen of Morgagni hernia		

  - Thymoma expands the differential diagnosis to include thymic cyst, thymic carcinoma, and thymic hyperplasia; teratoma expands the differential to include malignant germ cell tumors (seminoma and non-seminoma); and thyroid expands the differential to include parathyroid adenoma or carcinoma.
  - If these are ruled out, then the consideration should be for a connective tissue tumor.

- Middle mediastinal tumors
  - Given the number of tissue types in the middle mediastinum, lesions in this space have a broad differential diagnosis.
  - Tumors may arise from the major organs of this compartment such as the heart, trachea, bronchus, and esophagus.
  - Masses may also arise from lymphatic tissue (lymphoma), nerves (neurogenic tumor), and connective tissue.

- Posterior mediastinal tumors
  - Almost exclusively neurogenic in nature of which there are a variety of tissue types.

Clinical Presentation

Mediastinal masses are commonly found incidentally in asymptomatic patients on imaging such as chest radiograph, computed tomography scan (CT), or magnetic resonance imaging (MRI), obtained for other indications.

- In patients who are symptomatic, symptoms are related to mass effect on nearby structures, paraneoplastic syndromes, or systemic symptoms.
- Mass effects
  - Airway: dyspnea, cough, stridor, or wheeze
  - Esophagus: dysphagia
  - Heart: hypotension, palpitations
  - Superior vena cava: facial and upper extremity swelling
  - Recurrent nerve: hoarseness
  - Phrenic nerve: shortness of breath
  - Sympathetic chain: Horner syndrome
  - Spinal cord: lower extremity weakness
- Paraneoplastic syndromes such as myasthenia gravis, hypogammaglobulinemia, and Cushing's syndrome are associated with thymic neoplasms.
- Systemic symptoms due to advanced malignancy or B symptoms of night sweats, weight loss, fever, or fatigue, related to lymphoma.
- If the mass is malignant, the patient is more likely to be symptomatic.
- Clinical presentation specific to each pathology is further discussed below.

Workup

Anterior Mediastinum

- History and physical examination.
- Indicated labs include CBC, AFP, b-HCG, LDH, Calcium, PTH, and thyroid function.
- If myasthenia gravis is suspected, testing is indicated to rule in/out acetylcholine receptor antibodies, muscle-specific tyrosine kinase antibodies, EMG, and Tensilon test.
- CT chest with IV contrast (CTA).
- MRI
  - Can confirm benign thymic etiology such as thymic cystic or thymic hyperplasia.
  - For thymic cysts, the cystic nature may not be obvious on CT scan if the fluid is thick and proteinaceous but would be bright on T2-weighted MRI image (Fig. 40.2).

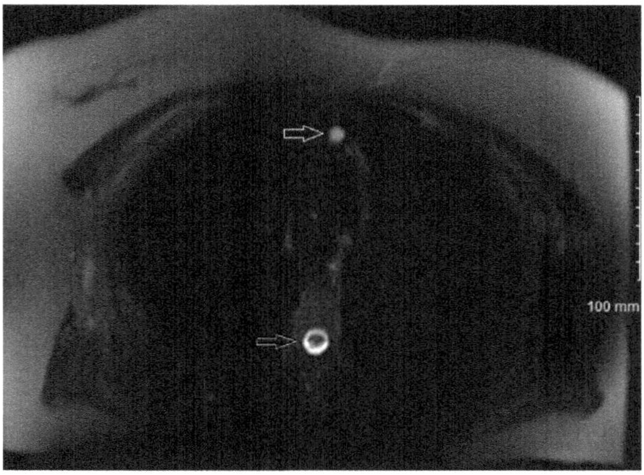

Fig. 40.2 MRI of a thymic cyst bright on T2-weighted image (white arrow); similarly the spinal canal also had bright areas as it contains cerebrospinal fluid (red arrow)

  - MRI is also helpful to assess adjacent vital structures such as the great vessels or heart.
- Nuclear medicine scan
  - If intrathoracic/substernal thyroid is the leading diagnosis, then technetium-99 scan may be used for diagnosis but is not always required as thyroid etiology is usually obvious on CT imaging.
  - Parathyroid sestamibi scan is indicated if parathyroid pathology is suspected.
- Biopsy
  - Tissue diagnosis is not necessary for clearly benign lesions, such as thymic hyperplasia, thymic cysts, thyroid goiter, teratoma, schwannoma, or parathyroid adenoma.
  - In cases of suspected thymoma, if early stage (no invasion into adjacent structures), then can proceed to surgery without biopsy as there is a risk of capsule breach resulting in pleural spread and needle tract seeding with needle biopsy of thymoma.
  - Tissue diagnosis is indicated for locally advanced or suspected malignant lesions.
  - Biopsy techniques

    Initial consideration is by CT-guided core needle.

    If CT-guided biopsy is nondiagnostic or not technically possible, then surgical biopsy can be by anterior mediastinotomy (Chamberlain procedure) or thoracoscopy.

Middle Mediastinum

- History and physical examination.
- CT scan with IV contrast.

- MRI can confirm diagnosis of bronchogenic cysts, pericardial cysts, or esophageal cysts, as the cystic nature of these lesions may not be obvious on CT scan if the fluid is thick and proteinaceous but would be bright on T2-weighted MRI image.
- Biopsy
  - Indicated for suspected malignant pathologies.
  - For clearly benign lesions such as bronchogenic cyst, pericardial cyst, or esophageal cyst, biopsy should be avoided due to the risk of introducing infection into the cyst.
  - Percutaneous image-guided needle biopsy of the middle mediastinum is difficult, due to the surrounding vital structures.
  - Bronchoscopy/endobronchial ultrasound (EBUS) with transbronchial biopsy can be considered if the pathology abuts the airway.
  - Upper endoscopy/endoscopic ultrasound (EUS) with transesophageal biopsy can be considered for lesions adjacent to the esophagus.
  - Surgical biopsy of the middle mediastinum is performed via cervical mediastinoscopy or thoracoscopy.

Posterior Mediastinum

- History and physical examination.
- CT scan with IV contrast.
- MRI, if tumor is near the spinal foramen, to rule out intraspinal extension (dumbbell tumor).
- If symptoms of catecholamine excess (hypertension, headache, palpitations, anxiety, diaphoresis, weight loss) are present, then obtain urine or serum catecholamine testing for extra adrenal pheochromocytoma (rare).
- Biopsy
  - Often not necessary as diagnosis based on imaging is usually clear.
  - Biopsy is indicated if diagnosis is not clear or if tumor appears invasive/malignant.
  - Biopsy is by CT-guided needle or surgical by thoracoscopy if necessary.

Management of Specific Mediastinal Pathologies

- Thymus (discussed in Chap. 40)
- Esophagus (discussed in Chaps. 31 and 33)
- Trachea (discussed in Chap. 36)

Mediastinal Thyroid

- Clinical presentation
  - Asymptomatic goiter, located in the anterior mediastinum (Fig. 40.3a) or the middle mediastinum (Fig. 40.3b).
  - Symptoms from compression of adjacent structures, most notably the trachea, causing shortness of breath, stridor, or wheezing.
  - If toxic multinodular goiter, then symptoms of hyperthyroidism.
  - Hoarse voice raises concern for malignancy with recurrent laryngeal nerve invasion.
- Workup
  - CT scan with IV contrast
  - Thyroid scan: may be helpful if diagnosis is still in doubt despite CT scan
  - Thyroid function tests if indicated
  - CT- or ultrasound-guided needle biopsy: not routine, difficult to biopsy intrathoracic component, may be indicated if malignancy is suspected
- Management
  - All patients should undergo full evaluation by a thyroid surgeon to help determine management.
  - Surgical resection is indicated if symptomatic, if there is growth, or if there is a concern for malignancy or proven malignancy.
  - If asymptomatic, surgery can still be considered to prevent future complications, but observation can also be appropriate for poor surgical candidates or the elderly.
  - Surgical resection

    The cervical and mediastinal components can often be resected via cervical collar incision alone, as substernal thyroids are supplied by the inferior thyroid artery and thus do not usually have thoracic blood supply (unless true ectopic thyroid).

    If necessary, a thoracic approach with sternotomy (partial or full), thoracotomy, thoracoscopy, or robotic may be added to facilitate safe resection.

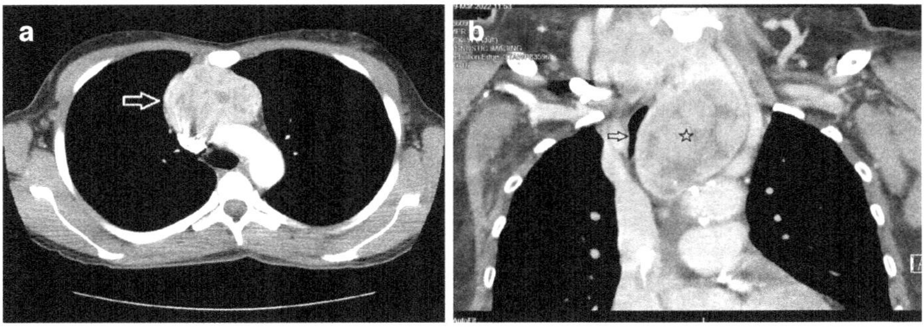

Fig. 40.3 CT scan of substernal or intrathoracic goiter. (**a**) Thoracic component in the anterior mediastinum (arrow); (**b**) thoracic component in the middle mediastinum (star) with tracheal deviation and compression (arrow)

Mediastinal Parathyroid

- Clinical presentation
  - Incidental finding on imaging done for other reasons in an asymptomatic patient
  - Found on workup for hypercalcemia, with symptoms referred to as "stones, bones, groans and psychiatric overtones"

    Flank pain from nephrolithiasis
    Bone pain from pathologic fractures or osteoporosis
    Gastrointestinal symptoms such as constipation, abdominal pain, decreased appetite, nausea, and vomiting
    Psychiatric symptoms such as confusion, psychosis, depression, and memory loss

  - Ectopic mediastinal gland found on imaging after cervical exploration for hyperparathyroidism fails to find the responsible gland or fails to cure the disease
- Workup
  - Laboratory tests such as PTH, phosphate level, vitamin D level, and urine calcium; these results along with the clinical evaluation will establish the diagnosis of primary, secondary, or tertiary hyperparathyroidism.
  - Localization tests such as 4D contrast CT scan (Fig. 40.4a) and/or parathyroid sestamibi scan (Fig. 40.4b).
  - Biopsy is usually not necessary as the diagnosis is often clear; also biopsy is difficult due to small size and location.

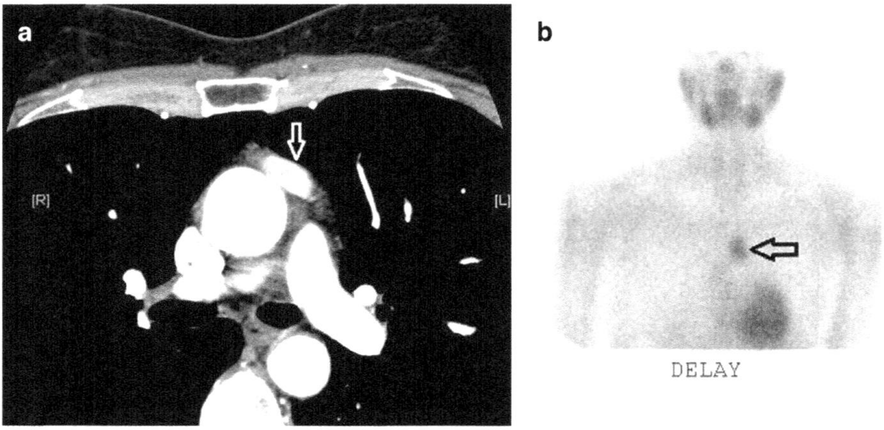

Fig. 40.4 Mediastinal parathyroid adenoma. (**a**) 4D contrast CT scan showing lesion in the anterior mediastinum with intense enhancement (arrow); (**b**) parathyroid sestamibi nuclear scan showing lesion in the anterior mediastinum (arrow)

- Management
  - All patients should be fully evaluated by a parathyroid surgeon to determine management.
  - Surgical resection is indicated for symptomatic patients or if malignancy (rare) is suspected.
  - For asymptomatic patients, options are resection versus observation; therefore, discussion with an endocrine surgeon is necessary to determine management.
  - Approach for parathyroid glands resection

    Transcervical approach can be successful for parathyroid glands within the thymus, especially those superior to the aortic arch.
    Otherwise, a minimally invasive approach by thoracoscopy or robotic can be utilized for resection of ectopic glands within the mediastinum.

  - Intraoperative monitoring of PTH level to confirm success

    Pre-incision PTH is sent as a baseline and again at 10 min after parathyroid excision with the goal of greater than 50% drop from baseline.

  - Intraoperative frozen sections can also be obtained to confirm resection of parathyroid tissue.

Mediastinal Germ Cell Tumors

- Types: mature teratoma, immature teratoma, seminoma germ cell tumor, and non-seminomatous germ cell tumor (choriocarcinoma, yolk sac tumor, embryonal carcinoma, teratocarcinoma).
- Mature teratomas (Fig. 40.5)
  - Clinical presentation

    Benign, slow-growing, therefore commonly found incidentally when asymptomatic.
    If symptomatic, symptoms are related to compression or erosion of adjacent structures or complications of the tumor itself such as infection.

  - Workup

    CT scan with IV contrast (Fig. 40.5a) demonstrates an anterior mediastinal mass that may contain density of fat, cartilage, or calcifications (possibly of teeth or bone).
    MRI may be performed if there is concern for invasion of major structures.
    Biopsy is often not necessary as diagnosis is usually clear.
    CT-guided biopsy if there is a question regarding the diagnosis or if malignancy is suspected.

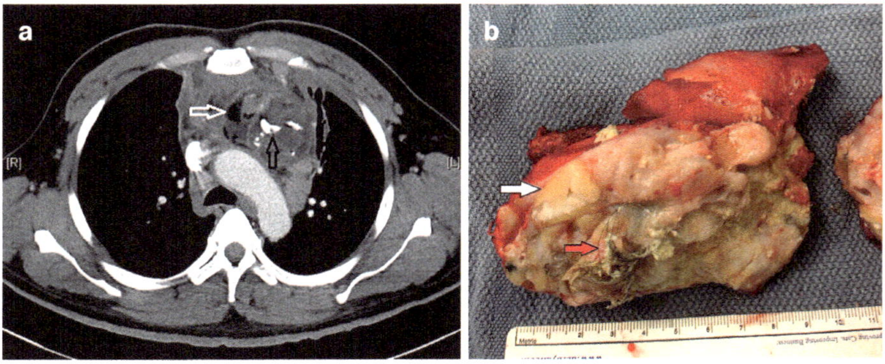

Fig. 40.5 Mature teratoma. (**a**) CT scan showing fat density (white arrow) and calcification (black arrow), with stranding surrounding the mass due to infection of the teratoma; (**b**) gross pathology of the resected teratoma showing fat (white arrow) and hair with sebaceous material (red arrow) within the mass

- Management

  Surgical resection

  - By sternotomy or minimally invasive (thoracoscopy/robotic) approach.
  - Resection specimens may include all three germ cell layers (ectoderm, mesoderm, endoderm) and a variety of tissues such as bone, teeth, cartilage, fat, pancreas, hair, etc. (Fig. 40.5b).

- Immature teratomas
  - Rare, more aggressive behavior than mature teratoma
  - Presentation, workup, and management similar to mature teratoma but with the consideration for chemotherapy
- Seminomas
  - Clinical presentation

    Classically, in a young male patient
    Symptoms related to compression or invasion into adjacent structures
    Constitutional symptoms: fevers, chills, and weight loss

  - Workup

    CT scan with IV contrast
    For male patients, a testicular exam and ultrasound to rule out testicular primary cancer.
    b-HCG may be normal or slightly elevated; AFP levels should be normal.
    Biopsy by CT-guided core needle.
    If necessary, surgical biopsy by anterior mediastinotomy or thoracoscopy.

- Management

  Chemotherapy is the mainstay of treatment, the addition of radiation may be considered in certain circumstances, and surgical resection is almost never indicated.

- Non-seminomatous germ cell tumor
  - Clinical presentation

    Classically, in a young male patient
    Symptoms related to compression or invasion into adjacent structures.
    Constitutional symptoms: fevers, chills, and weight loss
    May have symptoms specific to the site of metastasis (metastatic disease is common presentation)
    Associated with gynecomastia, Klinefelter's syndrome, and hematologic malignancies

  - Workup

    CT scan with IV contrast.
    AFP and b-HCG are elevated.
    For male patients, a testicular exam and ultrasound to rule out testicular primary cancer.
    Biopsy by CT-guided core needle.
    If necessary, surgical biopsy by anterior mediastinotomy or thoracoscopy.

  - Management

    Chemotherapy is the mainstay of treatment.
    Consider surgical resection.

    - If after chemotherapy, b-HCG and AFP normalize, but a residual mediastinal mass remains, then resection is indicated as this mass may represent teratoma which can grow or undergo malignant degeneration.

Bronchogenic Cyst

- Clinical presentation
  - Most commonly an asymptomatic, incidental finding.
  - Symptoms may occur, related to compression or erosion into adjacent structures, most commonly the tracheobronchial tree (cough, dyspnea).
  - Symptoms related to complication of the cyst such as infection or bleeding (rare).

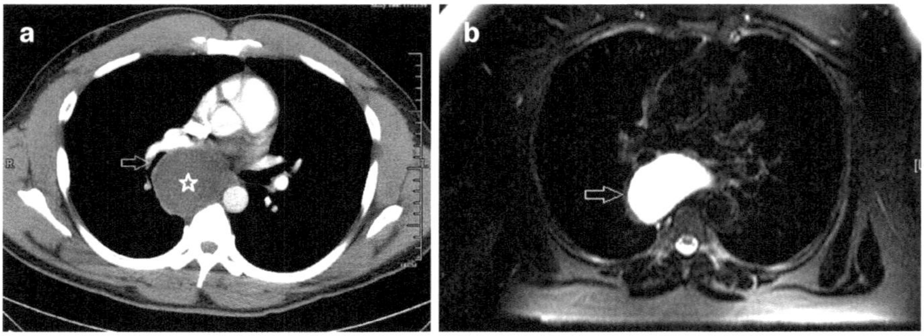

Fig. 40.6 Bronchogenic cyst. (**a**) CT scan showing a mass with fluid density (star) that compresses the bronchus intermedius (arrow); (**b**) MRI shows the lesion to be bright on T2-weighted image, confirming the lesion to be totally cystic in nature

- Workup
  - CT scan with IV contrast (Fig. 40.6a).
  - If the cystic nature is not clear on CT scan (often due to thick proteinaceous cyst content), then obtain an MRI (bright T2-weighted image; Fig. 40.6b) or EBUS/EUS to confirm.
  - If the lesion is purely cystic in nature, then avoid biopsy as this can introduce infection.
- Management
  - Observation is an option if asymptomatic, especially in high-risk patients or the elderly/frail.
  - Surgical resection if symptomatic, or in the asymptomatic low-risk patient, to prevent future growth and/or complications.

    Approach preferably by minimally invasive techniques with thoracoscopy or robotic.

    Total cyst excision is the goal; however, if the cyst is densely adherent to vital structures, rather than risk injury, resect the non-adherent portion of the cyst, and ablate the lining of the adherent portion with energy mechanically or chemically.

Pericardial Cysts

- Clinical presentation
  - Most commonly an asymptomatic, incidental finding.
  - Large cysts may cause symptoms related to compression against adjacent structures (chest pain, dyspnea, palpitation).
  - Rarely, symptoms may be related to secondary complications, such as infection or bleeding, or cyst rupture.

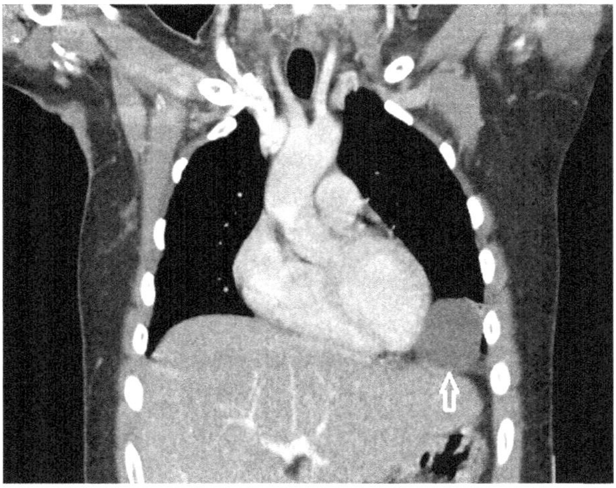

Fig. 40.7 Coronal CT scan showing a fluid-density lesion in the left cardiophrenic angle, consistent with a pericardial cyst

- Workup
  - CT scan with IV contrast, finding cyst commonly located at the cardiophrenic angle (Fig. 40.7).
  - If the cystic nature is not clear on CT scan (often due to thick proteinaceous cyst content), then obtain an MRI (bright T2-weighted image) to confirm.
  - If the lesion is purely cystic, then avoid biopsy as this can introduce infection.
- Management
  - Asymptomatic cysts can be observed, but can consider resection of large cysts in low-risk surgical candidates to prevent future complications.
  - Symptomatic cysts should be resected as drainage often results in recurrence.

Neurogenic Mediastinal Tumors

- Clinical presentation
  - Most commonly, asymptomatic incidental finding.
  - Symptoms related to compression or erosion into adjacent structures such as the spinal cord, spinal nerves, or lung.
  - Rarely, symptoms of catecholamine excess.
- Workup
  - CT scan with IV contrast (Fig. 40.8a).
  - If the lesion is near the spinal foramen, then obtain an MRI (Fig. 40.8b) to determine the extent of neural involvement within the foramen and/or spinal canal (dumbbell tumor).
  - Urine or serum catecholamine tests if symptoms of catecholamine excess are present.

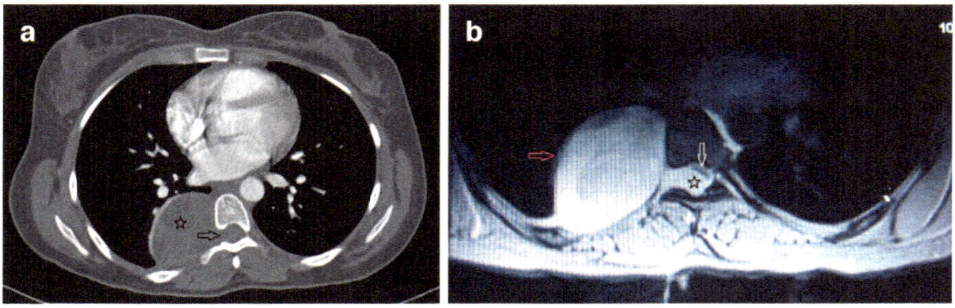

Fig. 40.8 Dumbbell neurogenic tumor. (**a**) CT scan showing paraspinal mass with widening of the spinal foramen suspicious for intraspinal extension; (**b**) MRI showing the paraspinal mass (red arrow) along with much more detail of the intraspinal component (star) causing spinal cord compression (white arrow)

- Biopsy is often not necessary as diagnosis is usually clear on imaging.
- CT-guided biopsy if diagnosis is in question or malignancy is suspected.

• Management

- Surgical resection is the mainstay of treatment; however, as the overwhelming majority of neurogenic tumors in adults are benign, observation is an option for asymptomatic patients, especially in high-risk patients.
- For tumors not near the spinal foramen, surgical resection with minimally invasive techniques by thoracoscopy or robotic approach is preferred, and open approach by thoracotomy can be utilized if necessary.
- For tumors with extension into the spinal foramen or with intraspinal extension (dumbbell tumor)

  Full evaluation by spine surgery is required, as a two-specialty approach is required, with the spine surgeon operating first to minimize risk of injury to the spinal cord.

  The operation begins with a posterior approach, often by laminectomy in the prone position by the spine surgeon, to resect the intraspinal and foraminal component.

  Followed by thoracic surgery, to resect the intrathoracic component by minimally invasive techniques (thoracoscopy or robotic approach), or by thoracotomy if necessary.

Key Reference

• Taka M, Kobayashi S, Mizutomi K, Inoue D, Takamatsu S, Gabata T, Matsumoto I, Ikeda H, Kobayashi T, Minato H, Abo H. Diagnostic approach for mediastinal masses with radiopathological correlation. Eur J Radiol. 2023;162:110767.

Further Reading

Chen X, Ma Q, Wang S, Zhang H, Huang D. Surgical treatment of posterior mediastinal neurogenic tumors. J Surg Oncol. 2019;119(6):807–13.

Fievet L, Gossot D, de Lesquen H, Calabre C, Merrot T, Thomas P, Becmeur F, Grigoroiu M. Resection of bronchogenic cysts in symptomatic versus asymptomatic patients: an outcome analysis. Ann Thorac Surg. 2021;112(5):1553–8.

Gawrychowski J, Kowalski GJ, Buła G, Bednarczyk A, Żądło D, Niedzielski Z, Gawrychowska A, Koziołek H. Surgical management of primary hyperparathyroidism-clinicopathologic study of 1019 cases from a single institution. J Clin Med. 2020;9(11):3540.

Hu J, Ngiam KY, Parameswaran R. Mediastinal parathyroid adenomas and their surgical implications. Ann R Coll Surg Engl. 2015;97(4):259–61.

Khayata M, Alkharabsheh S, Shah NP, Klein AL. Pericardial cysts: a contemporary comprehensive review. Curr Cardiol Rep. 2019;21(7):64.

Rosti G, Secondino S, Necchi A, Fornarini G, Pedrazzoli P. Primary mediastinal germ cell tumors. Semin Oncol. 2019;46(2):107–11.

Simó R, Nixon IJ, Vander Poorten V, Quer M, Shaha AR, Sanabria A, Alvarez FL, Angelos P, Rinaldo A, Ferlito A. Surgical management of intrathoracic goitres. Eur Arch Otorhinolaryngol. 2019;276(2):305–14.

Index

A

Abdominal esophagus, 345, 346
Ablative treatment, 167
Achalasia, 324–327
Acquired resistance, 159
Activating mutation, 156
Active bleeding, 426
Acute cellular rejection (ACR), 295
Acute respiratory distress syndrome (ARDS), 289
Adenoid cystic carcinoma (ACC), 409
Adenoma, 340
Advanced practitioners, vi
Airway injury, 267
Airway obstruction, 218
Albright's syndrome, 434
American Joint Committee on Cancer (AJCC) staging, 465
Analgesia
  acetaminophen, 33
  erector spinae plane block, 36
  intercostal nerve block, 36
  ketamine, 33
  NSAIDs, 33
  opioids, 33
  pain anatomy, 32–33
  paravertebral nerve block, 35
  regional techniques, 34, 35
  single injection intrathecal (spinal) injections, 35
  TEA, 35
Anesthesia
  advanced age, 28
  airway anatomy, 29–31
  airway management
    bronchial blockers, 38–40
    DLETT, 37, 38
    endotracheal tube, 40
    single lung ventilation, 36, 37
  analgesia
    acetaminophen, 33
    erector spinae plane block, 36
    intercostal nerve block, 36
    ketamine, 33
    NSAIDs, 33
    opioids, 33
    pain anatomy, 32–33
    paravertebral nerve block, 35
    regional techniques, 34, 35
    single injection intrathecal (spinal) injections, 35
    TEA, 35
  cardiac complications, 29
  COPD, 28, 29
  ERAS/ERATS, 41–43
  fluid management, 31, 32
  hemodynamic monitoring, 31
  mediastinal masses, 43, 44
  preoperative evaluation, 27, 28
  preoperative renal dysfunction, 29
  single lung ventilation, 40–41
Angiography, 426
Antibody mediated rejection (AMR), 295
Asbestos, 142
Aspergillosis, 195, 196
Atypical carcinoid lung cancer, 104, 105

B

Barrett's esophagus, 299, 303, 306, 358, 359

T. Ng, T. Geraci (eds.), *Thoracic Surgery Clerkship*, Contemporary Surgical Clerkships, https://doi.org/10.1007/978-3-031-44645-0

Benign esophageal tumors
  anatomy, 337, 338
  clinical presentation, 338
  diagnosis, 338, 339
  incidence, 337
  intraluminal tumors, 339, 340
  intramural tumors, 340–342
  periesophageal, 342, 343
Biphasic, 142
Blastomycosis, 194
Blebs, 223
Blunt cardiac injury, 263
Boerhaave syndrome, 346
Brachiocephalic artery, 416
Bronchial artery embolization, 183
Bronchial blocker, 180, 181
Bronchodilators, 221
Bronchogenic cyst, 487, 488
Bronchopulmonary sequestration, 203–205
Bronchoscopic lung volume reduction, 226, 227

C
Candidiasis, 197
Carcinoid tumor, 410
Cardiac surgery, v
Cardiopulmonary exercise testing (CPET), 79
Cardiopulmonary testing, 114
Caustic esophageal injury
  acid ingestion, 353
  alkali ingestion, 353
  long-term sequelae, 355, 356
  management, 353–355
  presentation, 353
Caustic ingestion, 347
Cervical esophageal cancer, 363
Cervical esophagus, 345, 346, 351
Cervical trachea, 416
Chemotherapy, 157
Chest tube, 234, 235
  contraindications, 16
  drainage systems, 20–22
  indications, 15, 16
  insertion technique
    large bore chest tube, 18, 19
    overview, 17, 18
    pigtail chest catheter, 19, 20
  selection, 16, 17
  tube removal
    complications, 24–26
    technique, 23, 24
    timing, 23
Chest wall deformity
  pectus carinatum
    curvature, 453, 454
    Poland syndrome, 454, 455
    sternal clefts, 455
    TOS, 455–458
    treatment, 454
  pectus excavatum
    cardiopulmonary morbidity, 449
    correction index, 450
    curvature, 447, 448
    definition, 447
    Haller index, 450
    interventions, 453
    Nuss procedure, 452, 453
    physical examination, 449
    presentation and work-up, 448, 449
    Ravitch procedure, 451, 452
    surgical repair, 451
    treatment and outcomes, 450, 451
Chest wall tumors
  benign tumors, 431, 432
    chondroma, 433
    desmoid tumor, 435
    eosinophilic granulomas, 436
    fibrous dysplasia, 434
  clinical presentation, 432
  history and physical examination, 432
  imaging, 432
  malignant tumors, 431, 432
    chondrosarcoma, 437
    Ewing's sarcoma, 438
    lymphoma, 440
    osteosarcoma, 438, 439
    soft tissue sarcomas, 439, 440
    solitary plasmacytomas, 438
  PFTs, 433
  secondary tumors, 431
  surgical treatment, 440–443
  tissue diagnosis, 433
Chondroma, 433
Chondrosarcoma, 437
Chronic lung allograft dysfunction (CLAD), 295
Chronic obstructive pulmonary disease (COPD), 28, 29, 74, 217, 231, 288
  clinical presentation, 219
  diagnosis, 219
  exacerbation, 222, 223
  medical management, 220, 221
  pathogenesis, 218, 219
Chylothorax, 249, 251, 252
  evaluation, 251, 252

pathogenesis, 249, 250
treatment, 252
Circular stapled anastomosis, 390, 391
Coccidiomycosis, 194
Collis gastroplasty, 319, 320
Colonic interposition, 385–387
Colorectal cancer (CRC), 136
Computed tomography angiography, 426
Concurrent chemoradiotherapy (CRT), 170
Congenital lobar emphysema, 208–210
Congenital pulmonary airway malformations, 200
anatomy, 200
imaging, 201
management, 202
stocker's classification, 200
Cryptococcus neoformans, 196
Cuffed tracheostomy tubes, 417
Cuffless tracheostomy tubes, 417

D

Decannulation, 425
Decortication, 145
DeMeester score, 303
Desmoid tumor, 435
Diaphragm injury, 264
Diffuse esophageal spasm, 328, 329
Diffusion capacity of the lung for carbon monoxide (DLCO), 112
Disease-free interval, 134
Donor evaluation, 292
Double lumen endotracheal tube (DLETT), 37, 38, 179
Dysplasia, 358

E

Electrocardiography (EKG), 259
En bloc total thymectomy, 472–475
Endobronchial ultrasound (EBUS), 86
Endovascular intervention, 428
Enhanced Recovery After Surgery (ERAS)/ Enhanced Recovery After Thoracic Surgery (ERATS), 41–43
Eosinophilic granulomas, 436
Epidermal growth factor receptor (EGFR), 82
Episodic bleeding, 426
Esophageal cancer, 375, 376
adenocarcinoma, 358
adjuvant therapy, 371
Barrett's esophagus, 358, 359
classification, 363, 364
clinical presentation, 359
epidemiology, 357
neoadjuvant therapy, 370, 371
staging, 364–368
T1bN0M0, 369
T2N0M0, 369, 370
T3N0M0, T4aN0M0 and TanyN1-3M0, 370
T4bNanyM0, 370
TisN0M0 and T1aN0M0, 369
treatment, 368, 369
TxNxM1, 370
work-up, 359–362
Esophageal injury, 265
Esophageal manometry, 304
Esophageal motility disorders, 323
Esophageal perforation
abdominal esophagus, 345, 346
cervical esophagus, 345, 346
evaluation, 347–350
pathogenesis, 346, 347
thoracic esophagus, 345, 346
treatment
endoscopic stenting, 352
initial management, 350
non-surgical, 350
surgical, 351, 352
Esophagectomy, 330
anastomosis, 389–391
anatomy, 373–375
colonic interposition, 385–387
complications
anastomotic leak, 393
anastomotic stricture, 394
chylothorax, 395
delayed gastric emptying, 394
gastric conduit necrosis, 394
recurrent laryngeal nerve injury, 395
reflux, 394
end-stage achalasia, 376
esophageal cancer, 375, 376
gastric conduit, 379, 385
history, 373
indications, 376, 377
jejunal conduit, 387, 388
surgical considerations, 391–393
surgical principles, 377–378
three-field esophagectomy, 384, 385
transhiatal esophagectomy, 381–383
transthoracic esophagectomy, 378–381
Ewing's sarcoma, 438
Extralobar sequestration, 204
Extrapleural pneumonectomy, 145

Exudative effusions, 239
Ex-vivo lung perfusion (EVLP), 295

F
Fenestrated tracheostomy tubes, 418
Fibrous dysplasia, 434
Fibrovascular polyps, 339
First rib resection and anterior scalenectomy (FRRS), 276
Focused abdominal sonography for trauma (FAST), 259
Foregut cysts, 205, 208
Foreign body ingestion, 347
Fresh tracheostomy, 424
Fundoplication, 317, 318

G
Gastric conduit, 379, 385
Gastroesophageal junction, 311
Gastro-esophageal junction (GEJ) cancer, 363
Gastrointestinal stromal tumor (GIST), 342
General surgery residents, vi
Germ cell tumors
  immature teratomas, 486
  mature teratomas, 485, 486
  non-seminomatous, 487
  seminomas, 486, 487
Glomus tumor, 410
Granular cell tumor, 340
Graves' disease, 463

H
Haller index, 450
Hand-sewn anastomosis, 389
Hemangioma, 339–340
Hemothorax, 261
Hiatal hernias
  anatomy, 311
  classification, 312, 313
  diagnosis, 314, 315
  fundoplication, 317
  operative technique, 318–320
  physiology, 311
  postoperative care, 320
  postoperative complications, 321
  presentation, 314
  treatment, 316
Histoplasma capsulatum, 193
Horner's syndrome, 93
Hypercarbia, 41
Hyperhidrosis, 281
  pathophysiology, 282
  presentation, 282
  treatment, 283

I
Immature teratomas, 486
Immune checkpoint blockade, 160
Immunotherapy, 82
Induction therapy, 87
Inflammatory pseudotumor, 340
Innominate artery, 416, 427
Innominate artery reconstruction, 428
Intensity-modulated radiation treatment (IMRT), 167
Interstitial lung disease (ILD), 289
Intralobar sequestration, 203–204
Intraluminal tumors, 339, 340

J
Jejunal conduit, 387, 388
Jugular venous distention (JVD), 258

L
Langerhans cell histiocytosis, 436
Large cell neuroendocrine carcinoma (LCNEC), 105–106, 154
  epidemiology, 105
  pathologic diagnosis, 105
  presentation, 106
  staging, 106
  treatment, 106
  work up, 106
Leiomyomas, 340, 341
Linear stapled anastomosis, 390
Lower esophageal sphincter (LES), 297, 324
Lung abscess, 187–190
Lung allocation score (LAS), 291
Lung cancer, v, 73
  American Cancer Society 2022, 58
  clinical evaluation, 58
  clinical presentation, 74
  diagnosis
    biopsy techniques, 61–63
    pathologic cell types, 63, 64
  initial radiographic evaluation, 59–61
  invasive staging techniques, 68–71
  non-invasive staging tests, 67, 68
  preoperative evaluation, 79, 80
  prevention and screening, 76

risk factors, 75
TMN staging, 64–67
workup and staging, 77, 79
Lung cancer screening
benefits, 53
clinical trials, 52, 53
epidemiology, 48
low-dose CT (LDCT), 76
potential harm, 53, 54
risk factors, 48
screening guidelines, 48–51
Lung isolation, 179
Lung-RADS classification system, 49, 50
Lung transplantation, 227
candidate selection, 290, 291
contraindications, 289–290
emerging technology/techniques, 295
history, 287
indications, 287–289
outcomes, 294
surgical technique, 293
survival, 295
Lung volume reduction surgery (LVRS), 224, 225
Lymphangiography, 252
Lymphoma, 440

M
Malignant pleural effusion, 243–246
Malignant pleural mesotheliomas (MPM)
chemotherapy, 146, 147
clinical presentation, 142
diagnosis and staging, 143
epidemiology, 142
pathogenesis, 141
prognosis, 147
treatment, 145
Manometry, 329
Masoaka Thymoma Staging, 466
Massive hemoptysis, 175, 177
anatomy, 176–178
definitive management, 183
initial management, 178, 179
Massive hemorrhage, 426
Mature teratomas, 485
Mediastinal lymphadenectomy, 128
Mediastinal tumors
anatomy, 477, 478
anterior mediastinum, 480, 481
bronchogenic cyst, 487, 488
clinical presentation, 480
differential diagnosis, 478, 479
germ cell tumors
immature teratomas, 486
mature teratomas, 485, 486
non-seminomatous, 487
seminomas, 486, 487
management, 482
middle mediastinum, 481, 482
neurogenic, 489, 490
parathyroid, 484, 485
pericardial cyst, 488, 489
posterior mediastinum, 482
thyroid, 483
Mesothelioma, 164
Minimally invasive esophagectomy (MIE), 377–378
Mucoepidermoid tumor, 410
Mucormycosis, 197, 198
Multidrug-resistant TB (MDR-TB), 190
Multimodality treatment, 85, 87
Multiple papillomatosis, 410
Myasthenia gravis
en bloc total thymectomy, 472–475
neuromuscular junction, 471
outcomes, 472
presentation and diagnosis, 471
treatment, 472
Mycobacterium avium complex (MAC), 191

N
National Comprehensive Cancer Network (NCCN), 77
National Lung Screening Trial (NLST), 76
Neoadjuvant therapy, 87, 95
Neurogenic mediastinal tumors, 489, 490
Non-fenestrated tracheostomy tubes, 418
Non-small cell lung cancer (NSCLC), 154
early-stage, 170
Non-tuberculous mycobacterial (NTM), 191, 192
Nuss procedure, 452, 453

O
Oligo-metastatic disease, 161, 172
Oncogene-targeted drugs, 157
Open tracheostomy, 422, 423
Oral endotracheal intubation, 424
Osteosarcoma, 438, 439

P
Paget-Schroder's syndrome, 457

Palliative drug therapy, 156
Pancoast tumor, 91, 92
Paracoccidiodomycosis, 195
Paraesophageal hernia, 312
Parapneumonic effusion, 240, 241
Parathyroid, 484, 485
Particle radiation treatment (PRT), 168
Pectus carinatum
  curvature, 453, 454
  Poland syndrome, 454, 455
  sternal clefts, 455
  TOS
    anatomy, 455
    arterial, 458
    neurogenic, 455–457
    venous, 457, 458
  treatment, 454
Pectus excavatum
  cardiopulmonary morbidity, 449
  correction index, 450
  curvature, 447, 448
  definition, 447
  Haller index, 450
  interventions, 453
  Nuss procedure, 452, 453
  physical examination, 449
  presentation and work-up, 448, 449
  Ravitch procedure, 451, 452
  surgical repair, 451
  treatment and outcomes, 450, 451
Penetrating cardiac injury, 262
Percutaneous tracheostomy, 421, 423–424
Pericardial cyst, 488, 489
Peroral endoscopic myotomy (POEM), 327
Phrenoesophageal membrane, 311, 313
Pleomorphic adenoma, 410
Pleural effusion (PE), 239, 250
Pleural empyema, 237, 238
Pleurectomy, 235
Pleurodesis, 235
Pneumocystis, 198
Pneumonectomy, 117, 128
Pneumothorax, 223, 260–261
  anatomy, 229
  history, 232
  imaging, 233
  immediate treatment, 234
  pathogenesis, 230
  physical examination, 232
  primary spontaneous, 230
  secondary spontaneous, 231
Poland syndrome, 454, 455
Posterolateral thoracotomy, 122
Preoperative evaluation, 115
Presentation, 201
Primary graft dysfunction (PGD), 294
Primary hyperhidrosis, 281
Prophylactic cranial irradiation (PCI), 171
Proton pump inhibitor, 301
Pulmonary arteriovenous malformation (PAVM), 211, 212
Pulmonary assessment
  age and frailty, 116
  interstitial lung disease, 117
  minimally invasive surgery, 117
  pneumonectomy, 117
  smoking, 116
Pulmonary fibrosis, 289
Pulmonary function, 217
Pulmonary function testing (PFTs), 111–113, 433
Pulmonary metastasis
  diagnosis, 135
  histologic subtypes, 135, 136
  imaging, 134
  nonsurgical therapies, 138
  pathophysiology, 133
  presentation, 134
  prognosis, 139
  surgical metastasectomy, 137, 138
Pulmonary rehabilitation, 221
Pulmonary resection, 28
  complications, 130
  indications, 121
  lobectomy/bilobectomy, 126
  mediastinal lymphadenectomy, 128
  minimally invasive approaches, 123, 124
  pneumonectomy, 127
  segmentectomy, 125
  sleeve lobectomy, 126
  wedge resection, 125
Pulseless electrical activity (PEA), 230

R

Radiation sensitization, 162
Radiofrequency ablation (RFA), 139
Radiotherapy, 167
Ravitch procedure, 451, 452
Renal cell carcinoma (RCC), 136
Rigid bronchoscopy, 179, 181
Routine tracheostomy, 425

S

Salmon-coloured tongues, 359
Sarcomatoid, 142

Secondary hyperhidrosis, 282
Secondary spontaneous pneumothorax, 231
Segmentectomy, 125
Seminomas, 486, 487
Sensitizing mutation, 154
Shunt, 40–41
Siewert classification, 363, 364
Sleeve obectomy, 126
Small cell lung cancer (SCLC), 107, 154, 171
Small cell neuroendocrine carcinoma, 105
Smoking cessation, 221
Soft tissue sarcomas, 439, 440
Solitary brain metastasis, 86, 88
Solitary fibrous tumor of pleura, 147, 148, 150
Solitary plasma cell tumor myeloma, 438
Solitary plasmacytomas, 438
Spirometry, 220
Split lung function, 115
Spontaneous pneumothorax, 235
Squamous cell carcinoma (SCC), 409
Squamous papilloma, 339
Stereotactic body radiation therapy (SBRT), 73, 82, 138, 167
Sternal clefts, 455
Stocker's classification, 200–201
Subglottic stenosis, 403, 404
Superior sulcus tumor, 91
  anatomy, 92
  clinical outcomes, 99
  complications, 98
  diagnosis, 94
  presentation, 93, 94
  staging, 94
  treatment, 94–97
Surgical resection, 73, 79
Sweating, 281, 283
Symptomatic advanced disease, 172

T

Targeted therapy, 82
Thoracic duct, 249, 253
Thoracic epidural analgesia (TEA), 35
Thoracic esophageal cancer, 363
Thoracic esophagus, 345, 346
Thoracic imaging
  chest wall, 13, 14
  computed tomography scan (CT), 2
  fluoroscopy, 2, 3
  lungs
    diffuse lung disease, 7
    pulmonary nodules and masses, 4–6
    trauma, 6, 7
  magnetic resonance imaging (MRI), 3
  mediastinum, 11–13
  nuclear medicine, 3, 4
  pleura
    effusion, 8
    infection, 9
    masses, 11
    trauma, 9, 10
  radiography, 2
  ultrasound (US), 3
Thoracic oncology, 153
Thoracic outlet syndrome (TOS), 269
  anatomy, 269, 455
  arterial, 458
  differential diagnosis, 274
  epidemiology, 271
  neurogenic, 272, 455–457
  pathogenesis, 271
  physical exam, 273
  surgical options, 276, 277
  surgical outcomes, 278
  testing, 275
  treatment, 275
  venous, 272, 457, 458
Thoracic trachea, 416
Thoracic trauma
  airway injury, 257, 267, 268
  blunt aortic injury, 265–267
  breathing, 258
  chest wall, 255
  circulation, 258
  diaphragm injury, 264
  disability, 258
  esophageal injury, 265
  esophagus, 257
  exposure, 258
  heart and great Vessels, 256
  hemothorax, 261
  lungs and pleura, 256
  penetrating cardiac injury, 262, 263
  pneumothorax, 260, 261
  rib fractures, 259, 260
  secondary survey, 259
  thoracic outlet, 257
  trachea, 257
Thoracic/abdominal esophagus, 351
Thoracotomy, 138
Three-Dimensional conformal radiation therapy (3D-CRT), 167
Thymic carcinoid tumors
  classification, 469
  incidence, 469
  outcomes, 470, 471
  presentation and diagnosis, 470
  treatment, 470, 471

Thymic carcinomas, 163
outcomes, 469
presentation and diagnosis, 468, 469
staging, 468
treatment, 469
Thymic cysts, 463, 464
Thymic hyperplasia
CT imaging, 462, 463
surgical resection, 463
types, 462
Thymic neoplasms
thymic carcinoid tumors
classification, 469
incidence, 469
outcomes, 470, 471
presentation and diagnosis, 470
treatment, 470, 471
thymic carcinomas
outcomes, 469
presentation and diagnosis, 468, 469
staging, 468
treatment, 469
thymic cysts, 463, 464
thymolipomas, 463, 464
thymomas, 465, 466
outcomes, 468
presentation and diagnosis, 465–467
staging, 465, 466
treatment, 467, 468
Thymic pathology, 462
Thymolipomas, 463, 464
Thymomas, 163, 465, 466
outcomes, 468
presentation and diagnosis, 465–467
staging, 465, 466
treatment, 467, 468
Thymus gland, 461, 462
Thyroid, 483
Total parenteral nutrition (TPN), 252
Trachea
anatomical relationships with, 416
anatomy, 415, 417
innominate artery (brachiocephalic artery), 416
vascular anatomy, 416
Tracheal malignancy
benign tumors, 410
clinical presentation, 407
complications, 412
diagnosis, 408, 409
incidence, 407
primary malignant tumors
ACC, 409
carcinoid tumors, 410
management, 411, 412
mucoepidermoid tumor, 410
SCC, 409
secondary tumors, 410
survival outcomes, 413
unresectable tumors, 412, 413
Tracheal stenosis
anatomy, 397, 398
epidemiology, 398
history, 399
imaging and workup, 399, 400
non-neoplastic cause, 397
physical examination, 399
prognosis, 405
treatment
non-surgical, 400, 401
surgical resection, 401–404
Tracheoesophageal fistula (TEF), 213–215
Tracheoinnominate fistula (TIF), 184
clinical presentation, 425, 426
diagnosis, 426
endovascular intervention, 428
initial main objectives during massive bleeding, 427
innominate artery reconstruction, 428
pathogenesis, 425
postoperative complications, 428
prognosis, 428
resect and ligate innominate artery, 427
risk factors, 426
tracheal defect management, 428
Tracheostomy
airway protection, 420
benefits, 420
contraindications to, 421
history, 421
specific to percutaneous tracheostomy, 421
cuffed tubes, 417, 418
cuffless tubes, 417, 418
decannulation, 425
early complications, 424
fenestrated tubes, 418, 419
indications, 420
inner cannula, 419
intraoperative complications, 424
key points, 422
late complications, 424
non-fenestrated tubes, 418, 419
obturator, 419
open tracheostomy, 423
open tracheostomy technique, 422

outer cannula with flange, 419
patient positioning, 422
percutaneous tracheostomy, 423, 424
physical examination, 421
postoperative management, 424, 425
preparation for procedure, 422
timing for respiratory failure, 420
upper airway obstruction, 420
variations of, 422
weaning strategies, 425
Transudative effusions, 239
Triglycerides, 249, 252
Tuberculous mycobacterial infections, 190, 191
Typical carcinoid lung cancer, 101–104

V
Venous drainage, 416
Venous thoracic outlet syndrome (vTOS), 271
Video-assisted thoracoscopic surgery, 135

W
Wedge resection, 125
World Health Organization Thymoma Classification, 466

Z
Zenker's diverticulum, 331–333, 335

GPSR Compliance

The European Union's (EU) General Product Safety Regulation (GPSR) is a set of rules that requires consumer products to be safe and our obligations to ensure this.

If you have any concerns about our products, you can contact us on ProductSafety@springernature.com

In case Publisher is established outside the EU, the EU authorized representative is:

Springer Nature Customer Service Center GmbH
Europaplatz 3
69115 Heidelberg, Germany

Batch number: 10256220

Printed by Printforce, the Netherlands